Lung Disease Associated with Rheumatoid Arthritis

Takahisa Gono • Hitoshi Tokuda
Fumikazu Sakai • Tamiko Takemura
Editors

Lung Disease Associated with Rheumatoid Arthritis

Springer

Editors
Takahisa Gono
Department of Allergy and Rheumatology
Nippon Medical School
Graduate School of Medicine
Tokyo
Japan

Fumikazu Sakai
Department of Diagnostic Radiology
Saitama International Medical Center
Saitama Medical University
Hidaka, Saitama
Japan

Hitoshi Tokuda
Department of Respiratory Medicine
JCHO Tokyo Yamate Medical Center
Tokyo
Japan

Tamiko Takemura
Department of Pathology
Japanese Red Cross Medical Center
Tokyo
Japan

ISBN 978-981-10-6749-5 ISBN 978-981-10-6750-1 (eBook)
https://doi.org/10.1007/978-981-10-6750-1

Library of Congress Control Number: 2017964232

Printed on acid-free paper

This Springer imprint is published by Springer Nature
The registered company is Springer Nature Singapore Pte Ltd.
The registered company address is: 152 Beach Road, #21-01/04 Gateway East, Singapore 189721, Singapore

Preface

Recent advances in the treatment strategy of rheumatoid arthritis (RA), including novel biological disease-modifying antirheumatic drugs (bDMARDs) and conventional synthetic DMARDs (csDMARDs), have revolutionized its management, resulting in the successful control of joint inflammation in a majority of patients and a significant improvement in their prognosis.

As a systemic inflammatory disease, RA frequently affects not only synovial joints but also various extra-articular organs. These extra-articular manifestations (EAMs) are the most serious predisposing factor for morbidity and mortality of RA patients. According to recent epidemiological studies, these EAMs are decreasing with the introduction of novel therapeutics, which would explain the improvement in prognosis. However, pulmonary involvements are an exception; they are becoming more and more serious and now are the major obstacles to the successful treatment of RA.

In the prebiologics era, lung diseases caused serious problems in the management of RA as well. As shown in a large-scale cohort study conducted in Japan, they were the major cause of death of RA patients, together with malignancy. Lung diseases comprise infection, interstitial lung disease (ILD), and drug-induced pneumonia.

With the introduction of novel DMARDs in the 2000s, severe pulmonary infections and drug-induced lung disease, along with exacerbations of preexisting ILD, began to occur with considerable frequency as adverse events of this therapy.

A Japanese cohort study conducted recently reported that among RA patients undergoing biologics therapy, nearly 50% of the fatalities were attributable to lung diseases such as respiratory infections and ILD. This means that one of the most vital challenges in the current treatment of RA is the control of lung complications.

The risk factors for such severe lung complications under the novel DMARD treatments have been enthusiastically screened and surveyed by many investigators. However, treatment strategies to address such complications have not been established in a sufficient manner.

How should we confront these situations? Should patients with risk factors for such complications be excluded from beneficial treatment in this novel era? What should we do to diagnose and treat each lung complication, sometimes in slowly progressive disease and sometimes in acutely developing illness? Except for tuberculosis, no practical guidelines have been formulated so far. In this book, we aim to answer these questions at the best level possible, on the basis of knowledge obtained from our recent investigations along with the current best evidence available.

First, we clarify the pathogenesis and clinical implications of the lung diseases directly associated with RA (pulmonary EAMs), including airway diseases and ILD, from various aspects: clinical, radiological, and pathological.

We emphasize the importance of airway disease, as one of the major risk factors of infections in RA patients. Also, we show that it can ultimately progress to respiratory failure due to obstruction of the peripheral airways. A new pathological classification of obliterative bronchiolitis is also presented.

We also introduce a new insight into the pathogenesis of honeycombing seen in RA-ILD, the so-called UIP (usual interstitial pneumonia) type. We clarify that this cystic structural derangement is caused by persistent inflammatory destruction derived from RA in the peripheral airways. From this insight, a possible treatment strategy is proposed against the progression of RA-ILD.

For ILD itself, clinical, radiological, and pathological problems are discussed, with a few of our original insights inserted among the established knowledge.

Lastly, we discuss the diagnosis and treatment of lung infections and their cognate disorders, including organizing pneumonia and acute diffuse lung disease along with *Pneumocystis* pneumonia and drug-induced pneumonia. Here, we propose specific and practical procedures to handle these complicated conditions.

We believe that the discussions presented here, which contain many of our new ideas and concepts, will be useful and beneficial for rheumatologists, pneumologists, and radiologists confronted with this vital clinical challenge, the diagnosis and treatment of lung diseases associated with RA.

Tokyo, Japan Takahisa Gono
Tokyo, Japan Hitoshi Tokuda
Saitama, Japan Fumikazu Sakai
Tokyo, Japan Tamiko Takemura

Contents

Part I

Introduction

Overview: Clinical Significance of Lung Disease Associated with Rheumatoid Arthritis

1

Takahisa Gono

Abstract

Rheumatoid arthritis (RA) is an immune-mediated disease that primarily affects joints. In the 2000s, numerous novel antirheumatic agents, called biological disease-modifying antirheumatic drugs (bDMARDs) as well as methotrexate, have becom available worldwide. These developments in treatment have resulted in RA remission or low disease activity in greater than 50% of RA patients. This recent progress has allowed RA patients attain improved physical function and prognosis. However, treatment-related events, such as infections, have occurred and occasionally caused severe or fatal outcomes in RA patients. Thus, clinicians must pay attention to complications during treatment with corticosteroids and/or DMARDs, especially bDMARDs. Approximately 50% of the causes of death in RA patients treated with bDMARDs involve respiratory disease, including pneumonia and interstitial lung disease. Therefore, clinicians should manage these pulmonary complications promptly. In this book, we will describe the current status of knowledge about lung disease in RA and would suggest the best form of management of lung disease in RA patients for clinicians, including general practitioners, rheumatologists, respirologists, radiologists, and pathologists. We hope that this book will prove helpful to all types of medical staff and clinicians who take care of RA patients.

Keywords

Rheumatoid arthritis • Lung disease • Management • bDMARDs

1.1 Introduction

Rheumatoid arthritis (RA) is an autoimmune disease that primarily affects joints. Recent advances in therapy for RA have been hugely beneficial in providing a better outcome in patients with arthritis. In the 2000s, numerous novel antirheumatic agents, called biological disease-modifying antirheumatic drugs (bDMARDs) as well as conventional synthetic DMARDs (csDMARDs), are now available worldwide as presented in Table 1.1 [1]. These developments in treatment have resulted in RA remission or low disease activity in greater than 50% of RA patients [2, 3]. This condition has allowed RA patients to achieve and

Table 1.1 List of antirheumatic agents

Conventional synthetic DMARDs	
	Methotrexate Sulfasalazine Leflunomide Hydroxychloroquine
Biological DMARDs	
TNF inhibitor	Adalimumab Certolizumab pegol Etanercept Golimumab Infliximab
Anti-B cell	Rituximab
Anti-T cell co-stimulation	Abatacept
Anti-IL-6R	Tocilizumab
Targeted synthetic DMARDs	
	Tofacitinib Baricitinib

DMARDs disease-modifying antirheumatic disease, *TNF* tumor necrosis factor, *IL-6R* interleukin 6 receptor

T. Gono, M.D., Ph.D.
Department of Allergy and Rheumatology, Nippon Medical School, Graduate School of Medicine, Tokyo, Japan
e-mail: t-gono@nms.ac.jp

T. Gono et al. (eds.), *Lung Disease Associated with Rheumatoid Arthritis*, https://doi.org/10.1007/978-981-10-6750-1_1

maintain better physical function in daily living. In this past decade, numerous studies and reports have been performed regarding arthritis in RA. Moreover, the American College of Rheumatology (ACR) and the European League Against Rheumatism (EULAR) have proposed guidelines or recommendations for the management of arthritis in patients with RA [4, 5]. Therefore, clinicians around the world can adequately understand how to manage patients who have joint symptoms in RA. This recent progress has allowed RA patients attain improved physical function and prognosis. However, treatment-related events, such as infections, have occurred not infrequently and occasionally caused severe or fatal outcomes in RA patients [6]. Thus, clinicians must pay attention to complications of adverse events or complications during treatment with corticosteroids and/or DMARDs, especially bDMARDs, which include tumor necrosis factor inhibitor (TNFi), anti-B cell or anti-T cell co-stimulation, and anti-interleukin 6 receptor (IL-6R). In addition, extra-articular lesions are frequently revealed and diverse in RA, as shown in Table 1.2 [7]. Mortality is increased in RA patients with extra-articular manifestations compared with those without. The age- and sex-adjusted mortality rate ratio is 2.49 (95% confidence interval (CI) 1.43–4.03) in RA patients with extra-articular manifestations compared with RA patients without [7].

Therefore, to improve the prognosis of RA patients, we must understand the causes of death and how to manage complications related to treatment or extra-articular RA disease. In particular, complications of pulmonary diseases, such as infection, RA-associated airway disease or interstitial lung disease (ILD), and drug-induced pneumonia, are critical issues in clinical practice for RA patients. Therefore, we focus here on the causes of death and pulmonary complications in RA.

Table 1.2 Extra-articular manifestations in RA

1.	Pericarditis
2.	Pleuritis
3.	Felty's syndrome
4.	Major cutaneous vasculitis
5.	Neuropathy
6.	Scleritis, episcleritis or retinal vasculitis
7.	Glomerulonephritis
8.	Vasculitis affecting other organs
9.	Amyloidosis
10.	Keratoconjunctivitis sicca
11.	Xerostomia
12.	Secondary Sjögren's syndrome
13.	Pulmonary fibrosis
14.	Organizing pneumonia
15.	Cervical myelopathy
16.	Subcutaneous rheumatoid nodules
17.	Rheumatoid nodules in other locations

RA rheumatic arthritis

1.2 Mortality and Causes of Death in RA

Life span is shortened by 15–20% in RA patients [8]. The median survival of RA patients is reduced by 10 years for men and 11 years for women compared with the general population [9]. In 1989, in Finland, the causes of excess mortality are cardiovascular disease in 40%, infections in 30%, and amyloidosis in 15% [8]. An inception cohort that was started in 1986 in the UK reported 459 deaths (32%) in 1429 patients recruited between 1986 and 1997 who were followed for up to 18 years. The standardized mortality ratio (SMR) was 1.27 (95% CI 1.04–1.46) [10]. In this cohort, the main causes of death were cardiovascular disease (31%), malignancy (25%), respiratory disease (22%), and cerebrovascular disease (10%), as shown in Fig. 1.1. Similarly, in the Institute of Rheumatology, Rheumatoid Arthritis (IORRA) cohort from Japan in 2010, the main causes of death in 289 RA patients were malignancy (24%), pulmonary disease (23%), and cardiovascular/cerebrovascular disease (22%), as shown in Fig. 1.2 [11]. Pulmonary disease included pneumonia (12%) and interstitial lung disease (11%). Pulmonary disease is one of the major causes of death in RA; however, its frequency is race dependent.

The risk factors for morality in the UK inception cohort included less favorable socioeconomic status, markers of RA disease severity, and diminished function within the first year [10]. The IORRA cohort demonstrated that the risk factors for mortality were associated with males, older age, worse physical disability, presence of rheumatoid factor (RF), corticosteroid use, and preexisting ILD. The risk factors for mortality in RA are presented in Table 1.3 and are reproduced from previous reports [10–13].

In addition, a study from Japan revealed that the SMR is 1.08 [95% CI 0.77–1.47] in patients treated with bDMARDs and 1.28 [95% CI 1.17–1.41] in those treated with conventional synthetic DMARDs (csDMARDs). Approximately 50% of the causes of death in RA patients treated with bDMARDs involve respiratory disease, including pneumonia and ILD (Fig. 1.3). Infection, malignancy, and vascular disease are also noted in ~10% of deaths in RA patients treated with bDMARDs [14].

Therefore, clinicians should manage these pulmonary complications promptly in RA patients, especially in patients who are treated with bDMARDs.

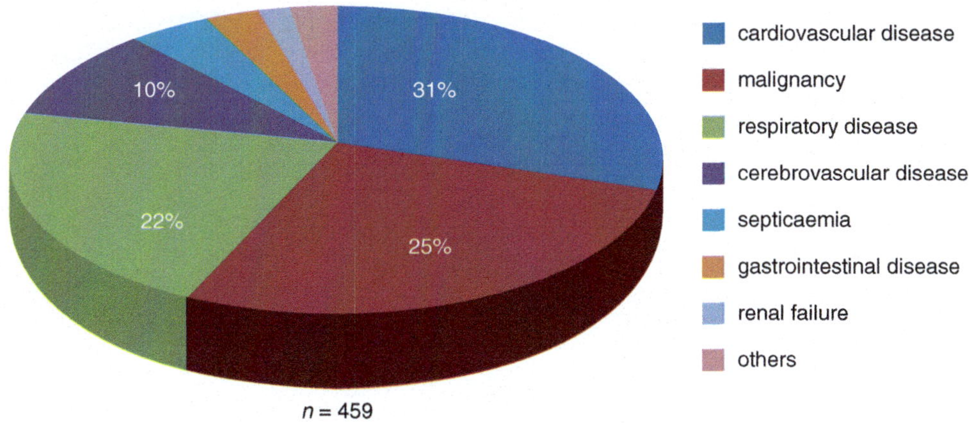

Fig. 1.1 Cause of death in RA patients from UK in 2007. *RA* rheumatoid arthritis, *UK* United Kingdom

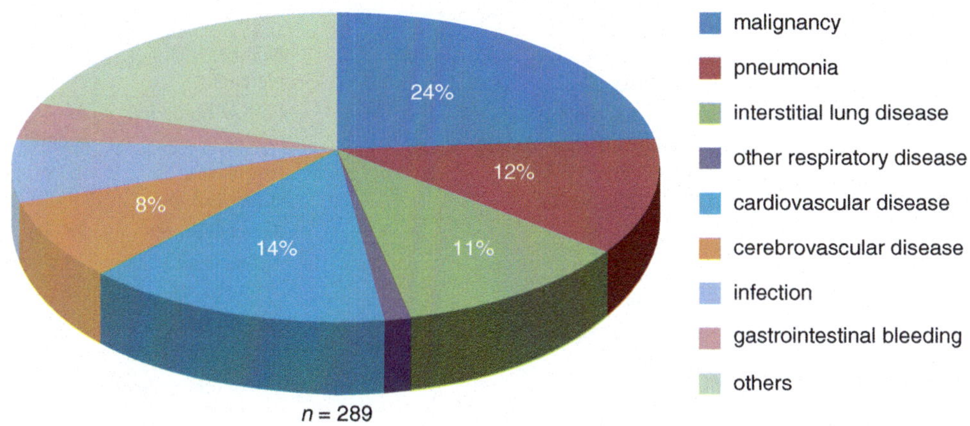

Fig. 1.2 Cause of death in RA patients from Japan in 2009. *RA* rheumatoid arthritis

Table 1.3 Risk factors for mortality in RA

Male
Older age
Lower socio-economic status
Smoking
Higher disease activity
Poor physical dysfunction
Presence of RF/ACPA
Carrying shared epitope of HLA-DRB1
Presence of bone erosion
Extra-articular features including ILD
High levels of ESR
Corticosteroid use

RA rheumatoid arthritis, *RF* rheumatoid factor, *ACPA* anti-citrullinated protein antibody, *HLA* human leukocyte antigen, *ILD* interstitial lung disease, *ESR* erythrocyte sedimentation rate

1.3 Pulmonary Complications in RA

In daily practice, we do not sufficiently know how to manage RA patients who have trouble in the lungs. Lung disease is a complication in approximately 5–60% of RA patients, depending on study design [15]. As shown in Table 1.4, the pulmonary manifestations revealed in RA are diverse [15]. Common pulmonary complications include RA-associated airway disease or ILD, infection, and drug-induced pneumonitis. How to manage each pulmonary complication will be described in detail in the relevant chapter.

1.4 bDMARDs and Pulmonary Complications in RA

In the Rochester cohort, RA patients were found to be at a higher risk of developing infection than non-RA subjects after adjusting for age, gender, smoking status, corticosteroid use, leukopenia, and diabetes mellitus [16]. This finding suggests that RA causes patients to be susceptible to infection. Although the precise reason remains unknown, sensitivities and excessive immune reaction or immune dysregulation to microorganisms might be involved in the occurrence of infections even without accounting for treatment with immunosuppressive agents such as bDMARDs.

According to a post-marketing survey from Japan, the rate of infection is 5–10% for the initial 6 months after the

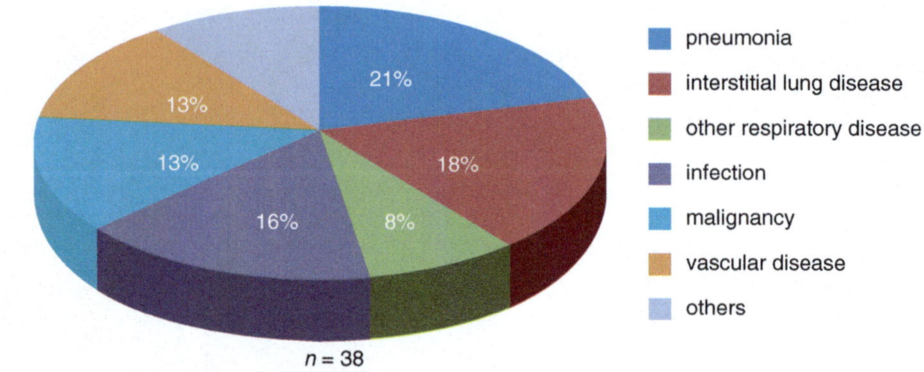

Fig. 1.3 Cause of death in RA patients treated with bDMARDs. *bDMARDs* biological disease-modifying antirheumatic disease

Table 1.4 Pulmonary manifestations in RA

RA-associated disease	
Airway	Bronchiectasis Bronchiolitis Emphysema
Parenchyma	Interstitial lung disease Organizing pneumonia Rheumatoid nodules
Pleura	Rheumatic pleuritis
Vascular	Vasculitis
Treatment-related disease	
	Infections
	Drug-induced pneumonitis
Others	
	Lung cancer Lymphoma

RA rheumatoid arthritis

Table 1.5 Frequency of infections and respiratory disease during treatment of bDMARDs in postmarketing surveys from Japan

	IFX	ETN	ADA	TCZ	ABA
Number of patients	5000	13,894	7740	7901	3985
Follow-up period	6 months	24 weeks	28 weeks	6 months	24 weeks
Respiratory comorbidity	4.7%	7.1%	13.4%	26.1%	13.5%
Adverse events	28%	27%	24%	38%	15%
The whole infections	18.4/100 per year	8.7%	7.0%	10%	5.9%
Pneumonia	2.2%	1.3%	1.3%	1.5%	0.7%
Tuberculosis	0.3%	0.07%	0.1%	0.05%	0.03%
Nontuberculosis mycobacteriosis	n.a	0.12%	0.1%	0.2%	0.05%
Pneumocystis pneumonia	0.4%	0.18%	0.34%	0.2%	0.1%
Aspergillosis	n.a	0.01%	0.03%	0.01%	0.03%
Cryptococcosis	n.a	0.01%	0.04%	n.a	n.a
Serious adverse events	6.2%	4.6%	4.5%	7.5%	2.5%
Infections	8.6/100 per year	2.4%	2.4%	3.6%	1.0%
Respiratory disease	1.7/100 per year	0.8%	0.7%	1.7%	0.3%

IFX infliximab, *ETN* etanercept, *ADA* adalimumab, *TCZ* tocilizumab, *ABA* abatacept, *n.a* not available

commencement of bDMARDs in RA patients [6]. The main sites of infection are the lung, urinary tract, and skin. The prevalence of each infection associated with the lung is presented in Table 1.5 [6, 17–20]. Pneumonia is noted in ~1% of RA patients treated with bDMARDs. Although the infection rate of mycobacterium and fungus is less than 1%, these infections frequently cause severe conditions and refractory or fatal outcomes. Therefore, the management and prevention of these infections are critical for clinicians who take care of RA patients. In addition, new events and acute exacerbation of ILD are also critical problems and occasionally cause mortality in RA patients treated with bDMARDs. It is occasionally difficult to determine whether the cause of ILD is the RA itself, the drugs used in treatment, an infection, or a combination of these factors.

1.5 Future Perspectives for Managing RA in Patients with Pulmonary Complications

Taking all of the findings mentioned above into considration, clinicians who take care of RA patients must learn how to prevent and manage these pulmonary complications in RA to improve the mortality and morbidity rates. However, there has been a lack of evidence regarding the pathophysiology and management of lung disease associated with RA. Therefore, in this book, we will describe the current status of knowledge about lung disease in RA and suggest the best form of management of lung disease in RA patients for clinicians, including general practitioners, rheumatologists, respirologists, radiologists, and pathologists. We hope that this book will prove helpful to all types of medical staff and clinicians who take care of RA patients. In the future, clinicians and researchers should continue to investigate more solutions regarding pulmonary issues in RA patients and establish more evidence in this regard. These continued efforts will thereby contribute to the improvement of outcome and prognosis in RA patients.

References

1. Smolen JS, Aletaha D, McInnes IB. Rheumatoid arthritis. Lancet. 2016;388:2023–38.
2. Haugeberg G, Hansen IJ, Soldal DM, Sokka T. Ten years of change in clinical disease status and treatment in rheumatoid arthritis: results based on standardized monitoring of patients in an ordinary outpatient clinic in southern Norway. Arthritis Res Ther. 2015;17:219.
3. Yamanaka H, Seto Y, Tanaka E, Furuya T, Nakajima A, Ikari K, Taniguchi A, Momohara S. Management of rheumatoid arthritis: the 2012 perspective. Mod Rheumatol. 2013;23:1–7.
4. Calabrese LH, Calabrese C, Kirchner E. The 2015 American College of Rheumatology guideline for the treatment of rheumatoid arthritis should include new standards for hepatitis B screening: comment on the article by Singh et al. Arthritis Rheumatol. 2016;68:1314–5.
5. Combe B, Landewe R, Daien CI, Hua C, Aletaha D, Álvaro-Gracia JM, Bakkers M, Brodin N, Burmester GR, Codreanu C, Conway R, Dougados M, Emery P, Ferraccioli G, Fonseca J, Raza K, Silva-Fernández L, Smolen JS, Skingle D, Szekanecz Z, Kvien TK, van der Helm-van Mil A, van Vollenhoven R. 2016 update of the EULAR recommendations for the management of early arthritis. Ann Rheum Dis. 2017;76(6):948–59.
6. Takayanagi N. Biological agents and respiratory infections: causative mechanisms and practice management. Respir Investig. 2015;53:185–200.
7. Turesson C, O'Fallon WM, Crowson CS, Gabriel SE, Matteson EL. Extra-articular disease manifestations in rheumatoid arthritis: incidence trends and risk factors over 46 years. Ann Rheum Dis. 2003;62:722–7.
8. Myllykangas-Luosujärvi R, Aho K, Kautiainen H, Isomäki H. Shortening of life span and causes of excess mortality in a population-based series of subjects with rheumatoid arthritis. Clin Exp Rheumatol. 1995;13:149–53.
9. Minaur NJ, Jacoby RK, Cosh JA, Taylor G, Rasker JJ. Outcome after 40 years with rheumatoid arthritis: a prospective study of function, disease activity, and mortality. J Rheumatol Suppl. 2004;69:3–8.
10. Young A, Koduri G, Batley M, Kulinskaya E, Gough A, Norton S, Dixey J, ERASE Group. Mortality in rheumatoid arthritis. Increased in the early course of disease, in ischaemic heart disease and in pulmonary fibrosis. Rheumatology (Oxford). 2007;46:350–7.
11. Nakajima A, Inoue E, Tanaka E, Singh G, Sato E, Hoshi D, Shidara K, Hara M, Momohara S, Taniguchi A, Kamatani N, Yamanaka H. Mortality and cause of death in Japanese patients with rheumatoid arthritis based on a large observational cohort, IORRA. Scand J Rheumatol. 2010;39:360–7.
12. Farragher TM, Goodson NJ, Naseem H, Silman AJ, Thomson W, Symmons D, Barton A. Association of the HLA-DRB1 gene with premature death, particularly from cardiovascular disease, in patients with rheumatoid arthritis and inflammatory polyarthritis. Arthritis Rheum. 2008;58:359–69.
13. Verstappen SM, Symmons DP. What is the outcome of RA in 2011 and can we predict it? Best Pract Res Clin Rheumatol. 2011;25:485–96.
14. Nakajima A, Saito K, Kojima T, Amano K, Yoshio T, Fukuda W, Inoue E, Taniguchi A, Momohara S, Minota S, Takeuchi T, Ishiguro N, Tanaka Y, Yamanaka H. No increased mortality in patients with rheumatoid arthritis treated with biologics: results from the biologics register of six rheumatology institutes in Japan. Mod Rheumatol. 2013;23:945–52.
15. Lake F, Proudman S. Rheumatoid arthritis and lung disease: from mechanisms to a practical approach. Semin Respir Crit Care Med. 2014;35:222–38.
16. Doran MF, Crowson CS, Pond GR, O'Fallon WM, Gabriel SE. Frequency of infection in patients with rheumatoid arthritis compared with controls: a population-based study. Arthritis Rheum. 2002;46:2287–93.
17. Koike T, Harigai M, Inokuma S, Ishiguro N, Ryu J, Takeuchi T, Tanaka Y, Yamanaka H, Hirose T, Yoshinaga T, Suzukawa M. Safety and effectiveness of 6 months' etanercept monotherapy and combination therapy in Japanese patients with rheumatoid arthritis: effect of concomitant disease-modifying antirheumatic drugs. J Rheumatol. 2013;40:1658–68.
18. Koike T, Harigai M, Ishiguro N, Inokuma S, Takei S, Takeuchi T, Yamanaka H, Haruna S, Ushida N, Kawana K, Tanaka Y. Safety and effectiveness of adalimumab in Japanese rheumatoid arthritis patients: postmarketing surveillance report of 7740 patients. Mod Rheumatol. 2014;24:390–8.
19. Koike T, Harigai M, Inokuma S, Ishiguro N, Ryu J, Takeuchi T, Takei S, Tanaka Y, Sano Y, Yaguramaki H, Yamanaka H. Effectiveness and safety of tocilizumab: postmarketing surveillance of 7901 patients with rheumatoid arthritis in Japan. J Rheumatol. 2014;41:15–23.
20. Takeuchi T, Tatsuki Y, Nogami Y, Ishiguro N, Tanaka Y, Yamanaka H, Kamatani N, Harigai M, Ryu J, Inoue K, Kondo H, Inokuma S, Ochi T, Koike T. Postmarketing surveillance of the safety profile of infliximab in 5000 Japanese patients with rheumatoid arthritis. Ann Rheum Dis. 2008;67:189–94.

Part II

Airway Disease in Rheumatoid Arthritis

Comprehensive Understanding of Airway Disease in Rheumatoid Arthritis

2

Hitoshi Tokuda

Abstract

Although the high prevalence of airway diseases in patients with rheumatoid arthritis (RA) has been recognized for decades, their clinical significance and treatment strategies have not been well discussed. With the introduction of potent disease-modifying treatments for RA, respiratory complications have emerged as the most important obstacle impeding the safe implementation of these therapies and improvement of patient prognosis. Along with interstitial lung disease, airway diseases are now regarded as one of the major risk factors of these lung complications and also result in their own problems such as airway obstruction and lung destruction. Bronchiectasis (BE) and bronchiolitis are well-known airway diseases that often develop concurrently. They are found in more than 10–30% of RA subjects and are thought to be caused by persistent inflammation of the airway attributed to the dysregulated immune response in RA. Not infrequently, airway inflammation may provoke destruction of the peripheral airway and lung parenchyma, leading to the formation of a honeycomb-like structure mimicking interstitial lung disease. Control of this inflammation is an urgent issue that needs to be addressed in the future.

Keywords

Rheumatoid arthritis • Airway disease • Bronchiectasis • Bronchiolitis • Respiratory infection

2.1 Introduction

The recent introduction of potent disease-modifying antirheumatic drugs (DMARDs), including methotrexate (MTX) and biologics, has revolutionized the treatment of rheumatoid arthritis (RA) and now allows almost complete control of joint inflammation in more than half of patients. However, we have yet to conclusively prove that they also improve patient prognosis.

A large-scale Japanese cohort survey in 2006 found that together with malignant tumors, respiratory diseases comprising pneumonia and interstitial lung disease (ILD) were the major causes of death in RA patients [1]. These data are derived from the prebiologics era (in Japan, biologics first became available in 2003). With the introduction of biologics, adverse events associated with these drugs were carefully studied in detail through clinical trials and postmarketing surveillance [2]. These studies elucidated that infections, specifically respiratory infections, were the most prominent issue among the various complications. Recently, a prospective, multicenter study was conducted in Japan to determine the prognosis of RA patients undergoing biologics therapy. Although treatment with biologics did not have a negative effect on overall outcomes, many fatalities occurred during this therapy, and in nearly 50% of the cases, death was attributed to respiratory diseases such as respiratory infections and ILD [3]. This means that one of the most vital challenges in current RA treatment,

H. Tokuda, M.D., Ph.D.
Department of Respiratory Medicine, Tokyo Yamate Medical Center, Japan Community Health Care Organization (JCHO), Tokyo, Japan
e-mail: tokuda@car.ocn.ne.jp

T. Gono et al. (eds.), *Lung Disease Associated with Rheumatoid Arthritis*, https://doi.org/10.1007/978-981-10-6750-1_2

particularly with biologics, is the control of respiratory complications and especially respiratory infections.

Until recently, the high incidence of respiratory infections in RA patients was attributed to the use of immunosuppressants such as corticosteroids [4]. However, this is not necessarily true under biologics therapy. For example, many autoinflammatory diseases are treated with biologics, but respiratory infections are only observed in RA at a high frequency, whereas they are not nearly as prevalent in inflammatory bowel disease. This suggests that factors unique to RA exist in the etiology of these infections. Attention is increasingly directed to underlying lung diseases, i.e., airway disease and ILD, as the major risk factors [5, 6].

In the past, studies on chronic lung complications of RA have focused primarily on ILD [7], and airway diseases have not been investigated nearly as thoroughly. However, within recent years, knowledge has been compiled on their incidence, pathogenesis, and effect on prognosis in RA patients [8–10].

Airway diseases are traditionally handled in two distinct entity, large airway disease and small airway disease. Large airway disease presents as bronchiectasis (BE), whereas small airway disease comprises various forms of bronchiolitis. Furthermore, we advocate here that bronchiolar dilatation should be added to this discussion as another peripheral type of airway disease (described below). These airway diseases all occur far more frequently in RA patients than in the general population, the fact of which urges us to assume that their etiology is closely related to the pathophysiology of RA [8, 11].

2.2 Bronchiectasis (BE)

2.2.1 Epidemiology

The frequency of BE in RA patients has been assessed in many studies using high-resolution computed tomography (HRCT) over the past two decades. Most of these studies report prevalence between 30 and 40% (Table 2.1) [12–19]. Early studies were retrospective and subject to selection bias, whereas the more recent studies are prospective and consecutively enrolled all RA patients who presented to a medical facility during a specified period. Given the large subject size of these studies, the results are highly reliable. Rheumatologists who have used chest radiography alone to assess their patients may find these figures as unacceptable. In a review of BE coexistence in RA patients, Wilczynska and colleagues pointed out that RA patients rarely complain of respiratory symptoms and also that chest radiographs lack the requisite sensitivity, declaring HRCT to be essential to provide an accurate assessment of BE [8]. Figure 2.1 illustrates a case in which chest radiography showed no remarkable findings, while an HRCT scan revealed widespread BE. There is no room for argument that HRCT scans are required in the diagnosis of BE.

There do not appear to be any national or racial differences in this frequency, nor does treatment history appear to be relevant. Mori and colleagues performed HRCT scans in 126 consecutive RA patients on their first visit, of which 41% had signs of BE [18]. This was observed not only in

Table 2.1 Reported prevalence of bronchiectasis in RA patients, literature review

Author	Country	Study type	*n*	Mean age (y)	Mean duration of RA (y)	Prevalence of bronchiectasis (%)	References
Perez T et al.	France	Prospective	50	57.8 ± 1.5	14.4 ± 1.3	30	Am J Resp Crit Care Med 1994 [12]
Cortet et al.	France	Prospective	68	58.8 ± 10.6	12 ± 9.2	31	Ann Rheum Dis 1997 [43]
Despaux et al.	France	Prospective	46	60.1 (30–85)	10.1(1–32)	41	Rev Rhum Engl Ed 1998 [13]
Mori et al.	Japan	Prospective	126	60.0 ± 12.4	0 or 11.8 ± 9.7[a]	41	J Rheumatol 2008 [18]
Wilsher et al.	New Zealand	Prospective	60	54 (26–76)	0.6(0–1)	35	Resp Med 2012 [17]
Remy-Jardin et al.	France	Retrospective	84	57 ± 9	12 ± 8	24	Radiology 1994 [12]
Tsuchiya et al.	Japan	Retrospective	144	65.2 ± 9.8	9.7 ± 12.0	22	Eur Respir J 2011 [19]
Akira M et al.	Japan	Retrospective	29	59 ± 11	n.a.	52	J Comput Assist Tomogr 1999 [15]
Terasaki H et al.	Japan	Prospective	34[b]	61(41–80)	12(0–39)	62	Radiat Med 2004 [16]

[a]Within 1 year in 65 patients and longer duration in 61 patients
[b]Subjects are limited to those with respiratory symptoms

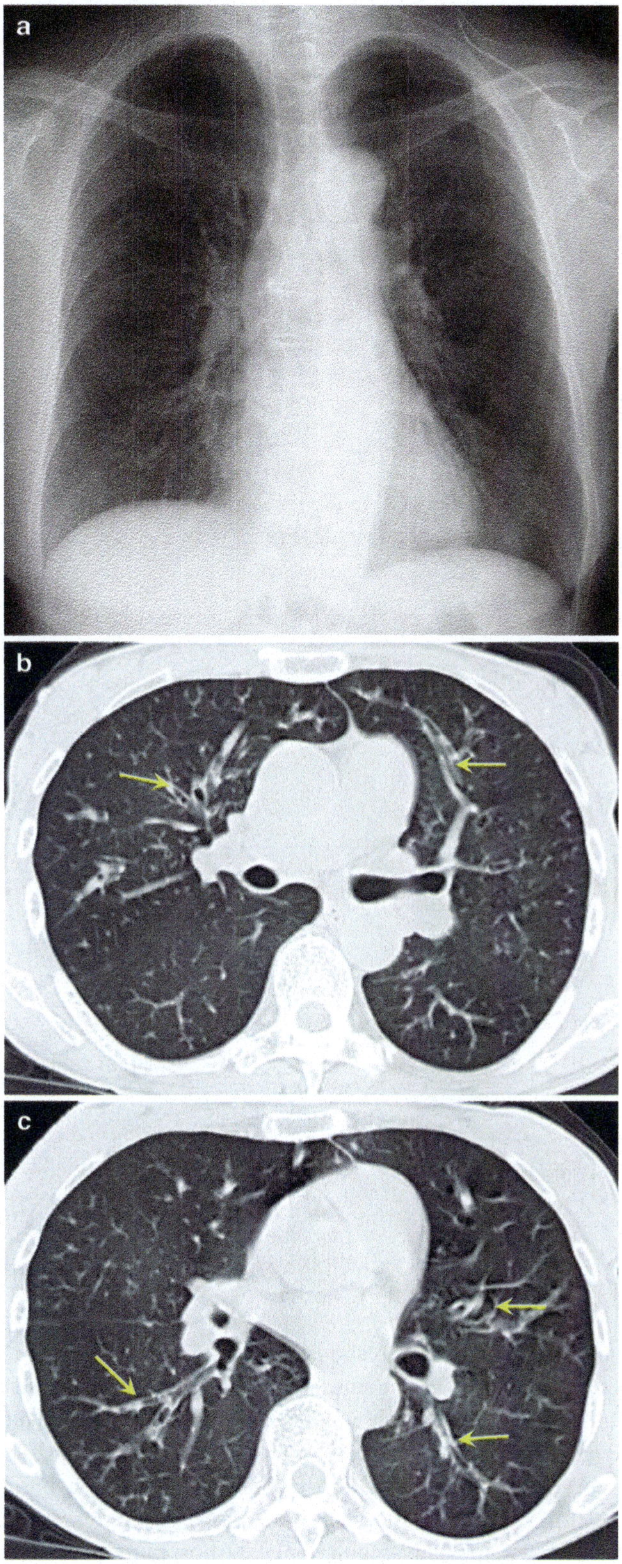

Fig. 2.1 Chest radiography is often powerless for detecting airway disease. (**a**) Chest radiograph in a 65-year-old woman with RA for 2 years. She complained of cough and sputum for several years. We cannot find any abnormality on this image. (**b, c**) HRCT reveals bronchiectasis with bronchial wall thickening distributed in every lobe (arrows), and also small nodules are scattered around. In this case, only HRCT can demonstrate these anatomic changes of the airway

patients with long-standing RA (49%) but also in 34% of patients with early RA. This high prevalence cannot be explained by the conventional hypothesis that BE is a result of repeated infection caused by immunosuppressive therapy. It is 10- to 20-fold higher than the prevalence in the general population [20], and it should be considered to be directly associated with RA itself.

2.2.2 Mechanism of Development

In non-RA subjects, BE is often attributed to a previous medical history of pneumonia or other infections during childhood or later years. This is, however, not true in those with RA. Detailed interviews prove that the majority had no history of major infectious episodes, whereas disease is often widespread with involvement of two or more pulmonary lobes at presentation.

In the general population, BE is considered to evolve through the following process (Fig. 2.2). Chronic neutrophilic inflammation in the airway persists and injures the supportive structure of the airway, that is, cartilage, elastic fibers and smooth muscle, causing fragility of the airway structure. There, negative pressure held inside the lungs causes airway dilatation. Edema of the submucosal layer, cellular infiltration, collagen deposition, and increases in bronchial glands then lead to thickening of the bronchial wall [21].

Recently, in addition to these morphological studies, immunological researches have been compiled and clarified the following scenario: macrophages and airway epithelial cells respond to the colonized bacteria such as *Streptococcus* or *Pseudomonas* and release cytokines such as IL-17, IL-8, and TNF-alpha, which drive neutrophils into action in the airway wall. Activation enzymes released from these neutrophils, such as elastase and matrix metalloproteinases, damage and destroy the supporting tissue of the bronchial wall as mentioned above (Fig. 2.3) [22–24].

In RA patients, it may be postulated that similar and more intense inflammation occurs in the airway, leading to the development of BE [11]. Unfortunately no studies have yet analyzed the inflammatory dynamics of the airway in patients with RA.

2.2.2.1 BE Appearing after RA Onset

BE may be observed to develop de novo in the course of RA. Figure 2.4 shows a case in which BE appeared in only a few years. This is a woman in her 60s with a 6-year history of RA. A CT scan performed 3 years ago for a mild productive cough revealed only a fibrotic scar in the middle lobe (Fig. 2.4a, b). Thereafter, she sometimes presented with a productive cough without any febrile episodes. At her presentation to our respiratory department, she complained of a

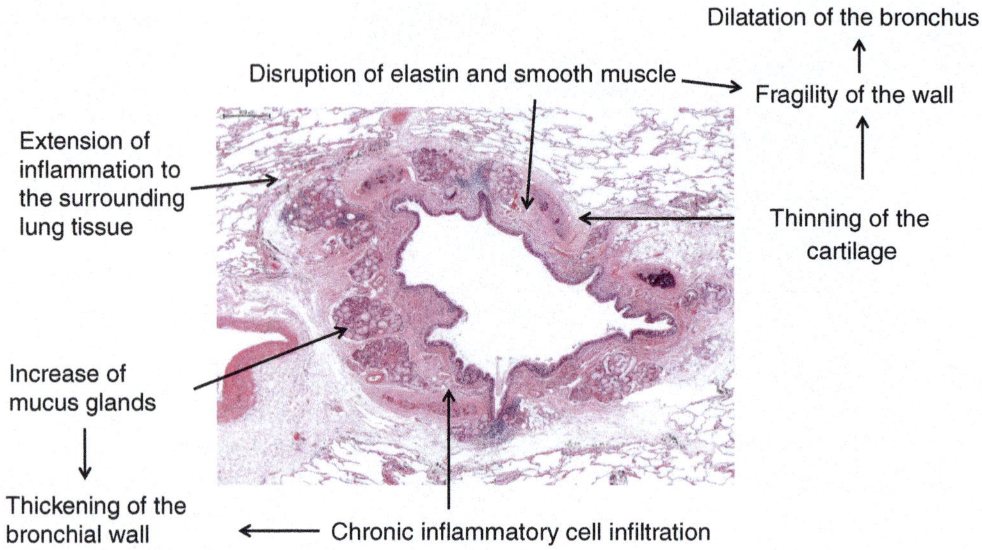

Fig. 2.2 Pathogenesis of bronchiectasis on a morphological basis. Chronic neutrophilic inflammation in the airway disrupts elastin, smooth muscle, and cartilage of the bronchial wall, leading to structural fragility and then dilatation of the bronchus. Thickening of the bronchial wall is also brought about by this chronic inflammation. Photomicrograph courtesy of Dr. T. Takemura

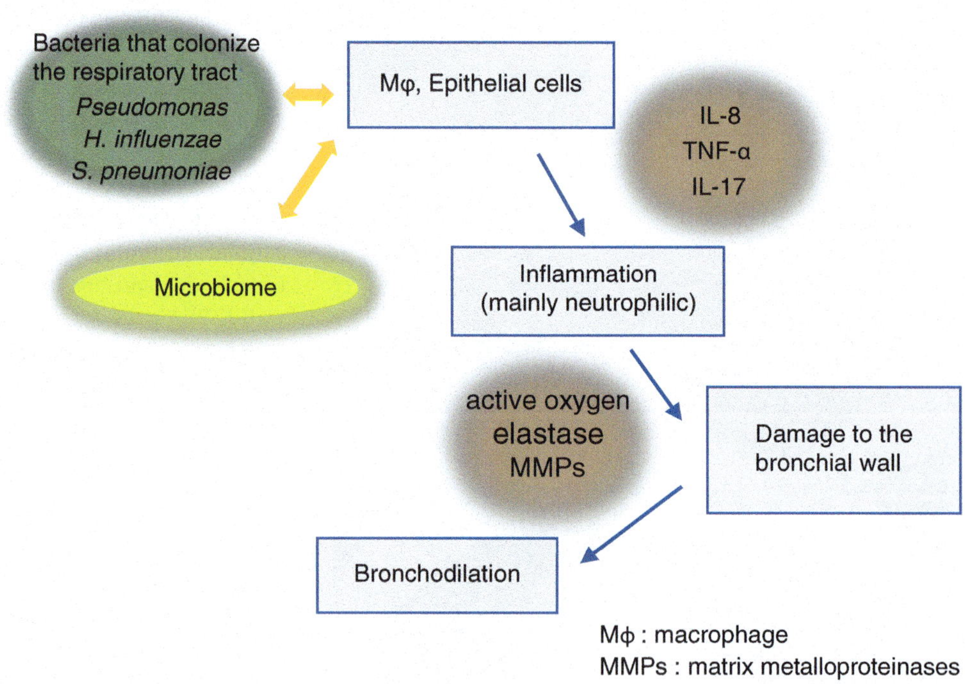

Fig. 2.3 Putative immunological pathogenesis of bronchiectasis in RA elucidated by clinical immunological studies over the recent decades. With the recognition of colonized bacteria, macrophages and epithelial cells release inflammatory cytokines such as IL-8, TNF-α, and IL-17, which induce persistent neutrophilic inflammation that leads to destruction of the bronchial wall. It has recently been postulated that this inflammatory process may be caused by dysbiosis of the microbiome in the airways and/or dysregulation of the host immune response, a subject that has attracted much attention in this decade

mild productive cough for 1 month and weight loss of 2 kg, and a CT scan was performed (Fig. 2.4c, d). BE has now become apparent in the right middle lobe over these 3 years. Fluoroquinolones were highly effective against symptoms in this patient and prevented further aggravation thereafter. This case clearly shows that BE may appear de novo during the course of RA. Importantly, in such cases, the signs or symptoms may be subtle or often absent. Physicians must be alert to this possibility.

BE also develops in patients with autoimmune diseases other than RA such as ulcerative colitis. How should we interpret this phenomenon? Boyton and colleagues, one of the leading investigators of the immunology of BE, postulate that in those patients with autoimmune diseases, an excessive and dysregulated immune response is the key concept [11, 25]. Recent advances in genome sequencing technology revealed that the respiratory tract, which was thought to be sterile until several years ago, harbors microorganisms that are not detected by standard culture techniques, forming a unique lung microbiome. In those autoimmune diseases, dysbiosis of this microbiome or dysregulation of the host immune response may evoke an exuberant immune response in the airway, leading to persistent inflammation and the development of BE (Fig. 2.3). Further research is awaited in this field.

2.2.2.2 BE Preceding RA Onset

As mentioned above, Mori and colleagues [18] found that 30% of patients showed signs of BE in HRCT during the

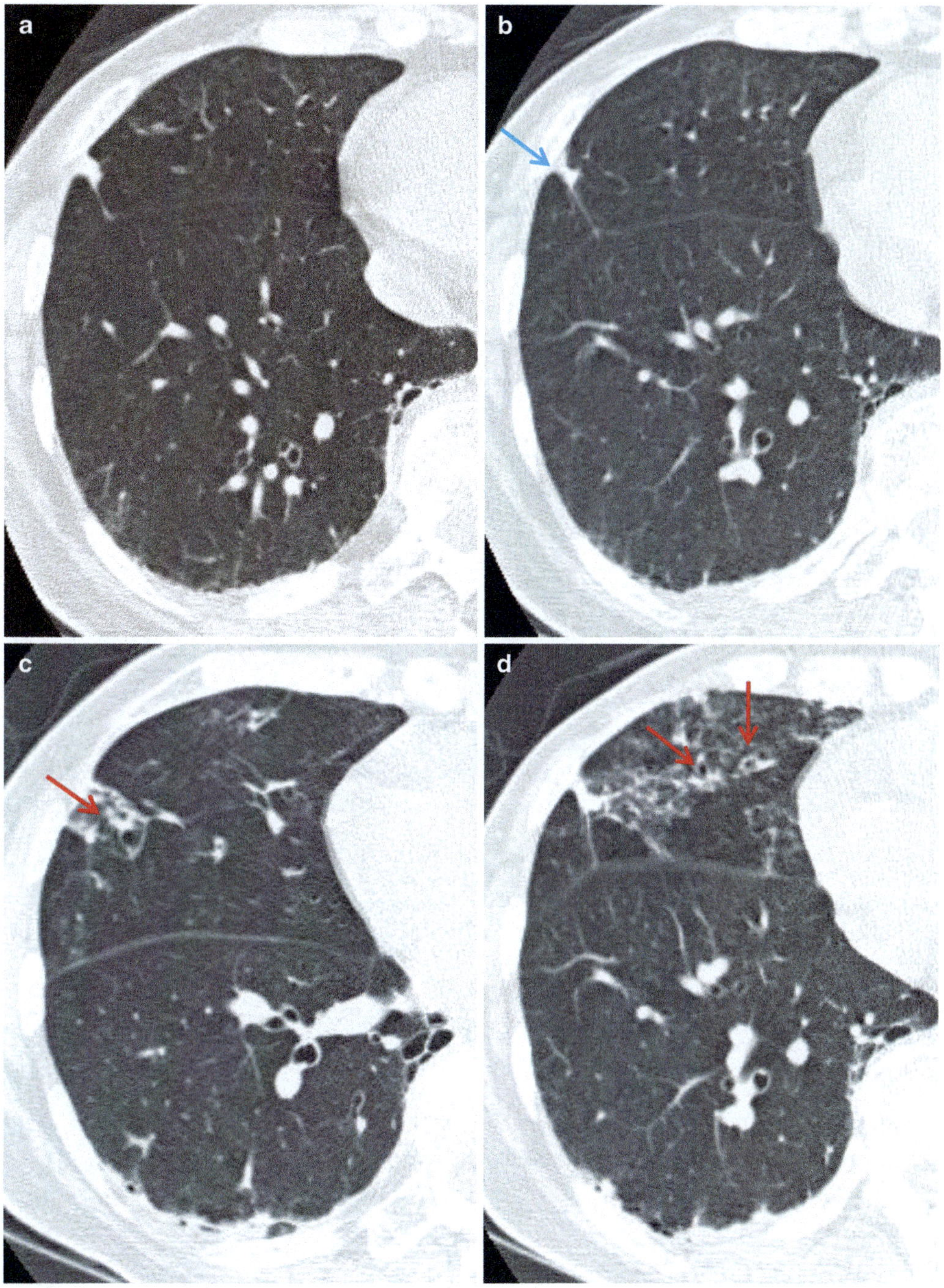

Fig. 2.4 A case of bronchiectasis in which its development was observed during the clinical course of RA. HRCT of a 67-year-old woman with RA of 6-year duration. (**a**, **b**) HRCT 3 years ago shows only fibrotic scarring in the right S^4 (blue arrow). No dilatation of the bronchi is visible. (**c**, **d**) Three years later, she complained cough, sputum, and weight loss. HRCT revealed newly developed bronchiectasis (red arrows) and micronodules surrounding these areas

early period of RA, suggesting the possibility of BE as concurrent or preceding disorder. In clinical experience, BE certainly precedes the onset of RA in a certain proportion of cases. We show a typical case of such a sequence in Fig. 2.5. A 55-year-old man who was diagnosed as RA 4 months earlier presented with a recurrent and prolonged productive cough. He had been diagnosed as having BE at his young age. In this patient, it is apparent clinically that BE preceded RA. CT scans revealed advanced BE in his middle and lower lobes. In the surrounding area, widespread micronodules are observed indicating bronchiolitis (Fig. 2.5a, b).

This sequence may have some relationship with the pathogenesis of RA. Demoruelle and colleagues examined HRCT findings in 42 subjects positive for RA-related autoantibody but who did not have inflammatory arthritis and found airway changes such as BE and bronchiolitis in 76% of them. Furthermore, five of those subjects later developed RA. They considered that an immune response at the mucosal site of the respiratory tract forms RA-related autoantibodies, particularly anti-CCP antibodies, which then reach the joints via the bloodstream and contribute to the development of RA. They postulated that the preclinical stage of RA

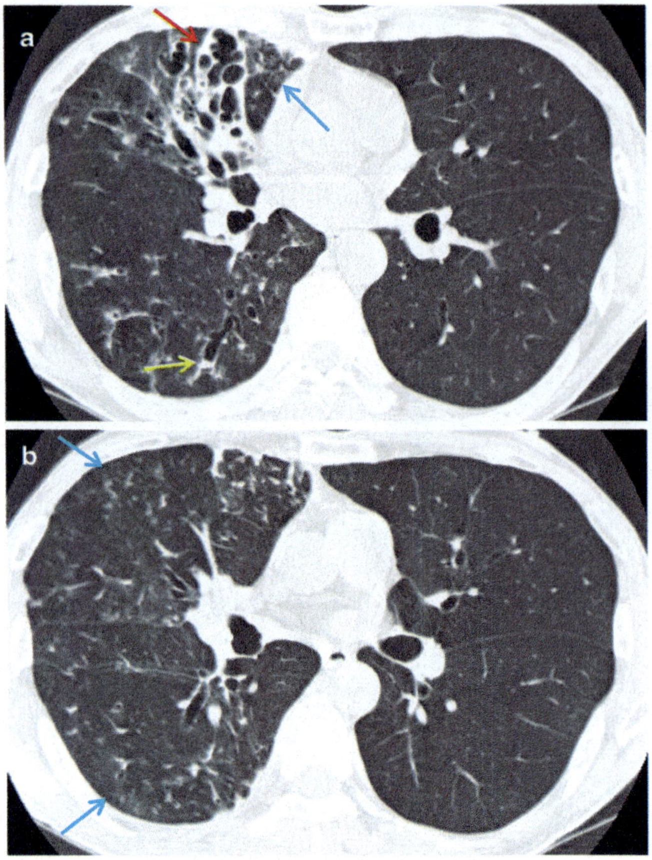

Fig. 2.5 A case of bronchiectasis that preceded the onset of RA. HRCT in a 55-year-old man with RA of 4-month duration. (**a**) Bronchiectasis with consolidation is conspicuous in the middle lobe (red arrow). (**b**) Bronchiectasis is also seen in the lower lobe (yellow arrow), and micronodules are scattered throughout the entire right lung (blue arrows). He was diagnosed as having BE at a younger age, that is, his airway disease preceded the onset of RA

may be chronic inflammation of the airway where interaction between the immune system and the altered microbiome may generate autoimmunity [26].

2.2.3 Imaging Findings

The diagnosis of BE on HRCT scans is detailed in Chap. 4. The criteria summarized and proposed by leading radiologist Naidich are easy to apply and are widely accepted [27].

The distribution of BE in RA patients is not necessarily limited to a single lobe. In nearly half of the patients, BE is found over two or more lobes and often in the entire lung including the upper lobes. Shrinkage of the affected lobe is common, which is thought to be a result of repeated bouts of inflammation. Findings indicating bronchiolitis such as centrilobular micronodules and branching opacities are often noted peripherally (Figs. 2.6 and 2.7).

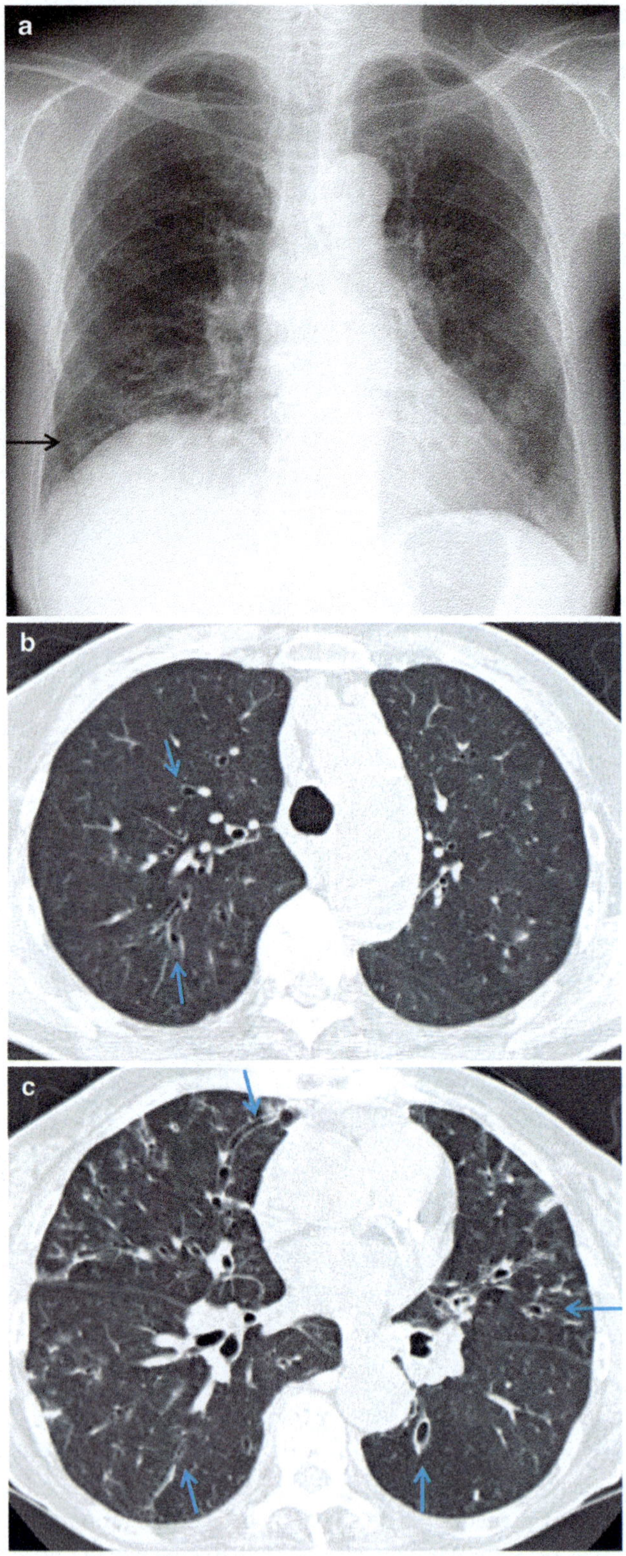

Fig. 2.6 Bronchiectasis distributed mainly in the lower lung field. (**a**) Chest radiograph in a 73-year-old woman with RA for 12 years. She had complained of a persistent productive cough for 2 years, with a weight loss of 4 kg. Reticular opacities are visible in the bilateral lung bases (arrow). In addition, shrinkage of the right lower lung is noted. (**b**) HRCT of the upper lung zone reveals mild bronchiectasis (blue arrows). (**c**) In the lower zone, diffuse bronchiectasis is visible with scattered micronodules in the surrounding area (blue arrows)

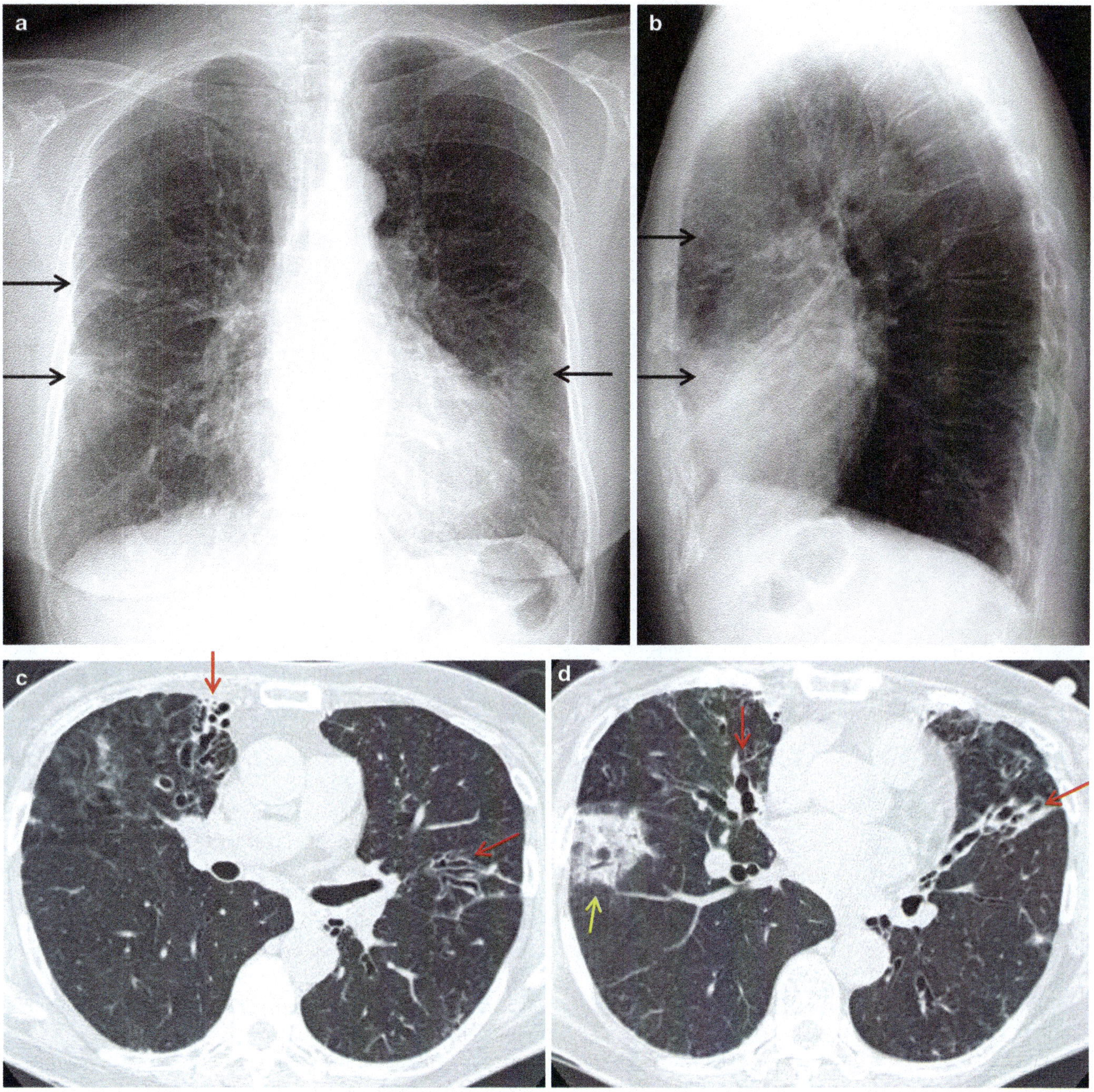

Fig. 2.7 Bronchiectasis with upper and middle lobe predominance. Chest radiograph of a 71-year-old woman. (**a**) In the posteroanterior radiograph, reticular shadows are visible in the middle and lower lung fields that mimic lung fibrosis (arrows). (**b**) In the lateral view, however, the shadows are extended to the ventral area in a segmental manner (arrow), suggesting upper and middle lobe distribution. (**c**, **d**) HRCT shows bronchiectasis distributed throughout the entire lung (red arrows). A focus of consolidation is seen in the right lower lobe (yellow arrow), indicating pneumonia

The primary clinical concern in BE is the risk of bacterial pneumonia [28, 29]. We show a case of pneumonia in Fig. 2.8. On the chest radiograph, a pneumonia shadow is visible in the right lower lung, and on HRCT, we recognize BE within the pneumonia and its adjacent area, indicating that BE is the predisposing factor for this pneumonia (Fig. 2.8b). RA patients with complications of BE are reported to have a poor prognosis because of repeated infection [30, 31]. This issue is detailed in Chap. 5.

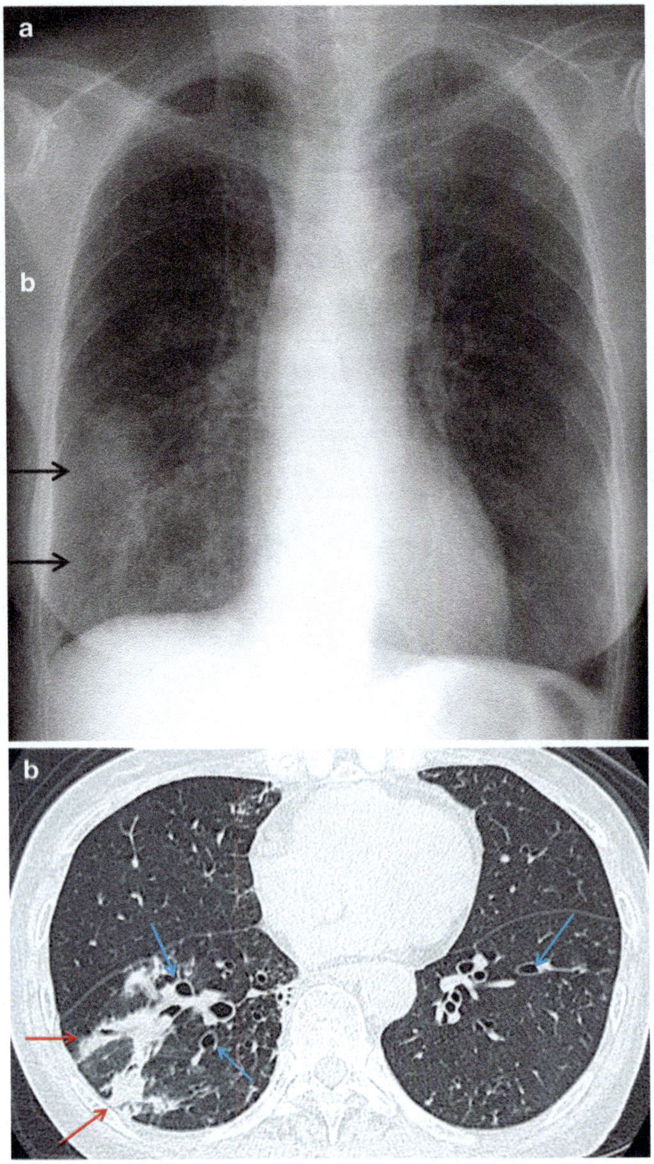

Fig. 2.8 Bronchiectasis complicated with pneumonia in a 72-year-old woman. She complained low-grade fever, cough, and sputum for several days. (**a**) This radiograph shows an infiltrative shadow in the right lower lung field (arrows). (**b**) HRCT shows an infiltrative shadow in the right lower lobe (red arrows). Bronchiectasis of a marked degree (blue arrows) is visible adjacent to those infiltrative shadow, suggesting that pneumonia has occurred at the base of bronchiectasis

2.3 Peripheral Airway Disease: Bronchiolitis

A great number of studies have been accumulated on the morphology and pathophysiology of bronchiolitis. They are detailed in Chap. 3. Here, we shall have a glance at these issues and consider their clinical significance.

2.3.1 Pathology of Bronchiolitis

Bronchiolitis in RA has been classified into several histopathological types [32] including (1) cellular bronchiolitis, (2) follicular bronchiolitis (FB), and (3) bronchiolitis obliterans (BO). We provide a simple overview below.

FB is observed in particular diseases such as RA or Sjögren's syndrome (Fig. 2.9b). FB is characterized by inducible bronchus-associated lymphoid tissue (iBALT) comprising mature B lymphocytes and plasma cells formed in the submucosal layer and outside the bronchial walls. In 2006, Rangel-Moleno and colleagues used modern immunohistological techniques to study the roles of these lymph systems and discovered that they produce various cytokines, chemokines, and anti-CCP antibodies that play major roles in the pathogenesis of RA. Of note, iBALT plays a harmful role to the surrounding lung tissue through these processes [33].

Agreement cannot be reached on the pathology of BO in RA [32]. BO is also often observed after transplantations, and there is controversy about whether BO in RA differs from post-transplant BO. In Japan, Homma and colleagues examined three BO patients with RA and described unique characteristics of these diffuse panbronchiolitis-like cases [34]. Hebisawa and colleagues reviewed many cases of BO and divided them into two categories. In one subtype, the structure of the airway wall is reserved, but the lumen is narrowed and obstructed by granulation tissue; they termed this "endobronchiolitis obliterans." This subtype is often found in patients after transplantation and is considered to be the same entity as conventional constrictive bronchiolitis. In the other subtype, inflammation extends to the entire airway wall, causing destruction and ultimate fibrosis of the wall that leads to constriction and obstruction of the lumen. They named the latter subtype "cellular and destructive bronchiolitis" (Fig. 2.9c). It is often seen in autoimmune diseases such as RA and Sjögren's syndrome and is accompanied by thickening and dilatation of the large airways [35]. These characteristics well match the clinical and radiological features of BO in RA [36].

In RA patients, two or more of these pathological types may coexist within the same patient's lungs [37]. A certain pattern may be prevailing at the biopsied site, but another pattern may prevail at another site; thence a diagnosis should not be based on this finding alone. Particularly in FB, several clinical and pathological reports handle this type as a distinct category [38]. Yet, on the basis of the above-mentioned reason, and because those reports failed to present distinct clinical features, the term "FB" should be used as a term for a pathological finding rather than an distinct clinicopathological entity.

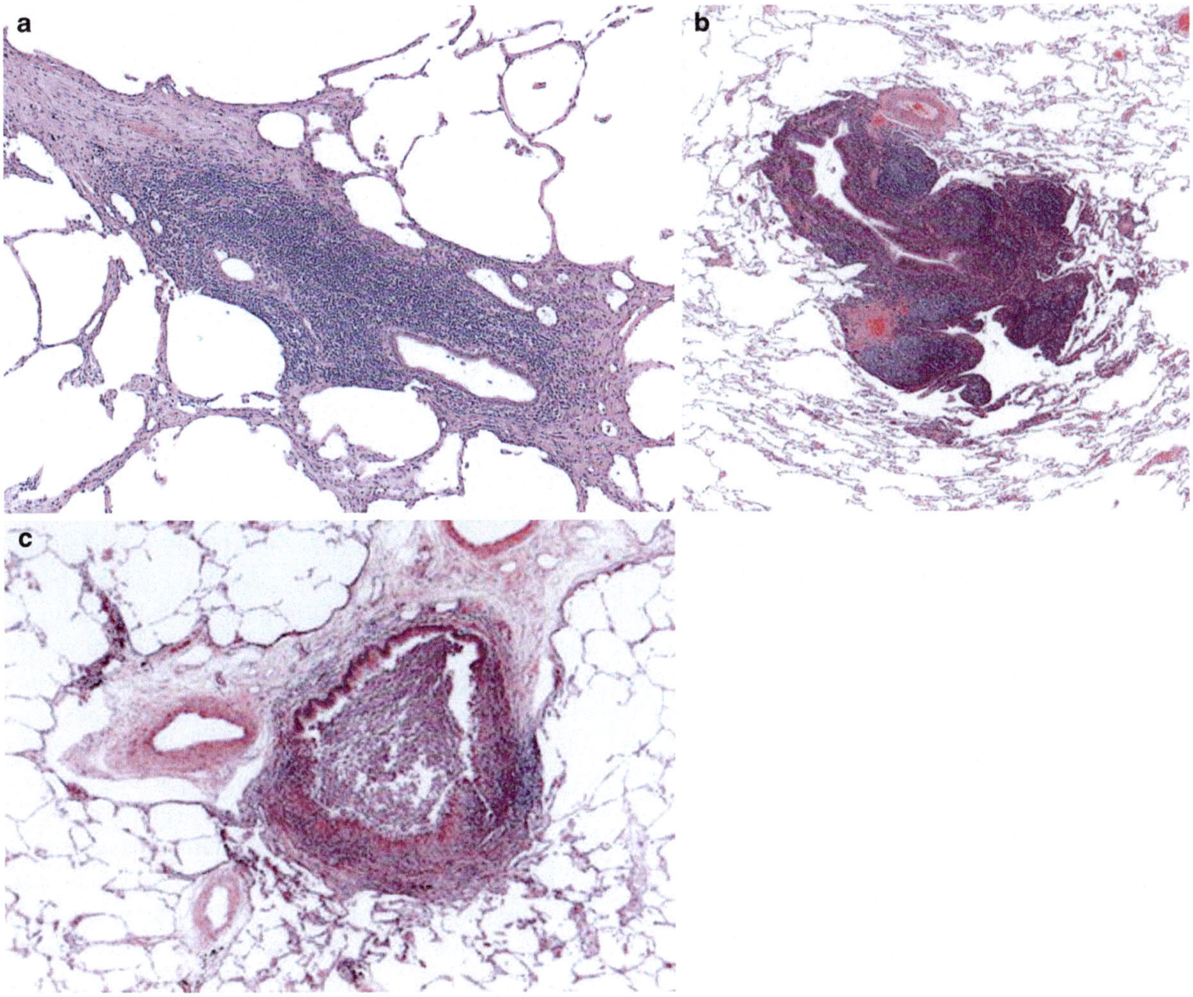

Fig. 2.9 Histological variations of bronchiolitis in RA. (**a**) Cellular bronchiolitis, (**b**) follicular bronchiolitis, and (**c**) cellular and destructive bronchiolitis (Photomicrograph in [**a**, **b**] courtesy of Dr. T. Takemura and that in [**c**] courtesy of Dr. A. Hebisawa)

How do the early stages of bronchiolitis look like? Figure 2.10 shows the histological findings of a surgical lung biopsy (SLB) specimen from an 18-year-old woman who developed RA 1 year ago. SLB was performed for suspicion of ILD. Cellular interstitial pneumonia was noted widely. At the site shown in this figure, a respiratory bronchiole is seen on a background of nearly normal lung. The walls are thickened due to inflammatory cell infiltration and collagen depo-

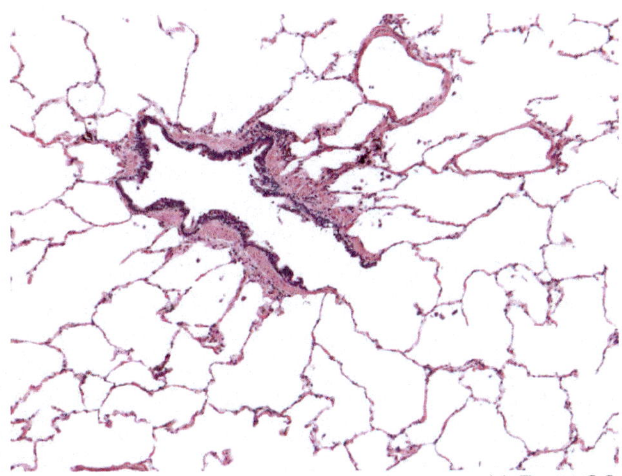

Fig. 2.10 Early stage of bronchiolitis in an 18-year-old woman with RA. Surgical lung biopsy was done for suspicion of interstitial pneumonia. In this almost normal lung, we see a respiratory bronchiole whose wall is thickened with inflammatory cell infiltration and collagen deposition. This patient has no respiratory symptoms (Photomicrograph courtesy of Drs. T. Takemura and H. Sugimoto)

sition and show the very early stages of bronchiolitis. This patient did not complain of any respiratory symptoms, indicating that bronchiolitis can develop from a very early stage in RA patients insidiously.

2.3.2 Epidemiology

The frequency of bronchiolitis among RA patients was investigated in various studies using HRCT, and a prevalence from 8 to 18% was reported [39, 40]. Takemura reported a prevalence of 61% in autopsied cases [41].

2.3.3 Imaging Findings

Centrilobular micronodules and branching opacities are thought to represent bronchiolitis on HRCT scans [37, 42]. The distribution is sometimes regional and sometimes diffuse. In BO, instead of the micronodular patterns, mosaic patterns may prevail in the lung field, which is shown more demonstrably in an expiratory CT scan. The details are discussed in Chap. 4.

2.3.4 How and When Does Bronchiolitis Appear and How Does It Progress in RA Patients?

No previous reports have tried to answer these questions. Below, we present some cases and discuss how and when bronchiolitis appears and how it persists or disappears in RA patients.

A case in which we fortunately witnessed the onset of bronchiolitis on sequential CT scans is shown in Fig. 2.11. The CT scan in Fig. 2.11a shows the first episode of pneumonia in a 49-year-old woman with RA of 15-year duration. The left lower lobe was consolidated with a marked loss of volume, inside of which dilated bronchi are visible. This was a case of pneumonia at the base of BE, which had progressed to organized pneumonia. This patient did not respond to antibiotics and required corticosteroids. At this point, there were no signs of abnormalities in the right lung.

Thereafter, MTX was restarted, and 4 months later, the patient had another episode of pneumonia. Along with the pneumonia in the left lower lobe, a chest radiograph revealed a newly developed granular opacity in the right lower lung (Fig. 2.11b), and HRCT scans confirmed a diagnosis of bronchiolitis (Fig. 2.11c). Thereafter, the patient suffered multiple recurrences of pneumonia, but each time, they were controlled with prompt administration of fluoroquinolones. Pharmacotherapy with MTX and biologics, essential to control her RA activity, was continued throughout the course of these episodes. Thanks to this persistence, the RA symptoms were stabilized, and she did not suffer recurrences of pneumonia thereafter. However, on the HRCT scan, micronodular opacities remained even after the successful disease course (Fig. 2.11d). A mild productive cough also persists. In this case, we observed the appearance of bronchiolitis, which was presumably formed through the spread of microorganisms from the left side during the second episode of pneumonia. We also learned through this case that once established, bronchiolitis would not disappear by any means.

A mild case of bronchiolitis in a woman in her 50s with RA for 10 years is shown in Fig. 2.12. Abnormal findings had been noted on chest radiography over the past 3 years (Fig. 2.12a). On HRCT, regional bronchiolitis is visible in the right upper lobe, and BE is noted in the left lingular division (Fig. 2.12b, c). During this period, the patient had suffered several episodes of mild respiratory tract infections. It was assumed that bronchiolitis had been formed through bacterial aspiration from the BE in the left side. Mycobacterial disease was ruled out with bronchoscopy. Over the next few years, this condition continued to wax and wane with aggravation and disappearance of the granular opacities on the images, which paralleled RA disease activity (Fig. 2.12d, e). A mild, productive cough was also noted during the periods of aggravation. This case shows that bronchiolitis, which began as an infectious type, may persist and fluctuate in parallel with RA disease activity in a patient with a mild disease course.

A 75-year-old woman with a chronic productive cough of a several years' duration and a 20-year history of RA is shown in Fig. 2.13. In chest images, widespread BE and bronchiolar disease were noted throughout the entire lung. Long-term therapy with macrolides had proven ineffective. Despite restrictive and occlusive mixed lung function impairment, the patients did not complain of dyspnea, presumably because of her low daily activity. This type of widespread broncho-bronchiolar disease is not infrequently seen in RA patients in clinical practice. Occasionally, this can be confused with diffuse panbronchiolitis in East Asia, but the distinct clinical course and the lack of response to macrolide therapy reveal a completely different disease profile.

Common to these cases presented here is the coexistence of BE at central side and bronchiolitis at peripheral side. Many CT studies report this coexistence, and also many studies using both HRCT and PFT have revealed a high prevalence of obstructive impairment in subjects with BE [17, 42, 43]. Airway inflammation in RA patients is not limited either to the central or peripheral airways, but it often involves the entire airway.

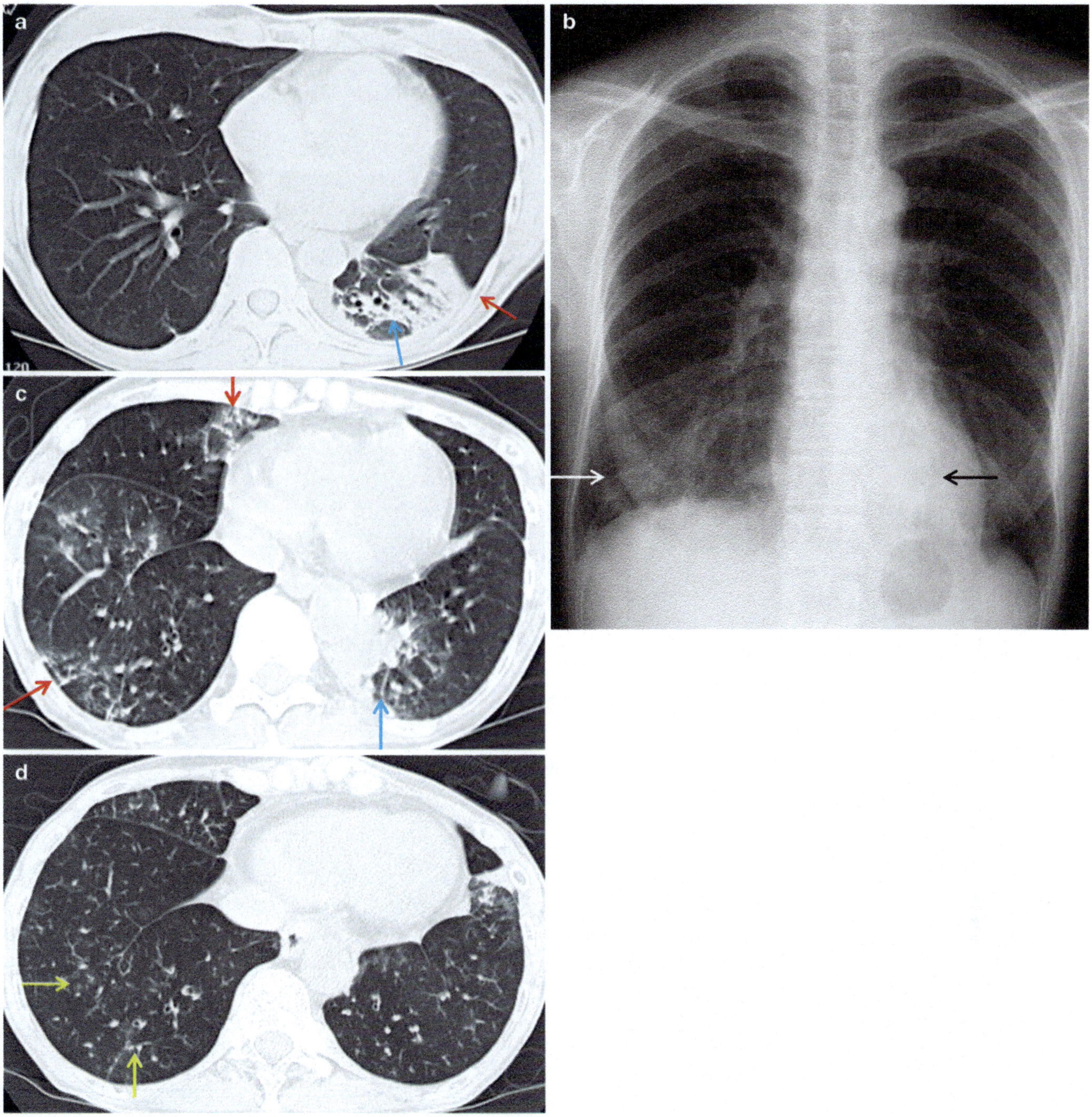

Fig. 2.11 Development of bronchiolitis observed in a 49-year-old woman with RA of 15-year duration. (**a**) HRCT at her first presentation for protracted pneumonia. The left lower lobe is collapsed and consolidated (red arrow), and dilated bronchial lumens are visible within it (blue arrow). This is the organized stage of pneumonia, which occurred at the base of bronchiectasis. Note that there are no abnormalities in the right lung. (**b**) The second episode of pneumonia after 4-month treatment of RA with MTX. The chest radiograph shows pneumonia in the left lower lung that obliterates the contour of the descending aorta (arrow). Disseminated granular shadows appear in the right lower lung field (white arrow). (**c**) HRCT scan shows pneumonia at S^{10} of the left lower lobe (blue arrow). Many micronodules are present in the right lower lobe and middle lobe (red arrows). (**d**) HRCT scan 4 years later shows micronodules and bronchiectasis remaining in the right lower lung field (yellow arrows). During this period, she suffered from several episodes of pneumonia, all of which were successfully controlled with the prompt use of fluoroquinolones. In the successive 5 years until now, she has not been troubled by pneumonia in accordance with good control of her RA disease activity. She still complains of cough and sputum, but it is tolerable

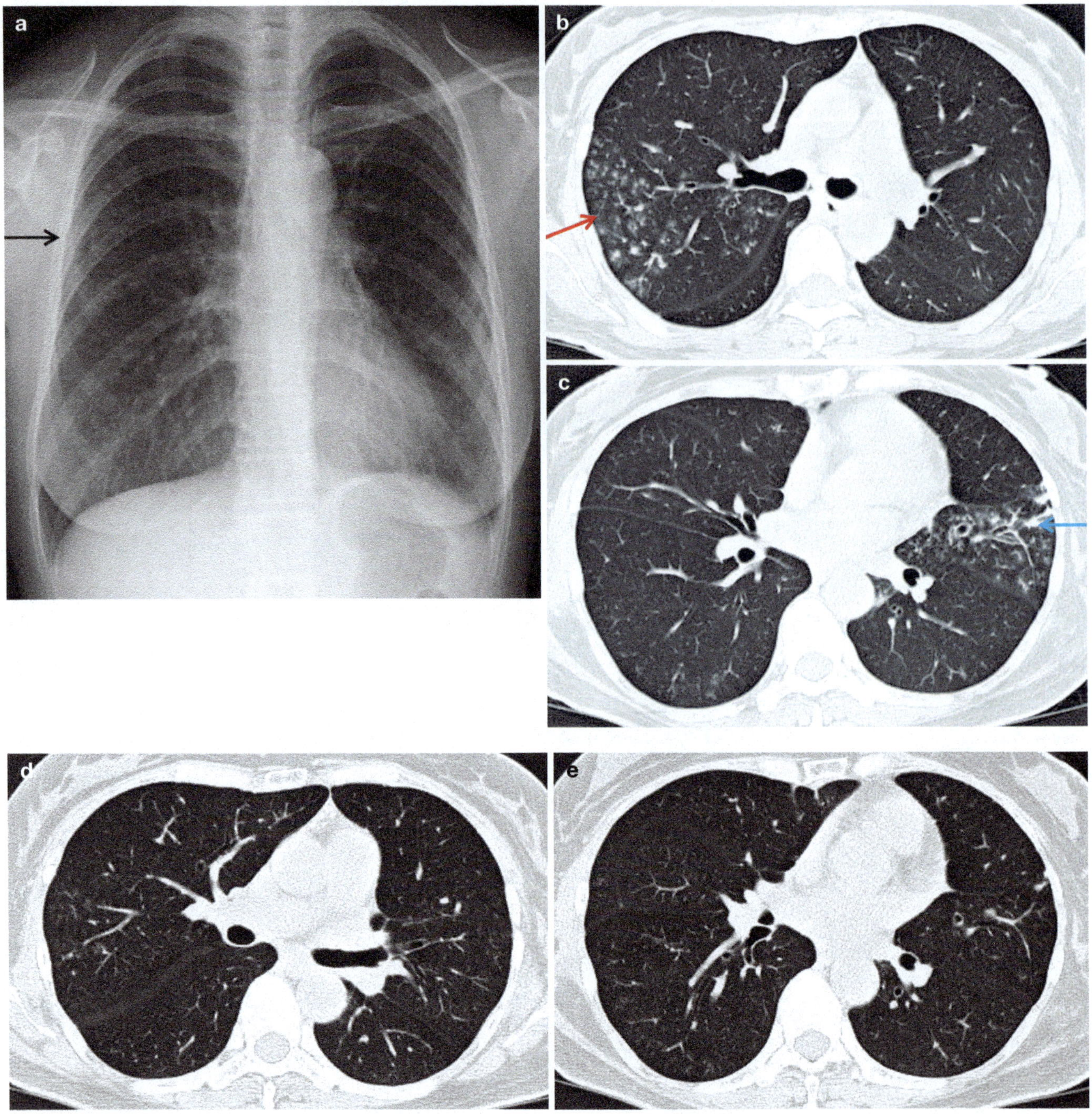

Fig. 2.12 Bronchiolitis in segmental distribution observed in a 57-year-old woman with RA for 10 years. (**a**) Chest radiograph shows a granular shadow in the right lung field (arrow), which had been pointed out for 3 years. Her RA disease activity is relatively low. (**b**) HRCT reveals centrilobular micronodules in S^2 of the right upper lobe (red arrow). (**c**) Bronchiectasis accompanied by micronodules is seen in the left lingular division (blue arrow), which is thought to be the origin of bacterial dissemination. This condition persisted for 3 years, with subtle respiratory symptoms. (**d**, **e**) Three years later, the micronodules have disappeared spontaneously without any specific therapy for this disorder. RA treatment was successfully conducted during this period

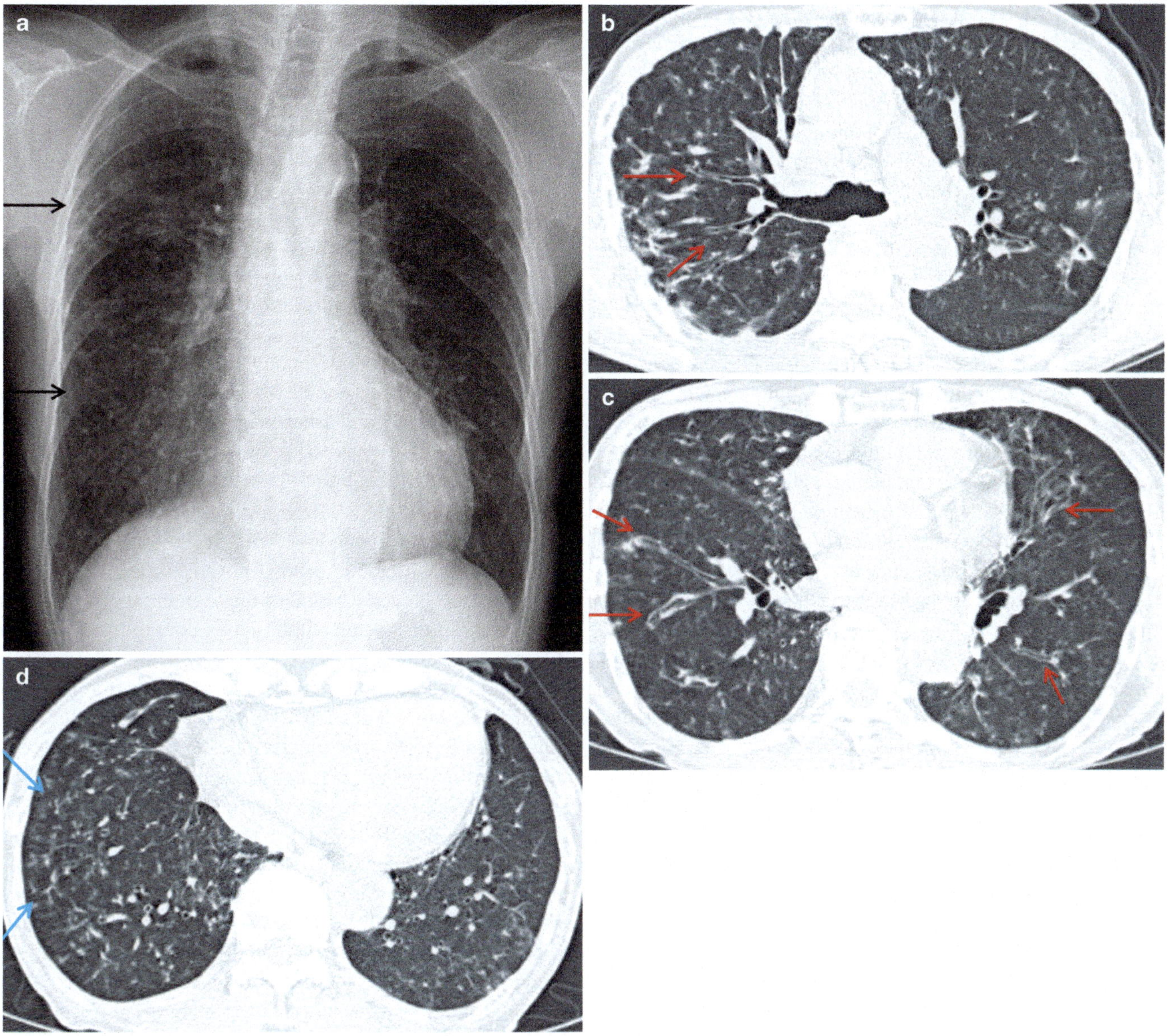

Fig. 2.13 Bronchiectasis and bronchiolitis diffusely distributed in the entire lung. (**a**) Chest radiograph of a 73-year-old woman with RA for 20 years shows a diffuse granular shadow (arrows). She complained of cough and sputum for several years, for which macrolides were prescribed with no effect. HRCT reveals prominent bronchiectasis in the upper lobes (**b**, red arrows) and also in the lower lobes (**c**, red arrows) with numerous centrilobular micronodules (**d**, blue arrows). These imaging findings closely resemble nontuberculous mycobacterial disease. However, the mycobacterium was not detected with repeated sputum examinations and with bronchoscopy. Thus, this condition was diagnosed as an advanced stage of RA-specific airway disease

2.4 Peripheral Airway Disease: Cystic Bronchiolectasis and Honeycomb-Like Structural Remodeling

As widely acknowledged, inflammation at the bronchiolar level leads to thickening of the bronchiolar walls and narrowing of the lumen; thereby, CT images show signs of centrilobular micronodular and branching opacities. Conversely, although relatively rare, the inflammatory process can destroy the bronchiolar wall and surrounding lung tissue, resulting in dilation of the bronchioles in patients with RA. In such cases, multiple cystic structures are formed along the stem bronchi or in subpleural region, revealing morphology similar to the honeycombing seen in chronic fibrotic interstitial pneumonia. These findings have never been described before and, in diagnostic imaging, have been most likely diagnosed as interstitial pneumonia, particularly ILD with usual interstitial pneumonia (UIP) pattern. We believe that this type of lung lesion is not rare in RA patients, and we would like to present our findings. Detailed pathological descriptions are provided in Chap. 7.

Case 1 (Fig. 2.14) A 75-year-old woman had a 30-year history of RA. She suffered from a chronic cough for several years, and reticular opacities are noted on her chest radiograph at the base of both lungs (Fig. 2.14a). Her coughing had worsened over the past 3 months, and because aggravation of ILD was suspected, she was referred to our respiratory department. Her main laboratory results were KL-6 813 IU/mL, ACPA 2530 U/mL, and RF 341 IU/mL. Arterial blood gas analysis showed mild oxygenation impairment. Bronchoscopy was performed, and bronchoalveolar lavage fluid revealed an increase in lymphocyte-predominant cells. On HRCT, we could see cysts of various sizes distributed in a segmental manner (Fig. 2.14b), which indicated a close relation to the airway. Lower lung slices showed clusters of cysts ranging from 5 to 10 mm in size arrayed contiguously in the subpleural area (Fig. 2.14c, d). These findings closely resemble the honeycombing seen in ILD with UIP pattern. In the pathological examination of the SLB specimen, a cystic structure is observed that involves an entire lobule (Fig. 2.14e, f). The walls of the cysts are made up of inflamed and disrupted bronchiolar walls. The surrounding alveolar tissue is also destroyed by inflammation and has disappeared. Histopathologically, these cysts are judged to be the result of inflammatory destruction and dilation of bronchioles. Notably, these changes were not accompanied by large airway disease in this case. When CT images in RA reveal clustered cysts in the subpleural area, radiologists commonly make a diagnosis of honeycombing, that is, ILD with UIP pattern. However, clinicians should note that similar findings might be produced by dilatation of bronchioles through intense inflammation owing to the RA.

Case 2 (Fig. 2.15) An 80-year-old woman was diagnosed as RA 4 years ago. On the same occasion, she was judged to have ILD based on CT findings. RA was treated with prednisolone and tacrolimus. She had no respiratory symptoms such as cough, sputum, or shortness of breath or any history of past pneumonia. The patient presented with a productive cough for 2 months, and a chest radiograph revealed a bilateral hilar infiltrative opacity that had expanded compared to previous films, and the patient was referred to our respiratory department. Her CRP was 2.5 mg/dL, KL-6 550 IU/mL, anti-CCP antibodies 362 U/mL, and results of PFT were within normal limits. She was diagnosed as having pneumonia at the base of BE, but antibiotics therapy failed to improve her condition. It was assumed the disease had developed into organized pneumonia, and she was started on 40 mg of prednisolone for 3 weeks, leading to successful resolution clinically and radiologically.

Chest radiographs showed a reticular opacity that predominated in the upper lobe with segmental distribution, indicative of bronchial origin, not ILD (Fig. 2.15a, b). HRCT scans showed dilation of the segmental bronchi with consolidation of the surrounding area containing countless dilated bronchi and cyst clusters (Fig. 2.15c, d). Consolidation in the surrounding areas showed a panlobular distribution, suggesting its airway origin. In the right lung, from S^2 to S^9, cyst clusters are formed along the segmental bronchi (Fig. 2.15e). Areas around these lesions showed the absence of reticular opacity, the sign of ILD, denying the possibility of traction bronchiectasis. These findings clearly ruled out ILD and led to the conclusion that all of these changes arose from an inflammatory process in the airway. Although lung biopsies were not conducted in this patient, the pathological findings of Case 1 help to imagine how these cyst clusters evolved (Fig. 2.15f, g). In inflamed lung tissue, respiratory bronchi arising from terminal bronchioles just adjacent to the membranous bronchioles are destroyed with the surrounding lung parenchyma. Inflammatory cell infiltration and fibrosis are also observed. From these findings, in such situation, we can postulate that small bronchi or bronchioles that branch off from the stem bronchus (so-called daughter branches) may form cysts, leading to the propagation of cysts such as is shown in Fig. 2.15c–e.

In summary, this is an example of extensive airway disease, not ILD, which has progressed insidiously. There were most likely several incidents of focal pneumonia that left organization after each episode, which ultimately created the consolidation around the bronchi. Concurrently, destruction and dilatation of the bronchi and bronchioles led to the formation of multiple cysts. These types of findings are relatively rare among RA patients, but they do occur and are the result of the intense inflammation of the airway characteristic in RA patients.

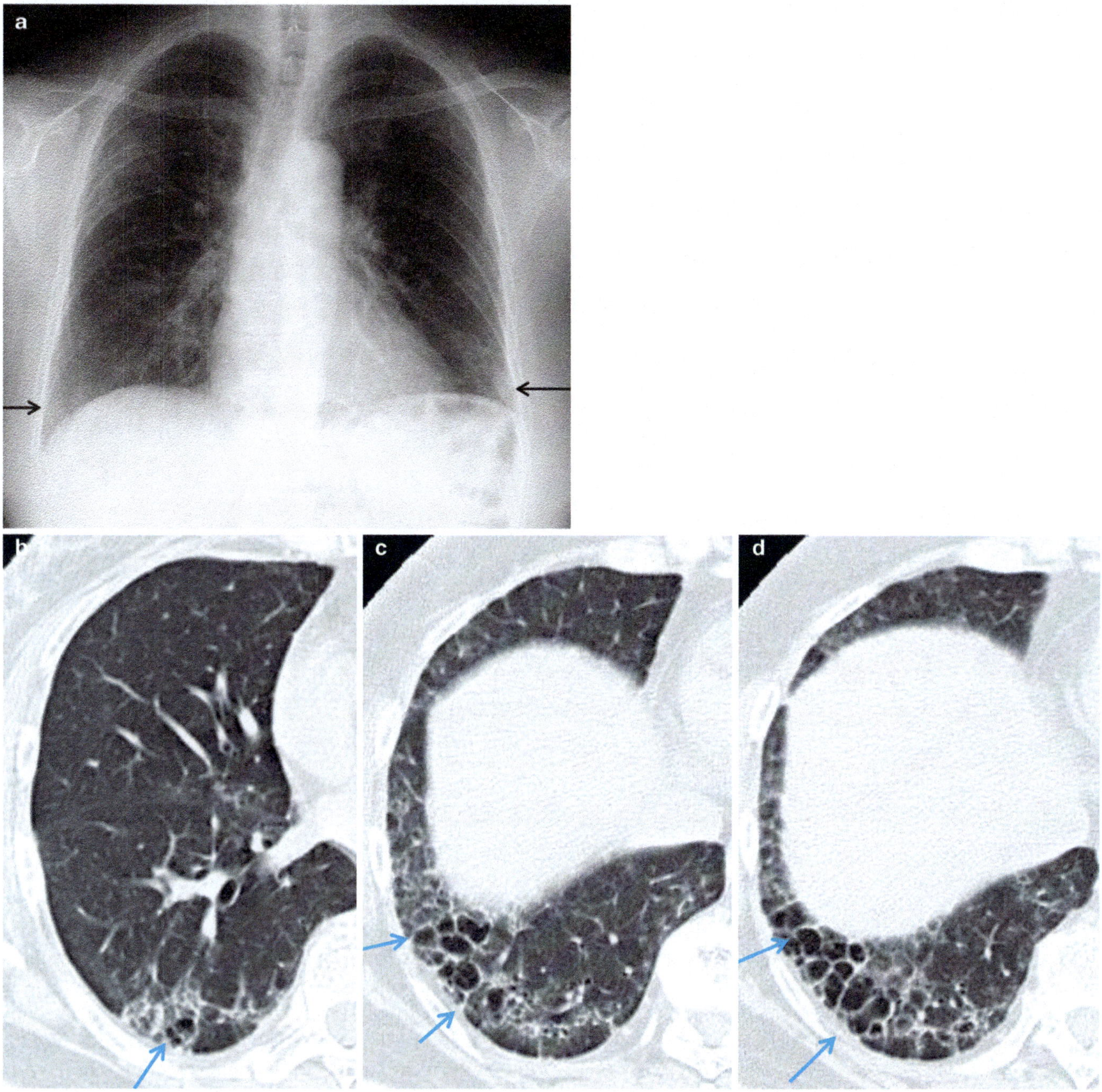

Fig. 2.14 Cystic bronchiolectasis mimicking honeycombing. (**a**) Chest radiograph of a 75-year-old woman with RA for 30 years. She complained of cough for 2 years, which had worsened over the recent 3 months. Tocilizumab had been given for 3 years. Reticular shadows are seen in the bilateral lung bases. (**b**) HRCT shows multiple cysts of various sizes distributed in a segmental manner (blue arrows). (**c**, **d**) Larger cysts are arrayed contiguously near the pleura that mimic a usual interstitial pneumonia (UIP) pattern (blue arrows). These cysts were proven to be dilated bronchioles histologically. Cystic bronchiolectasis was observed in the SLB specimen. (**e**) Panoramic view shows a cyst involving an entire lobule located slightly apart from the pleura (arrow). The cyst consisted of the destroyed and dilated bronchiole. (**f**) Cystic dilatation of bronchioles is visible in the inflammatory lesion (arrows). The wall of the cyst is composed of destroyed bronchiolar wall and the alveolar tissue around it, due to inflammatory destruction (Photomicrograph courtesy of Dr. T. Takemura)

These two cases share several clinical features. (1) KL-6, an important serum marker for ILD activity, was only slightly elevated, which is not compatible with ILD. KL-6 is also produced by the bronchiolar epithelium, making its slight elevation in these cases explicable [44]. (2) The symptoms were chronic cough and sputum presenting as of airway origin. (3) These airway symptoms were easily controlled with short-term fluoroquinolone therapy. These characteristics are all unlikely to occur in ILD. The details are described in Chap. 5.

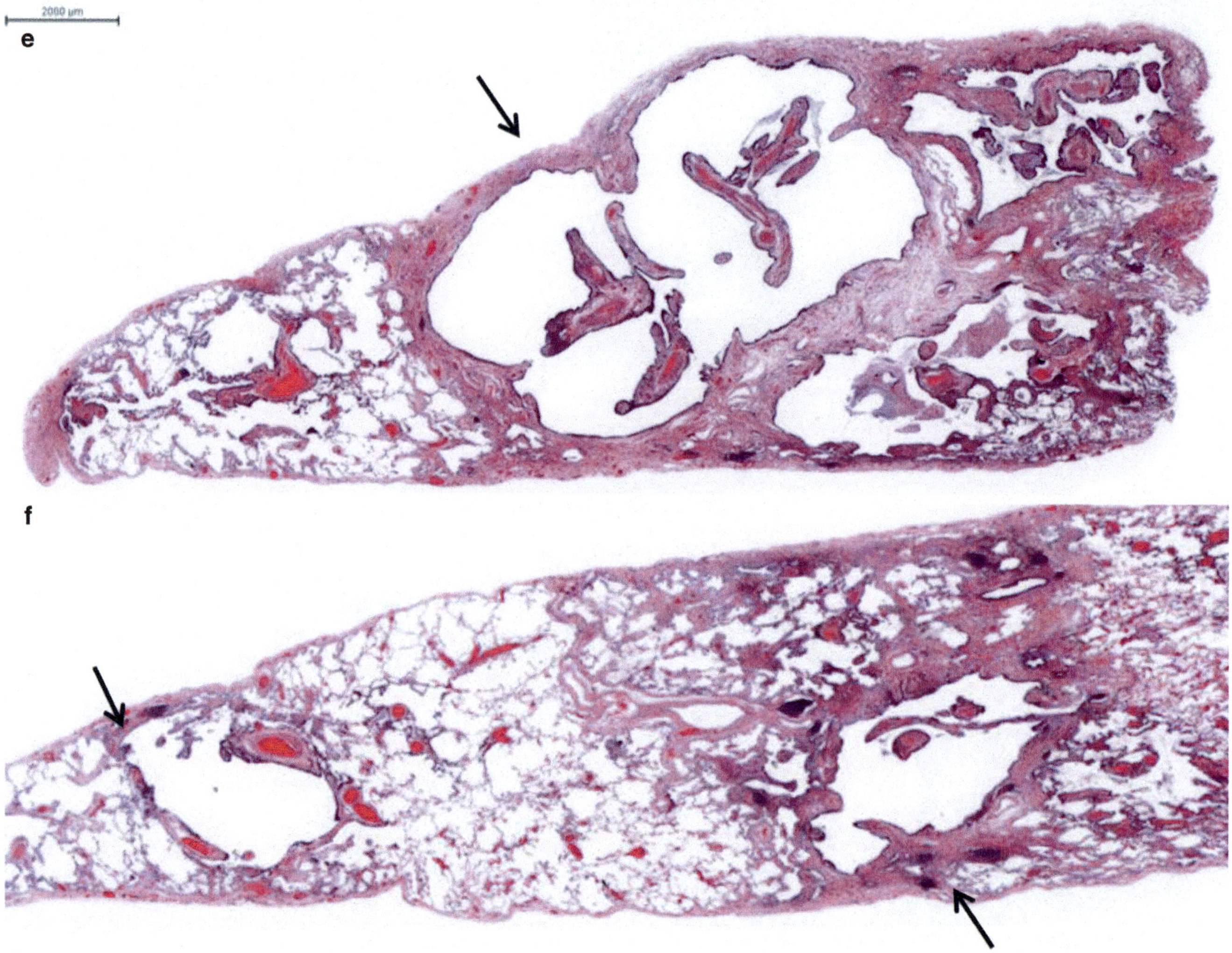

Fig. 2.14 (continued)

Case 3 In Fig. 2.16, we present a case with normal lungs at first in whom BE gradually developed and eventually progressed to honeycomb-like structures over 7 years of observation. At the time of first presentation, the patient was 50 years of age, with RA for 4 years, an ex-smoker (until age 30), and an office worker. Over the first 5 years, he experienced several episodes of pneumonia with hospitalization, and each time, antibiotics alone were not enough to cure, and he required additional corticosteroids. Over this period, BE emerged from an almost normal lung in the bilateral lower lobes (Fig. 2.16b–d). This emergence of BE can be attributed to the intense inflammation of the airway with repeated aggravation. Despite all treatment efforts over the next 2 years including biologics, his RA activity was difficult to control, and symptoms of chronic respiratory tract inflammation including productive cough also persisted. Two years later, a CT scan taken 7 years after the initial presentation revealed a new finding, the appearance of a honeycomb-like structure in the lingular division and lower lobes (Fig. 2.16e–h). Pathological studies on SLB specimens revealed that these cystic structures are formed through a destructive inflammatory process. The walls of the cysts are composed of the remaining bronchiolar wall and surrounding alveolar tissue that was destroyed by inflammation (Fig. 2.16i, j). In other words, although the findings appear similar to the honeycombing observed in ILD with UIP pattern (which is caused not by inflammation but by fibrosis), a completely different mechanism has created this structural remodeling, as shown in these sequences of CT images and the pathological findings. However, radiologists who interpret the last CT would likely make a diagnosis of ILD with honeycombing. We suspect that a certain proportion of RA patients diagnosed as having ILD of UIP pattern may in fact have airway disease formed through the process like this. RA patients with ILD with UIP pattern are reported to have poor prognosis. However, if a fair percentage of those were in fact airway diseases, then the treatment strategy would be entirely different. This is an important issue that should be addressed in the future.

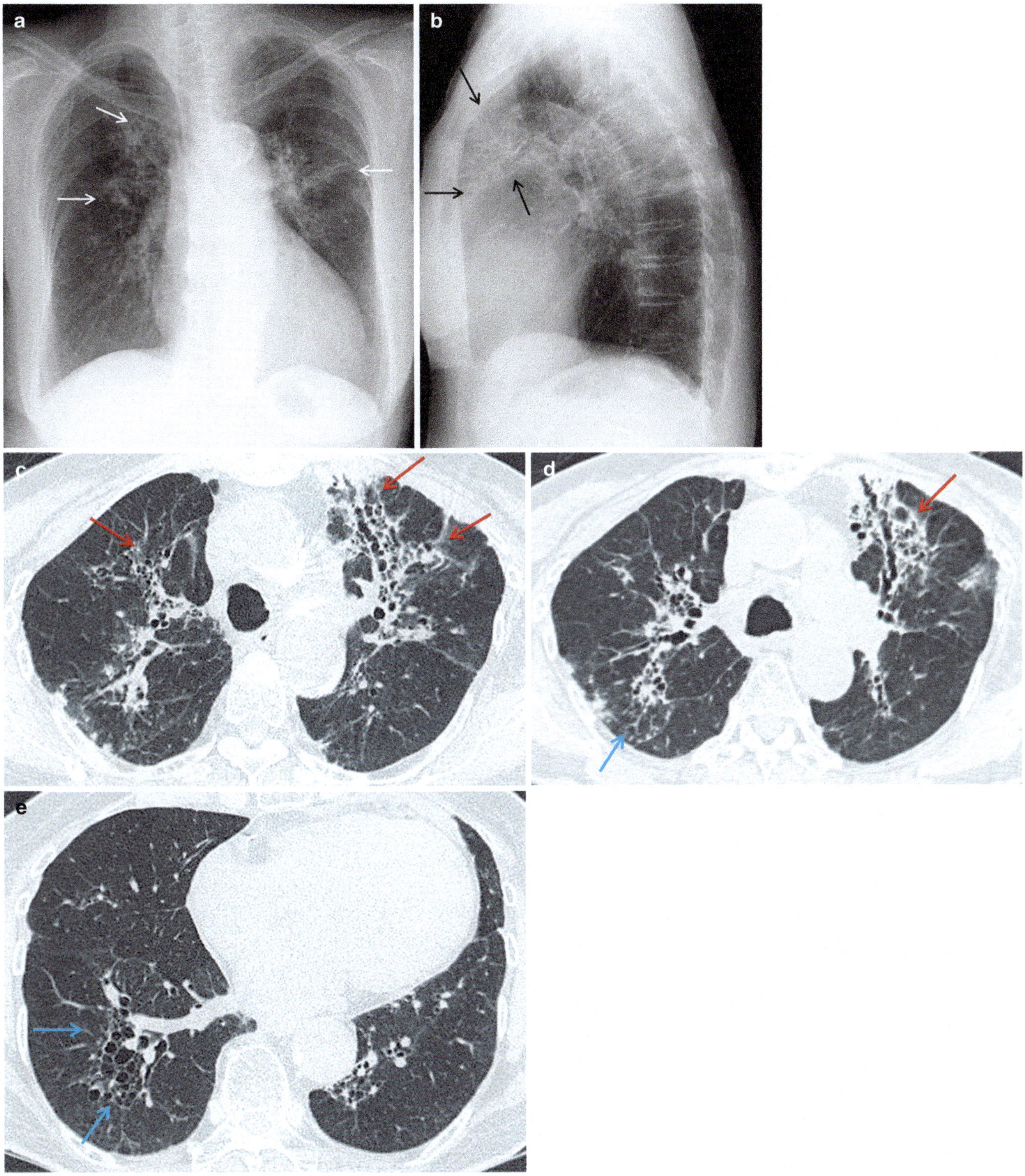

Fig. 2.15 (**a**) Posteroanterior chest radiograph in an 80-year-old woman with RA of 4-year duration. Infiltrative or reticular shadows are present in the bilateral hilar area (white arrows). (**b**) Lateral view shows segmental distribution of the reticular shadows (arrows). This pattern strongly suggests that the shadows are formed via the airway. (**c**, **d**) HRCT reveals multiple cystic lesions within the consolidated area around the dilated segmental-subsegmental bronchi (red arrows). (**e**) Clustered cysts are visible around B^9 and around B^2 (**d**) of the right lung (blue arrows). (**f**) Panoramic view of the SLB specimen of Case 1 and (**g**) a schema drawn by the inspecting pathologist would help to illustrate how all these abnormalities evolved. Both show structural remodeling in a lobule. Adjacent to the membranous bronchiole (red circle), cystic transformation of respiratory bronchioles arises from a terminal bronchiole, destroying the lung parenchyma in the vicinity. Chronic inflammatory cell infiltration and fibrosis are also noted. *Br* bronchiole (Photomicrograph and schema courtesy of Dr. T. Takemura)

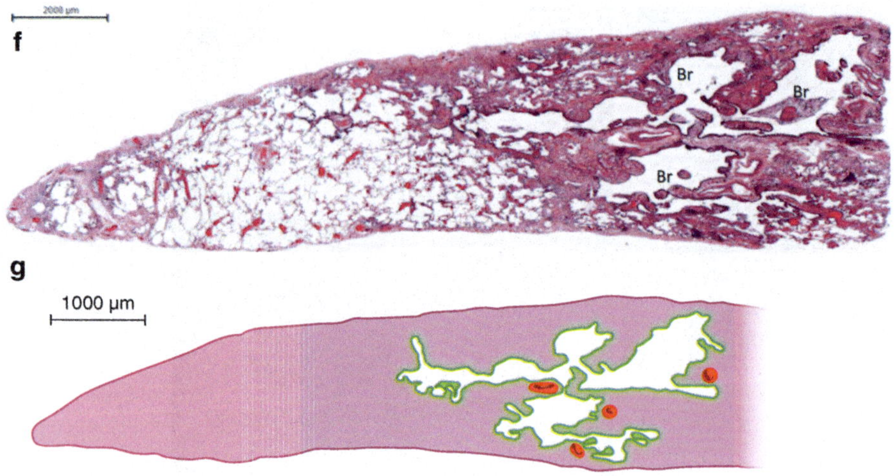

Fig. 2.15 (continued)

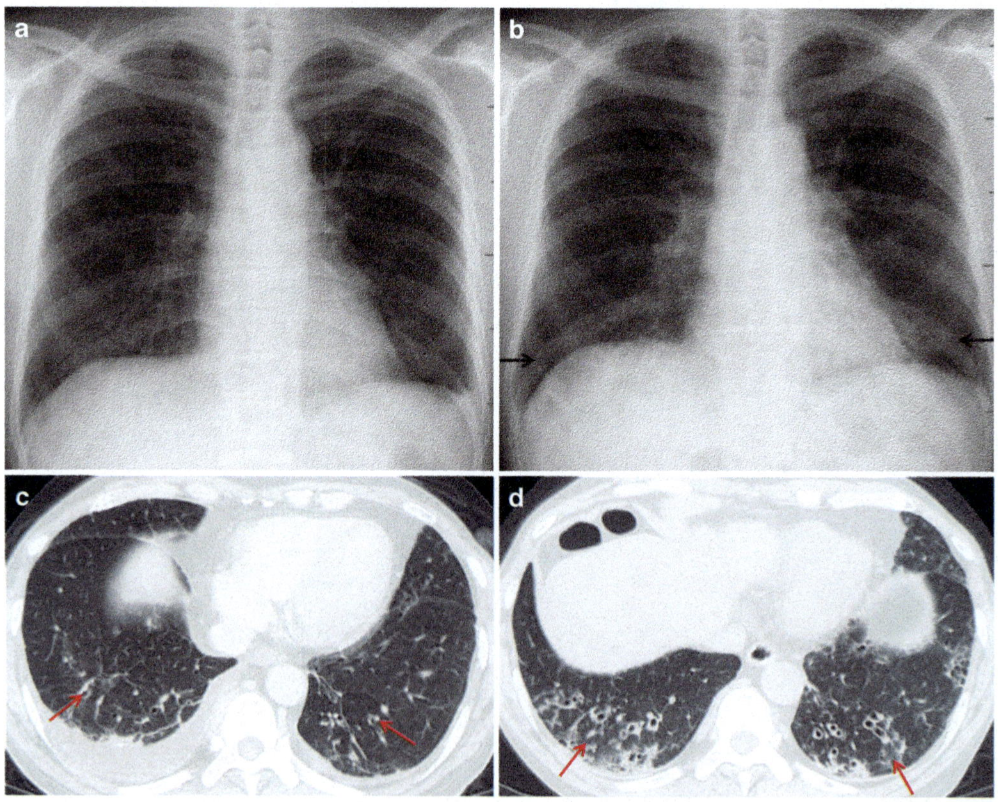

Fig. 2.16 (**a**) A case of uncontrollable airway disease observed for 7 years. Chest radiograph from a 50-year-old man with RA of 4-year duration at his first presentation to our respiratory department. The findings are almost normal except for pleural adhesion in the left costal phrenic angle. (**b**) Chest radiograph 5 years later. He had suffered from four recurrent episodes of pneumonia, all of which took a prolonged course that finally necessitated corticosteroid therapy. Reticular shadows appeared at the bilateral lung bases. (**c**) HRCT at the first presentation shows a small amount of pleural effusion, resolving pneumonia, and only a slight change in the bronchi (arrows). (**d**) HRCT 5 years later shows the emergence of many dilated bronchi with thickened walls in the bilateral lung base (arrows). These bronchial changes (bronchiectasis) are assumed to develop through repeated inflammation of the respiratory tract. Persistent inflammation of the airway ultimately caused bronchiolar destruction. (**e**) Chest radiograph 2 years later shows a reticular opacity at the left lung base (arrow), which has worsened compared with that in (**b**). (**f–h**) HRCT reveals multiple cyst formation along segmental and subsegmental bronchi (blue arrows) and a honeycomb-like appearance in the subpleural area (red arrows). This clinical course strongly suggests that the cysts are caused by persistent inflammation in the airway associated with RA. Histological findings in the SLB specimen. Panoramic view. (**i**) In addition to bronchiolar dilatation (red arrow), multiple cyst formation is visible (blue arrows).These cystic changes correspond to the honeycomb-like appearance found on HRCT. Infiltration of inflammatory cells is prominent around the cysts. (**j**) Magnified view of the box in (**i**). The walls of the cysts are composed of the remaining bronchiolar wall and surrounding alveolar tissue that was destroyed by inflammation. Although mimicking the honeycombing of ILD with UIP pattern, the pathogenesis of cyst formation is entirely different (Photomicrographs courtesy of Dr. T. Takemura)

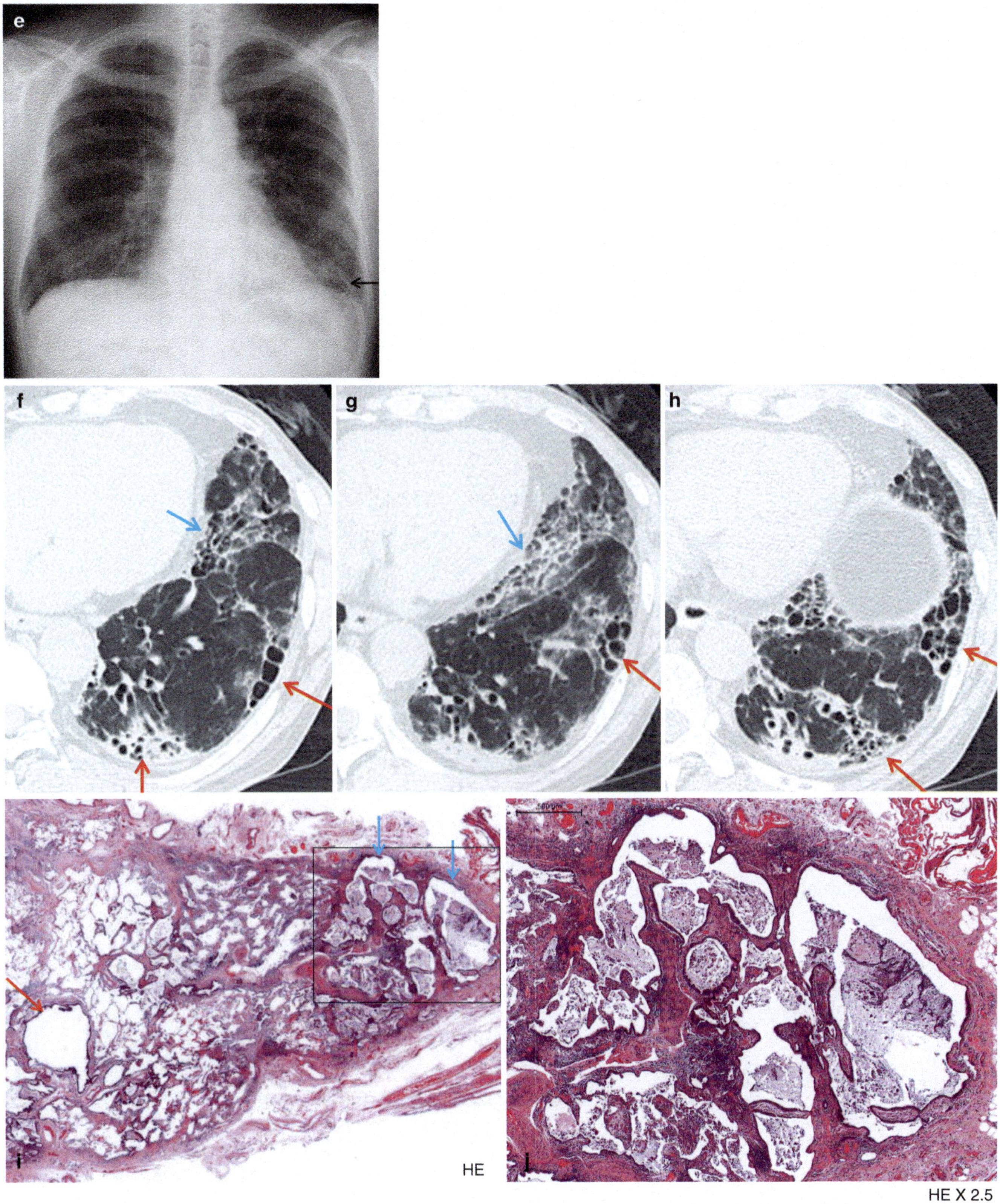

Fig. 2.16 (continued)

2.5 How to Understand and Confront Airway Diseases of RA Patients

We have discussed the high prevalence of airway diseases in RA patients and their significance in clinical settings of RA. Yet, questions remain: why are airway disorders formed so frequently, and how should we confront them?

Regarding the risk factors of airway disease in RA, Mori and colleagues have listed the clinical stage of RA and high titers of anti-CCP antibody and rheumatoid factor, whereas Nannini and colleagues have pointed out disease severity of RA (erythrocyte sedimentation rate, rheumatoid factor, necessity of DMARDs) [45, 46], both of which stress the importance of host factors.

From another viewpoint, the airway is an interface between the host and the external environment. It has a proper immune system in the submucosal zone in which an active immunological response is continuously in process with the microbiota, invading microorganisms, or inhaled particles (such as those of tobacco). It is hypothesized that in RA subjects, dysregulated and exuberant responses of this immune system occur, causing airway disorders [11, 46]. From this perspective, airway diseases of RA should be considered to be one of the extra-articular manifestations (EAM), pulmonary EAM. ILD, small airway disease, pleuritis, and rheumatoid nodules have been listed as pulmonary EAM [47], but the latter two are relatively rare and do not affect patient prognosis. Currently, airway diseases

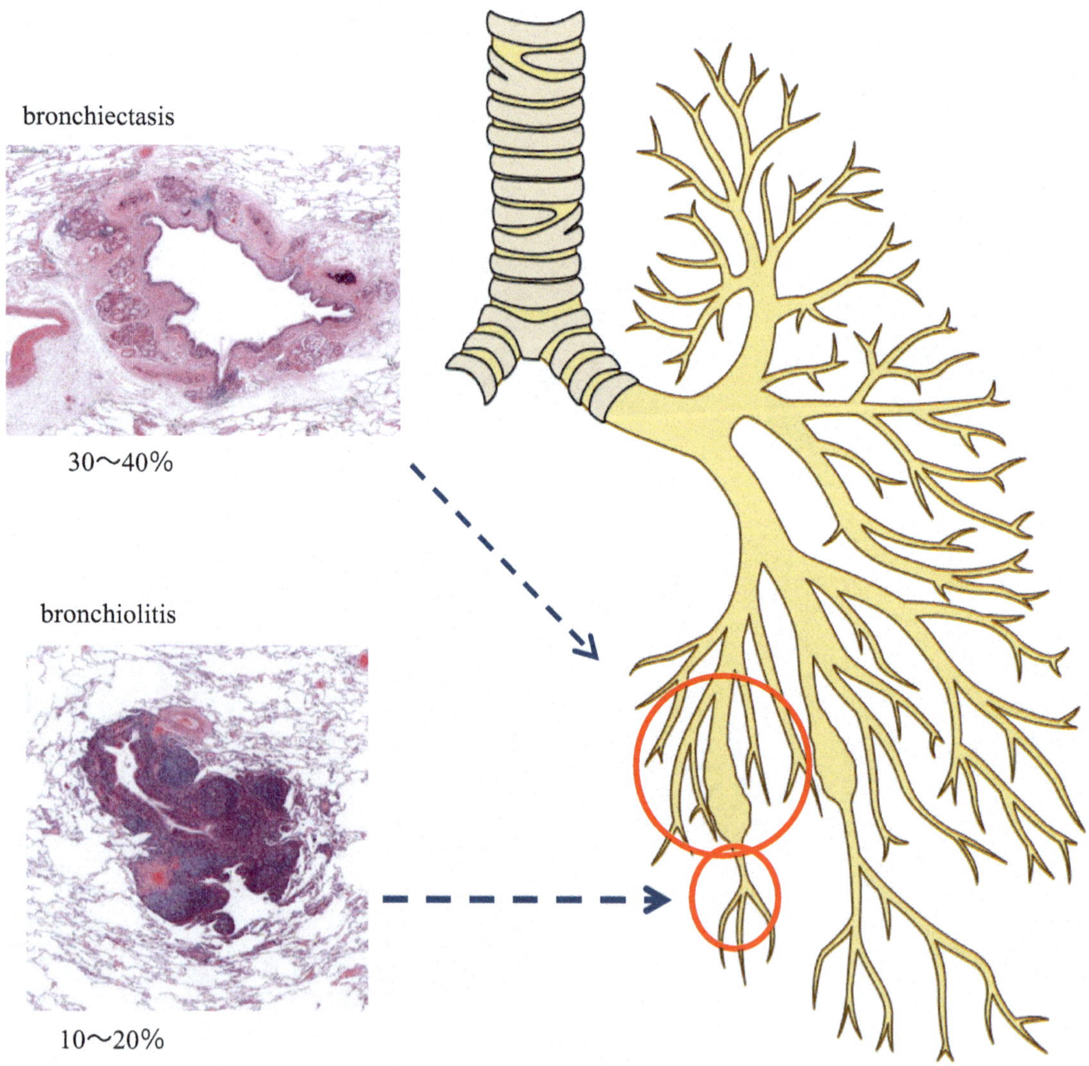

Fig. 2.17 How to understand airway diseases in RA patients? The airway is an interface between the host and the external environment. Various microorganisms may invade or colonize there, and inhaled particles such as those of tobacco could reach them. In RA patients, an exuberant host immune reaction might occur against these microorganisms and particles, leading to persistent inflammation and the formation of various airway disorders. Thus, these disorders should be considered as extra-articular manifestations of RA

including BE and ILD are considered to be the major pulmonary EAM [9, 46] (Fig. 2.17).

It is well acknowledged that the presence of EAM is associated with poor survival in RA patients [47, 48]. A recent epidemiological study of EAM conducted in the USA has revealed a steady, major decrease in vasculitis, carditis, and Felty's syndrome. These improvements are thought to be caused by the new disease-modifying RA treatments. The only exceptions are respiratory complications, which have conversely increased and threaten the lives of RA patients [49]. This tendency could be interpreted as follows: organs such as the heart, kidneys, and vasculature are closed systems and are benefitted by new-generation DMARDs without intervening factors. However, the lungs are exposed to the environment, and thereby, inhibition of the immune process with immune modulators would enhance vulnerability to infections or worsening of ILD. This could result in the destruction of lung structures, which would further aggravate the lung conditions, leading to a vicious cycle.

Taking these perspectives into consideration, we must manage to conquer lung complications, especially those originating from airway disorders, to successfully accomplish the control of RA and improve patient prognosis.

References

1. Nakajima A, Inoue E, Tanaka E, et al. Mortality and cause of death in Japanese patients with rheumatoid arthritis based on a large observational cohort, IORRA. Scand J Rheumatol. 2010;39:360–7.
2. Takeuchi T, Kameda H. The Japanese experience with biologic therapies for rheumatoid arthritis. Nat Rev Rheumatol. 2010;6:644–52.
3. Nakajima A, Saito K, Kojima T, et al. No increased mortality in patients with rheumatoid arthritis treated with biologics: results from the biologics register of six rheumatology institutes in Japan. Mod Rheumatol. 2013;23:945–52.
4. Doran MF, Crowson CS, Pond GR, O'Fallon WM, Gabriel SE. Frequency of infection in patients with rheumatoid arthritis compared with controls: a population-based study. Arthritis Rheum. 2002;46:2287–93.
5. Strangfeld A, Eveslage M, Schneider M, et al. Treatment benefit or survival of the fittest: what drives the time-dependent decrease in serious infection rates under TNF inhibition and what does this imply for the individual patient? Ann Rheum Dis. 2011;70:1914–20.
6. Koike T, Harigai M, Ishiguro N, et al. Safety and effectiveness of adalimumab in Japanese rheumatoid arthritis patients: postmarketing surveillance report of 7740 patients. Mod Rheumatol. 2014;24:390–8.
7. Wells AU, Denton CP. Interstitial lung disease in connective tissue disease—mechanisms and management. Nat Rev Rheumatol. 2014;10:728–39.
8. Wilczynska MM, Condliffe AM, McKeon DJ. Coexistence of bronchiectasis and rheumatoid arthritis: revisited. Respir Care. 2013;58:694–701.
9. Lieberman-Maran L, Orzano IM, Passero MA, Lally EV. Bronchiectasis in rheumatoid arthritis: report of four cases and a review of the literature—implications for management with biologic response modifiers. Semin Arthritis Rheum. 2006;35:379–87.
10. Tokuda H, Harigai M, Watanabe A, et al. Consensus statements for medical practice: biological agents and lung disease. Abridged English translation by the Japanese Respiratory Society. Respir Investig. 2017;55:229–51.
11. Boyton RJ, Altmann DM. Bronchiectasis: current concepts in pathogenesis, immunology, and microbiology. Annu Rev Pathol. 2016;11:523–54.
12. Remy-Jardin M, Remy J, Cortet B, Mauri F, Delcambre B. Lung changes in rheumatoid arthritis: CT findings. Radiology. 1994;193:375–82.
13. Despaux J, Manzoni P, Toussirot E, Augé B, Cedoz JP, Wendling D. Prospective study of the prevalence of bronchiectasis in rheumatoid arthritis using high-resolution computed tomography. Rev Rhum Engl Ed. 1998;65:453–61.
14. Perez T, Remy-Jardin M, Cortet B. Airways involvement in rheumatoid arthritis: clinical, functional, and HRCT findings. Am J Respir Crit Care Med. 1998;157:1658–65.
15. Akira M, Sakatani M, Hara H. Thin-section CT findings in rheumatoid arthritis-associated lung disease: CT patterns and their courses. J Comput Assist Tomogr. 1999;23:941–8.
16. Terasaki H, Fujimoto K, Hayabuchi N, et al. Respiratory symptoms in rheumatoid arthritis: relation between high resolution CT findings and functional impairment. Radiat Med. 2004;22:179–85.
17. Wilsher M, Voight L, Milne D, et al. Prevalence of airway and parenchymal abnormalities in newly diagnosed rheumatoid arthritis. Respir Med. 2012;106:1441–6.
18. Mori S, Cho I, Koga Y, Sugimoto M. Comparison of pulmonary abnormalities on high-resolution computed tomography in patients with early versus longstanding rheumatoid arthritis. J Rheumatol. 2008;35:1513–21.
19. Tsuchiya Y, Takayanagi N, Sugiura H, et al. Lung diseases directly associated with rheumatoid arthritis and their relationship to outcome. Eur Respir J. 2011;37:1411–7.
20. Weycker D, Edelsberg J, Oster G, Tino G. Prevalence and economic burden of bronchiectasis. Clin Pulm Med. 2005;12:205–9.
21. Whitwell F. A study of the pathology and pathogenesis of bronchiectasis. Thorax. 1952;7:213–39.
22. Morrissey BM. Pathogenesis of bronchiectasis. Clin Chest Med. 2007;28:289–96.
23. King PT. The pathophysiology of bronchiectasis. Int J Chron Obstruct Pulmon Dis. 2009;4:411–9.
24. Fuschillo S, De Felice A, Balzano G. Mucosal inflammation in idiopathic bronchiectasis: cellular and molecular mechanisms. Eur Respir J. 2008;31:396–406.
25. Boyton RJ, Reynolds CJ, Quigley KJ, Altmann DM. Immune mechanisms and the impact of the disrupted lung microbiome in chronic bacterial lung infection and bronchiectasis. Clin Exp Immunol. 2012;171:117–23.
26. Demoruelle MK, Deane KD, Holers VM. When and where does inflammation begin in rheumatoid arthritis? Curr Opin Rheumatol. 2014;26:64–71.
27. Naidich DP. Bronchiectasis. In: Naidich DP, Webb WR, Grenier PA, et al., editors. Imaging of the airway; functional and radiologic correlations. Philadelphia: Lippincott WW; 2005. p. 107–45.
28. Takayanagi N. Biological agents and respiratory infections: causative mechanisms and practice management. Respir Investig. 2015;53:185–200.
29. Doran MF, Crowson CS, Pond GR, O'Fallon WM, Gabriel SE. Predictors of infection in rheumatoid arthritis. Arthritis Rheum. 2002;46:2294–300.
30. Swinson DR, Symmons D, Suresh U, Jones M, Booth J. Decreased survival in patients with co-existent rheumatoid arthritis and bronchiectasis. Br J Rheumatol. 1997;36:689–91.

31. Puéchal X, Génin E, Bienvenu T, Le Jeunne C, Dusser DJ. Poor survival in rheumatoid arthritis associated with bronchiectasis: a family-based cohort study. PLoS One. 2014;9:e110066.
32. Colby TV, Travis WD. Bronchiolar disorders. In: Travis WD, Colby TV, Koss MN, et al., editors. Non-neoplastic disorders of the lower respiratory tract. Washington, DC: American Registry of Pathology and AFIP; 2002. p. 351–80.
33. Rangel-Moreno J, Hartson L, Navarro C, Gaxiola M, Selman M, Randall TD. Inducible bronchus-associated lymphoid tissue (iBALT) in patients with pulmonary complications of rheumatoid arthritis. J Clin Invest. 2006;116:3183–94.
34. Homma S, Kawabata M, Kishi K, et al. Diffuse panbronchiolitis in rheumatoid arthritis. Eur Respir J. 1998;12:444–52.
35. Sugino K, Hebisawa A, Uekusa T, Hatanaka K, Abe H, Homma S. Histopathological bronchial reconstruction of human bronchiolitis obliterans. Pathol Int. 2011;61:192–201.
36. Devouassoux G, Cottin V, Lioté H, et al. Characterisation of severe obliterative bronchiolitis in rheumatoid arthritis. Eur Respir J. 2009;33:1053–61.
37. Hayakawa H, Sato A, Chida K, Toyoshima M, Chida K, Iwata M. Bronchiolar disease in rheumatoid arthritis. Am J Respir Crit Care Med. 1996;154:1531–6.
38. Yousem SA, Colby TV, Carrington CB. Follicular bronchitis/bronchiolitis. Hum Pathol. 1985;16:700–6.
39. Mori S, Koga Y, Sugimoto M. Small airway obstruction in patients with rheumatoid arthritis. Mod Rheumatol. 2011;21:164–73.
40. Tanaka N, Kim JS, Newell JD, et al. Rheumatoid arthritis-related lung diseases: CT findings. Radiology. 2004;232:81–91.
41. Takemura T. Pathological features of the lung in rheumatoid arthritis. Nihon Kyoubu Rinsho. 2007;66:470–84. (in Japanese).
42. Tokuda H. Broncho-bronchial disorders in patients with rheumatoid arthritis. Jpn J Clin Radiol. 2015;60:1085–96. (in Japanese).
43. Cortet B, Perez T, Roux N, et al. Pulmonary function tests and high resolution computed tomography of the lungs in patients with rheumatoid arthritis. Ann Rheum Dis. 1997;56:596–600.
44. Kohno N, Kyoizumi S, Awaya Y, Fukuhara H, Yamakido M, Akiyama M. New serum indicator of interstitial pneumonitis activity. Sialylated carbohydrate antigen KL-6. Chest. 1989;96:68–73.
45. Mori S, Koga Y, Sugimoto M. Different risk factors between interstitial lung disease and airway disease in rheumatoid arthritis. Respir Med. 2012;106:1591–9.
46. Nannini C, Medina-Velasquez YF, et al. Incidence and mortality of obstructive lung disease in rheumatoid arthritis: a population-based study. Arthritis Care Res (Hoboken). 2013;65: 1243–50.
47. Turesson C. Extra-articular rheumatoid arthritis. Curr Opin Rheumatol. 2013;25:360–6.
48. Gabriel SE, Crowson CS, Kremers HM, et al. Survival in rheumatoid arthritis: a population-based analysis of trends over 40 years. Arthritis Rheum. 2003;48:54–8.
49. Bartels CM, Bell CL, Shinki K, Rosenthal A, Bridges AJ. Changing trends in serious extra-articular manifestations of rheumatoid arthritis among United State veterans over 20 years. Rheumatology (Oxford). 2010;49:1670–5.

3 Pathology of Airway Disease in Rheumatoid Arthritis

Akira Hebisawa, Masashi Kitani, Hirotoshi Matsui, and Atsuhisa Tamura

Abstract

This chapter describes the lesions in the airways of the lungs, particularly those observed in bronchiolitis obliterans, in patients with rheumatoid arthritis (RA). RA-associated bronchiolitis obliterans has two different morphological presentations: (1) endobronchiolitis obliterans (EBO), in which the lesions are primarily present in the lumen of the airway, with minimal destruction of the airway wall, and (2) cellular destructive bronchiolitis (CDB), in which transmural inflammation causes destruction of the airway wall. The clinical presentations of EBO are markedly different from those of CDB, and they are generally characterized by distinct pathologies. Notably, a few cases of RA-associated bronchiectasis have been found to represent secondary lesions of CDB.

Keywords

Bronchiolitis obliterans • Endobronchiolitis obliterans • Cellular destructive bronchiolitis • Follicular bronchiolitis

3.1 Introduction

The main bronchi branch repeatedly to form membranous bronchioles within the lobules of the lung. These membranous bronchioles branch further into respiratory bronchioles that further divide into the alveolar ducts and alveoli. Although the bronchi, membranous bronchioles, and respiratory bronchioles are a single continuous anatomical structure, their histological structures are significantly different. The inner surface of the bronchi is made of columnar epithelium, mainly ciliated columnar epithelium, and basement membrane, containing thick bundles of elastic fibers and smooth muscle bundles in its deeper regions. Under these layers, cartilage and bronchial glands are present (Fig. 3.1). The membranous bronchioles have thin walls with no cartilage or bronchial glands. Similar to the bronchi, however, they have an elastic lamina and a layer of smooth muscles in addition to the epithelial layer and basement membrane (Fig. 3.2). Respiratory bronchioles form a transition between the membranous bronchioles and the alveolar ducts, and their walls are made up of a membranous portion containing smooth muscle and elastic fibers as well as alveoli (Fig. 3.3).

RA-associated respiratory diseases that cause severe obstructive lesions may affect different parts of the lung airways; e.g., bronchiectasis affects the bronchi [1, 2] and bronchiolitis obliterans affects the membranous bronchioles. However, because the bronchi and the respiratory bronchioles are both part of a continuous structure, when lesions involve a part of airways, they spread to the others. Therefore, to understand the characteristics of obstructive airway diseases, it is important to study all the airways of the lung.

In this chapter, we describe the pathology of RA-associated airway disease, with a particular focus on bronchiolitis obliterans, which has recently become the subject of attention.

A. Hebisawa, M.D., Ph.D. (✉) • M. Kitani, M.D.
Division of Histopathology, National Hospiral Organization Tokyo National Hospital, Tokyo, Japan
e-mail: hebisawa-in@tokyo-hosp.jp

H. Matsui, M.D., Ph.D.
Clinical Research Center, National Hospiral Organization Tokyo National Hospital, Tokyo, Japan

A. Tamura, M.D., Ph.D.
Center for Respiratory Diseases, National Hospiral Organization Tokyo National Hospital, Tokyo, Japan

T. Gono et al. (eds.), *Lung Disease Associated with Rheumatoid Arthritis*, https://doi.org/10.1007/978-981-10-6750-1_3

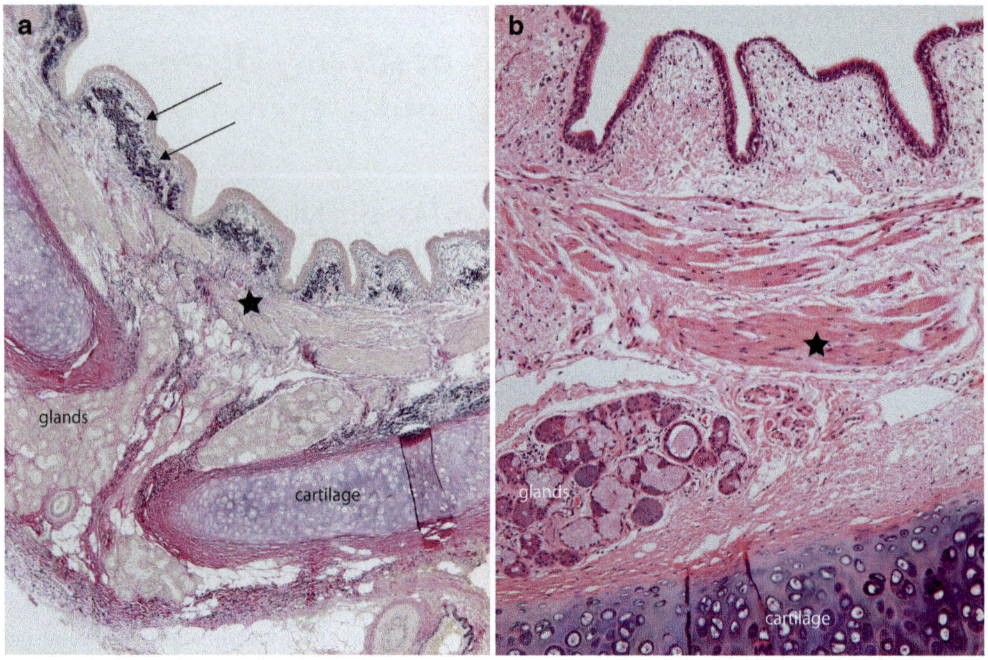

Fig. 3.1 Histology of the bronchus (**a**, elastic van Gieson stain; **b**, HE staining). Elastic fiber bundles (arrow) and fascicles of smooth muscles (asterisk) can be seen in the superficial layer of the bronchial wall, and bronchial glands and cartilage are observed in the deeper layers

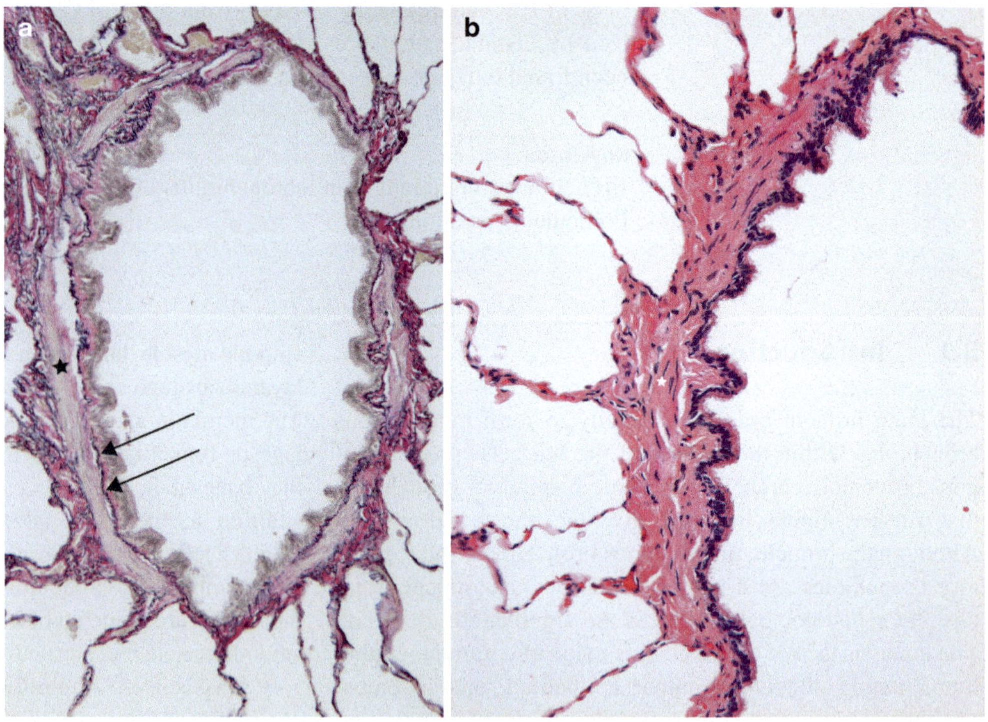

Fig. 3.2 Histology of a membranous bronchiole (**a**, elastic van Gieson stain; **b**, HE staining). An elastic fiber layer (arrow) can be seen immediately below the epithelium and basement membrane, below which is a thin smooth muscle layer (asterisk). No bronchial glands or cartilage are observed

3.2 Bronchiolitis Obliterans

3.2.1 Definition of Bronchiolitis Obliterans

"Bronchiolitis obliterans" was first described as a pathological condition by Lange [3] and is characterized by myxoid granulation tissue protruding in the form of polyps into the lumina of the terminal and respiratory bronchioles (Fig. 3.4). However, several studies have reported that the formation of such granulation tissue is not limited to the bronchiolar lumina, but is also found in the surrounding alveolar spaces; therefore, this condition is currently understood as a type of organizing pneumonia rather than bronchiolitis [4].

Bronchiolitis obliterans is currently defined as diffuse lesions affecting the membranous bronchioles that cause severe functional obstructive impairment [4, 5]. There are two pathological presentations of RA-associated bronchiolitis obliterans that fit this definition. The first is the obliterative bronchiolitis described by Geddes et al. [6]. This is the same condition as the "constrictive bronchiolitis" described by Colby et al. [5], in which

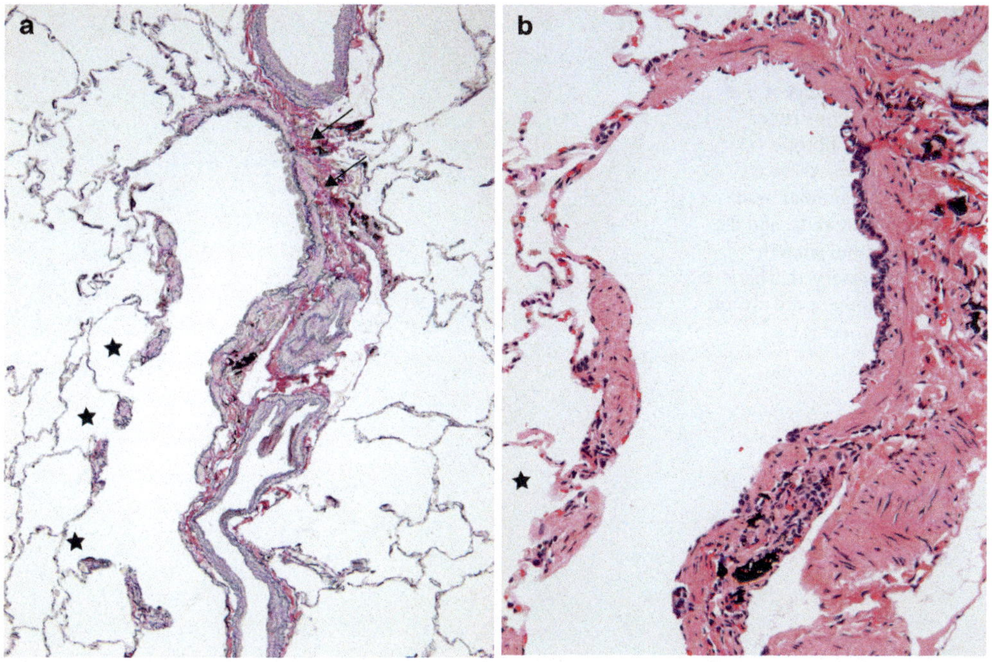

Fig. 3.3 Histology of a respiratory bronchiole (**a**, elastic van Gieson stain; **b**, HE staining). The respiratory bronchiole wall is composed of a membranous portion (arrow) with elastic fibers and smooth muscle, as well as alveoli (asterisk)

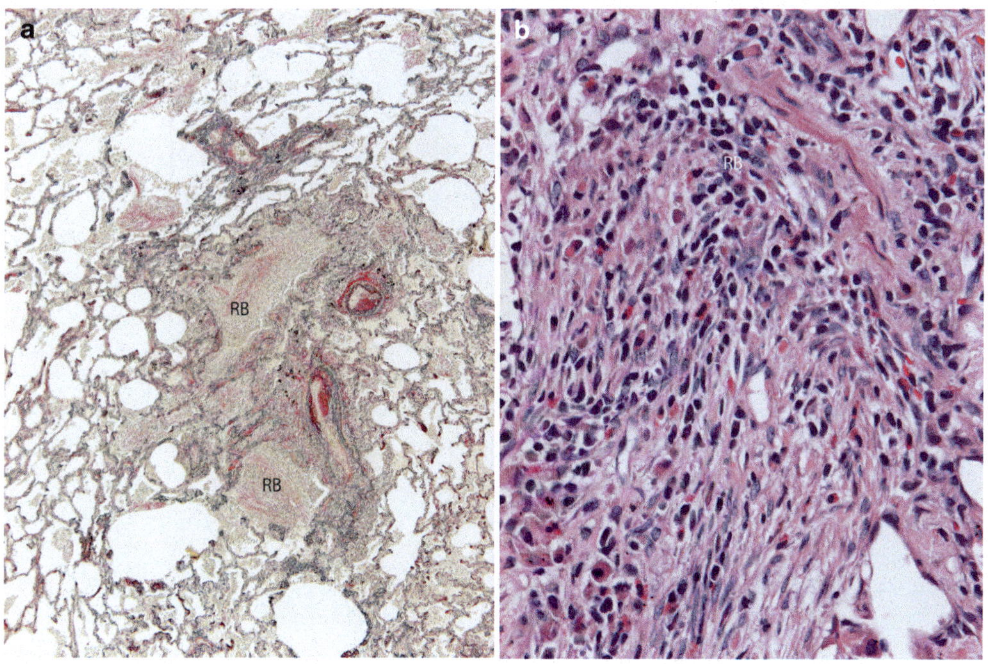

Fig. 3.4 Microscopic findings of bronchiolitis obliterans as described by Lange (**a**, elastic van Gieson stain; **b**, HE staining). Granulation tissue formed from the lumen of the respiratory bronchioles (RBs) to the alveolar spaces is observed. Small round cells, including plasma cells, have infiltrated the granulation tissue and the interstitium

emphasis is placed on the stenosis or obstruction of the airways by fibrous lesions protruding into the lumina of the bronchioles. Observation of these lesions with elastic fiber staining, however, reveals only mild inflammation of the airway wall and the preservation of elastic fibers and smooth muscle in the bronchiolar wall, demonstrating that the main cause of the obstruction are the lesions present in the airway lumina (Fig. 3.5). On the basis of these pathological characteristics, we preferred the term "endobronchiolitis obliterans (EBO)."

The other pathological presentation has been described as follicular bronchiolitis [7, 8] or cellular bronchiolitis [5, 9]. It has been reported that these lesions cause stenosis of the lumen by thickening of the airway wall as a result of severe inflammatory cell infiltration. Observation of these lesions with elastic fiber staining reveals severe destruction of the airway wall, with clear loss of the smooth muscle and elastic fibers (Fig. 3.6). Patients with destructive airway diseases often also exhibit other lesions showing even greater tissue breakdown. This type of lesion should therefore be termed "cellular destructive bronchiolitis" (CDB) to reflect its actual histology.

It is rare for EBO and CDB to coexist in the same patient with RA, and they also differ markedly in their clinical signs.

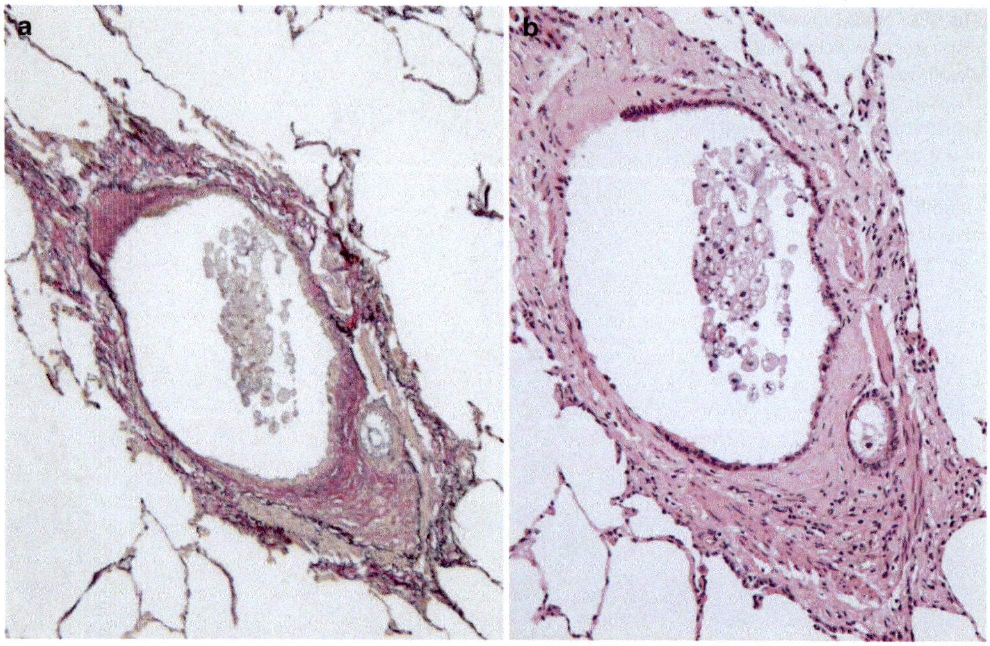

Fig. 3.5 Endobronchiolitis obliterans (EBO) (**a**, elastic van Gieson staining; **b**, HE staining). The lumina of the bronchiole are constricted with concentric fibrotic lesions. However, there is only slight inflammation of the bronchiolar walls, and the elastic fibers and smooth muscle are preserved. There is no inflammation of the alveoli around the bronchioles

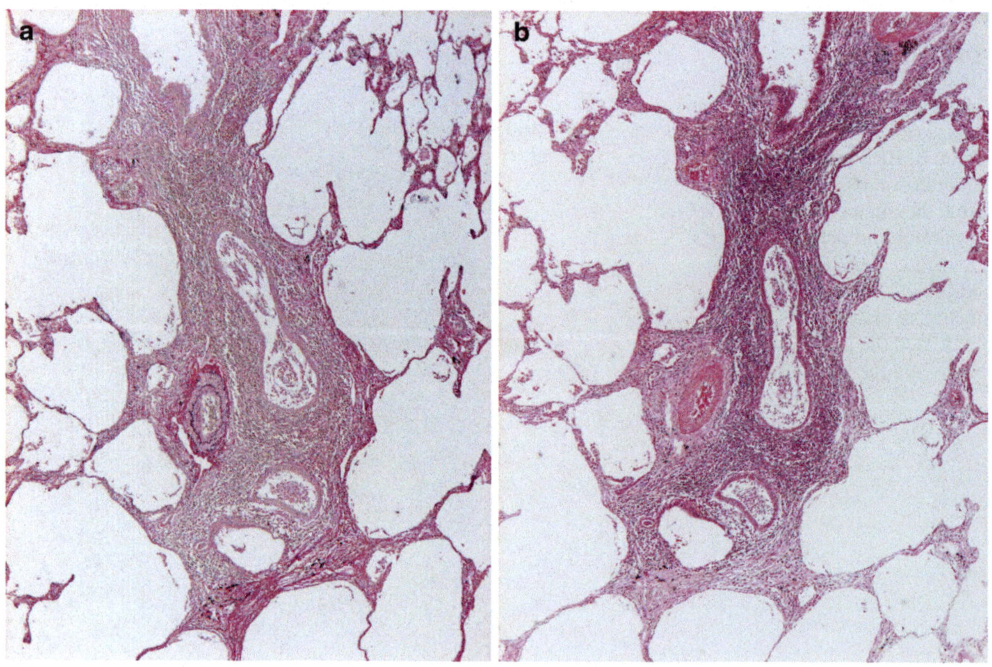

Fig. 3.6 Cellular destructive bronchiolitis (CDB) (**a**, elastic van Gieson stain; **b**, HE staining). There is severe small round cell infiltration of the bronchiolar walls, and the elastic fibers and smooth muscle have disappeared. Inflammatory cell infiltration has spread from the bronchiolar walls to the surrounding alveoli, and fibrosis is also present

3.2.2 Endobronchiolitis Obliterans (EBO)

RA-associated EBO is almost always found in women. Clinically, these patients exhibit acute to subacute airway obstructive disease. It is rare for purulent sputum to appear in this disease [6, 10], and in most cases, it is not associated with chronic sinusitis. In addition to RA, EBO may also be associated with post-transplant graft-versus-host disease, paraneoplastic pemphigus, or Stevens–Johnson syndrome, and drug-induced cases have also been reported [5, 9, 10]. However, irrespective of the underlying disease, the morphological features of EBO remain the same.

EBO is characterized by focal, multiple lesions, involving the membranous bronchioles, although it may also affect the small bronchi. Lesions causing obstructive disease extend from the submucosa into the airway lumen and are composed of granulation tissue with aggregations of foamy macrophages (Fig. 3.7) and/or edematous or dense fibrosis. In addition to concentric fibrosis, airway fibrosis may result in total occlusion of the airway lumen (Fig. 3.8), obliterating the lumen in the form of membranous fibrosis (Fig. 3.9), or protruding into the lumen in the form of polyps, and in many cases, more than one of these types of fibrosis are present. With the passage of time after onset,

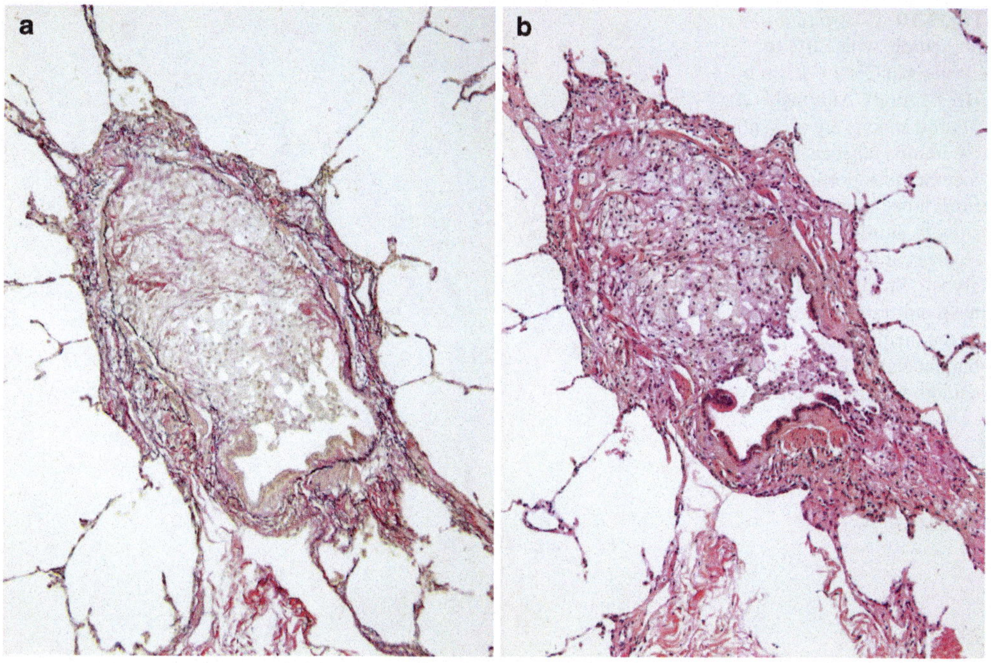

Fig. 3.7 EBO (**a**, elastic van Gieson stain; **b**, HE staining). Fibrosis with aggregations of foamy macrophages can be seen inside the lumina of the membranous bronchioles. There is slight infiltration of the bronchiolar walls by small round cells and foamy macrophages, and the elastic fibers and smooth muscle are preserved. There is only slight inflammation of the alveoli around the bronchioles

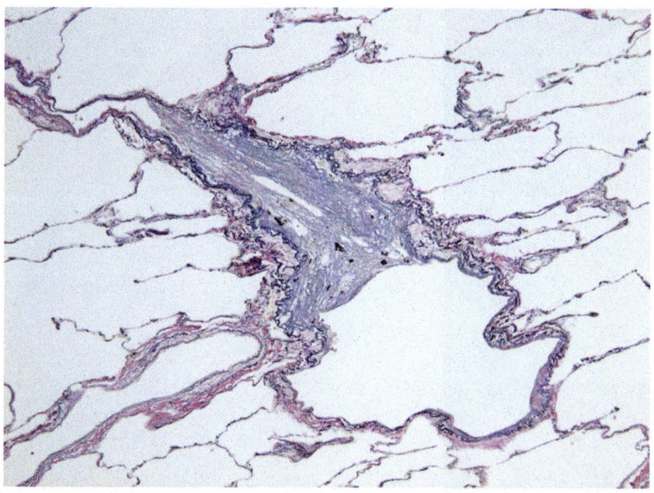

Fig. 3.8 EBO (elastic van Gieson stain). The lumina of the bronchioles are occluded by focal fibrosis. The concentration of fine elastic fibers increases within the fibrosis

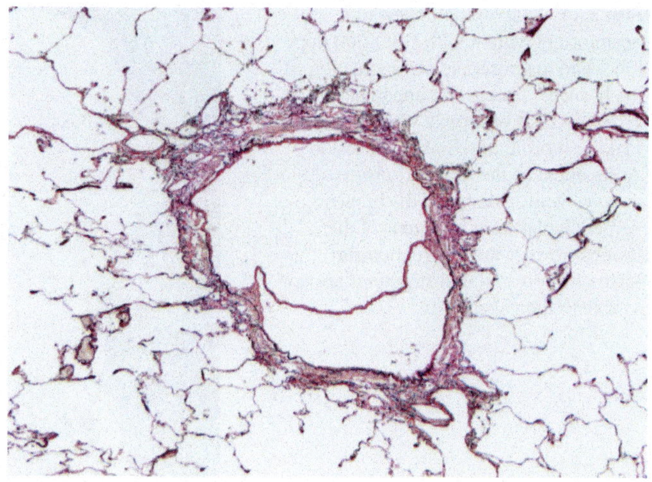

Fig. 3.9 EBO (elastic van Gieson stain). Membranous fibrosis has formed across the airway lumina

the amount of fine elastic fibers within the fibrosis increases. Inflammation of the airway wall is mild, and although mild infiltration by foamy macrophages or small round cells may occur, it is rare for this infiltration to involve lymph follicles. The elastic fibers and smooth muscles of the airway remain, and the alveoli around the airway are slightly inflamed.

The walls of the airways between the EBO lesions and those proximal to the EBO lesions undergo minimal changes. Although mucus may accumulate in the airway lumen, thickening of the wall is only mild, and inflammatory cell infiltration is minimal.

EBO of the respiratory bronchioles is rare. Even if these are affected, lesions are only formed in lumina adjacent to a membranous portion with smooth muscle (Fig. 3.10), and there is no inflammation of the alveolar area.

EBO is characterized by multiple lesions; however, these lesions are focal and almost entirely localized to the airway lumen, with no thickening of the airway wall and few lesions of other airways or alveolar tissue, making them difficult to observe with the naked eye (Fig. 3.11). To identify the affected region macroscopically, the specimen must be cut meticulously perpendicular to the long axis of the bronchi for visual assessment of the internal surface of the airways.

However, bronchiectasis may be observed in areas proximal to EBO if a secondary airway infection develops during the course of the disease. If a bronchial wall becomes dilated due to an airway infection, it is destroyed by fibrosis and

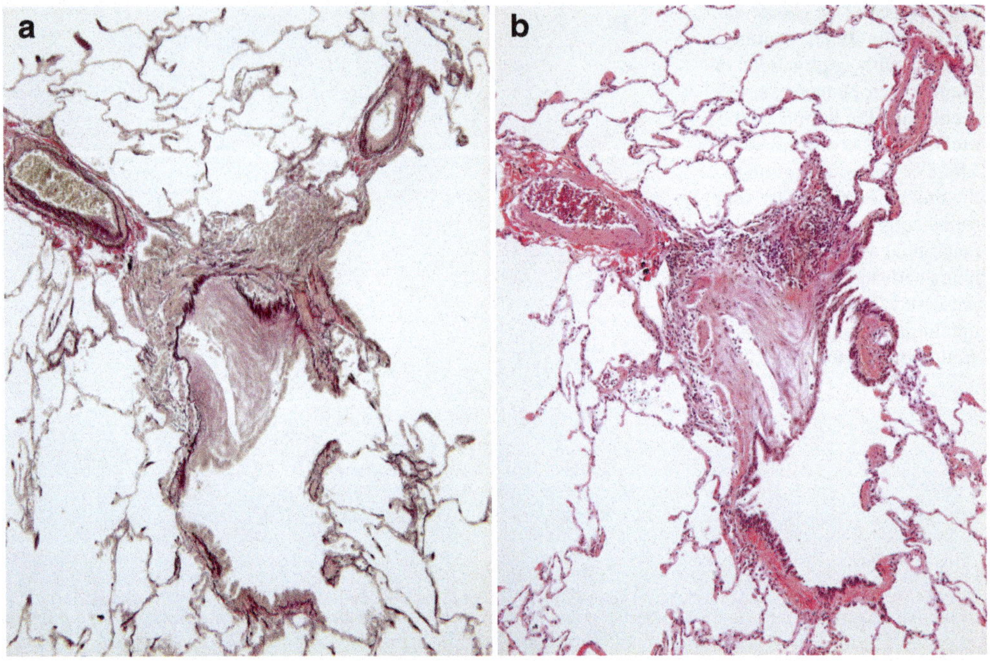

Fig. 3.10 A respiratory bronchiole with EBO (**a**, elastic van Gieson stain; **b**, HE staining). Although fibrotic lesions are present in the lumina adjacent to the membranous portion of the respiratory bronchioles with smooth muscle, no major changes are observed in the alveoli. Small round cells have infiltrated the outer layer of the membranous portion, but the elastic fibers and smooth muscle are preserved

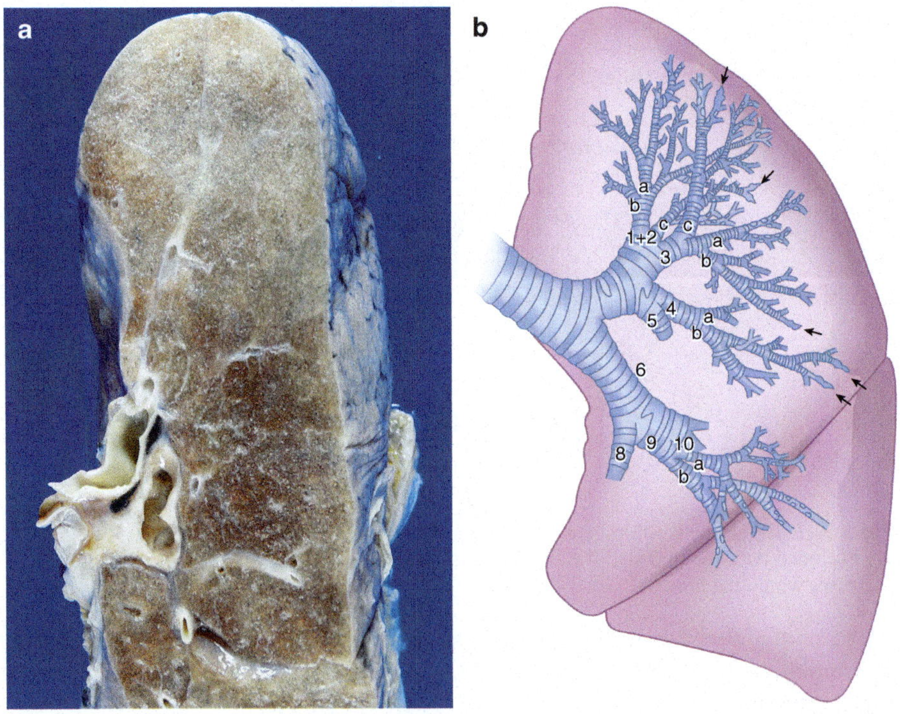

Fig. 3.11 Macroscopic view of a postmortem patient with EBO (left upper lobe) and macroscopic reconstruction of the bronchi. There is no apparent bronchiectasis or airway wall thickening, making it difficult to locate the lesion. Assessment of the internal surface of the airways while dissecting the bronchi perpendicular to its long axis of the bronchi reveals the obstruction site (arrow). More distal obstructions are not visible to the naked eye

inflammatory cell infiltration, resulting in loss of the elastic fibers and smooth muscles, which is not found in EBO. However, EBO can be confirmed by the presence of typical lesions at the distal edge of the bronchiectasis.

3.2.3 Cellular Destructive Bronchiolitis (CDB)

The exact incidence of CDB in the patients with RA has not been reported. There is no gender difference in the incidence of CDB in RA in our cohort [10]; CDB may also be associated with Sjogren syndrome or may be idiopathic. Cases of CDB may be subacute or chronic, with airway infection, and production of purulent sputum, occurring in the early stage of the disease. Many patients with CDB either suffer from chronic sinusitis or have a history of it [7, 10].

Similar to EBO, in CDB, the most severe stenotic lesions develop from the membranous bronchioles or the small bronchi. Most patients with CDB exhibit lesions with varying degrees of inflammatory cell infiltration and fibrosis.

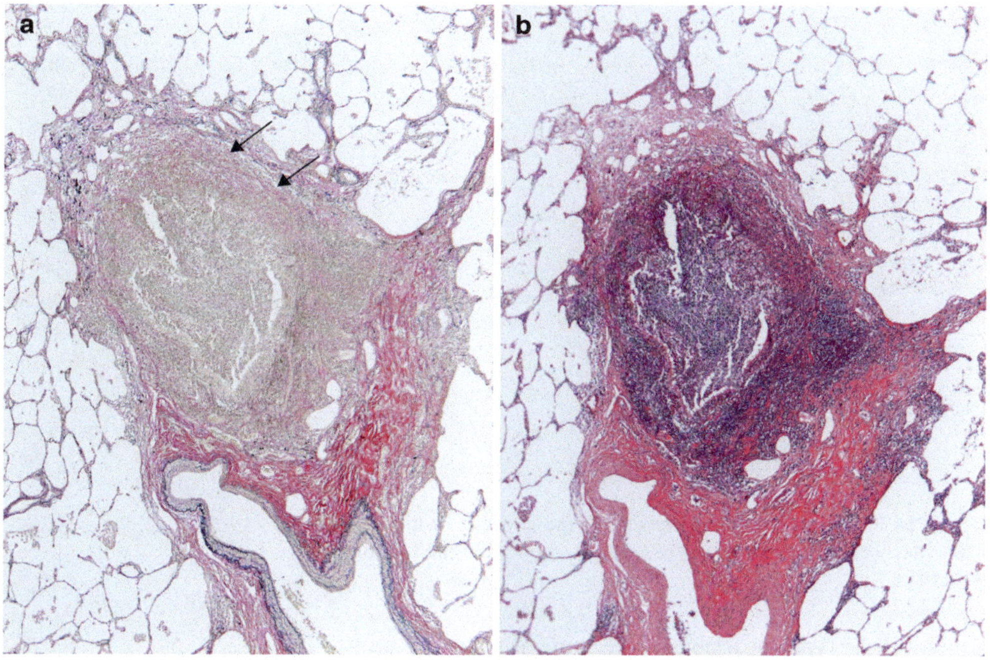

Fig. 3.12 CDB (**a**, elastic van Gieson stain; **b**, HE staining). In addition to lymphoid follicles and severe small round cell infiltration, granulation tissue (arrow) is also visible in the membranous bronchiolar walls, and the elastic fibers and smooth muscle have disappeared. Mucus and neutrophils are seen in the lumen. The inflammation also encompasses the surrounding alveoli

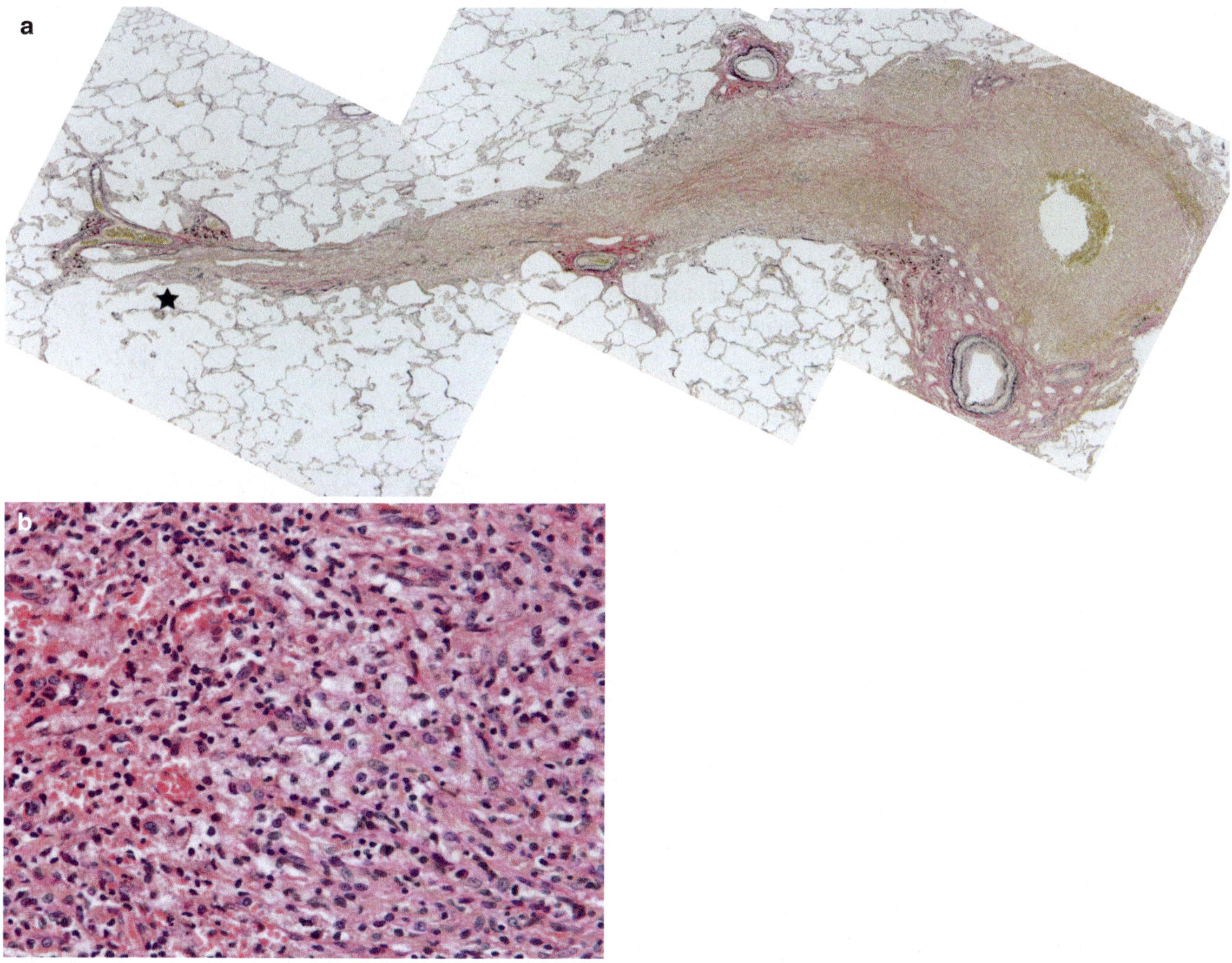

Fig. 3.13 CDB (**a**, elastic van Gieson stain; **b**, HE staining). Lesions are continuous from the membranous bronchioles to the respiratory bronchioles (asterisk) (**a**), and the airway walls are replaced by granulation tissue with foamy macrophages and small round cells (**b**). The structure of the membranous bronchiolar walls has been completely destroyed, but elastic fibers are still present in the respiratory bronchioles (**a**)

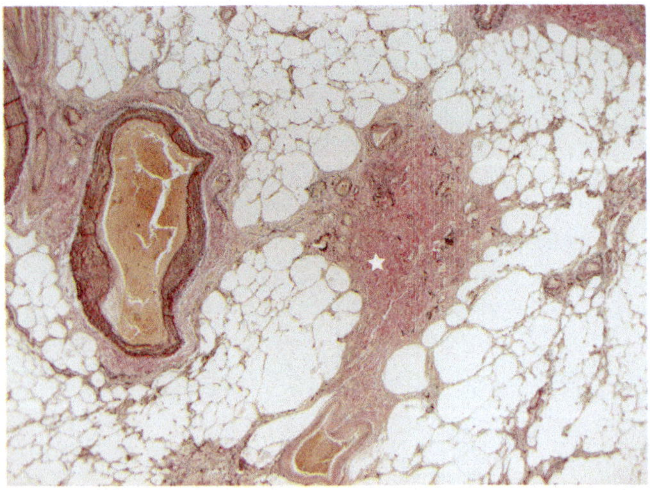

Fig. 3.14 CDB (elastic van Gieson stain). The structure of the bronchus has been completely destroyed and shows fibrotic scarring (asterisk)

One of these types of lesions is the same as follicular bronchiolitis [7, 8] or cellular bronchiolitis [9], characterized by severe inflammatory cell infiltration, erosion, or ulceration of the mucosa, increase in the number of lymphoid follicles, and lymphocyte infiltration of the entire thickness of the airway wall. However, this lesion also exhibits fibrosis and granulation tissue in addition to inflammatory cell infiltration, and these inflammatory responses cause the destruction of the structure of the airway wall, with the loss of elastic fibers and smooth muscle (Figs. 3.6 and 3.12). Most patients with CDB also have other airway lesions exhibiting even more severe tissue destruction, with signs that small bronchi and bronchioles have been replaced by granulation tissue containing aggregations of foamy macrophages (Fig. 3.13) or hyaline fibrosis (Fig. 3.14).

Unlike EBO, which causes focal, multiple lesions, in CDB, the occlusive or stenotic lesions affect the airway continuously from the small bronchi to the membranous bronchioles. Fibrosis and inflammatory cell infiltration may sometimes extend as far as the respiratory bronchioles and the surrounding alveoli (Fig. 3.13). However, tissue destruction in this region is less severe than that of lesions in the small bronchi and membranous bronchioles, and in most cases, the elastic fibers and smooth muscle of the respiratory bronchioles and alveoli are still present.

Most patients with CDB exhibit bronchiectasis of the bronchi proximal to the lesions of CDB (Fig. 3.15). The pattern of bronchiectasis varies in different patients and may be tubular, cystic, or mixed. Airway walls affected by bronchiectasis develop ulceration as well as inflammatory cell infiltration of varying degrees of severity and fibrosis with lymphoid follicles. As a result, the structure of the airway wall is destroyed, and the existing smooth muscle, elastic fibers, and even collagen and bronchial glands decrease or disappear.

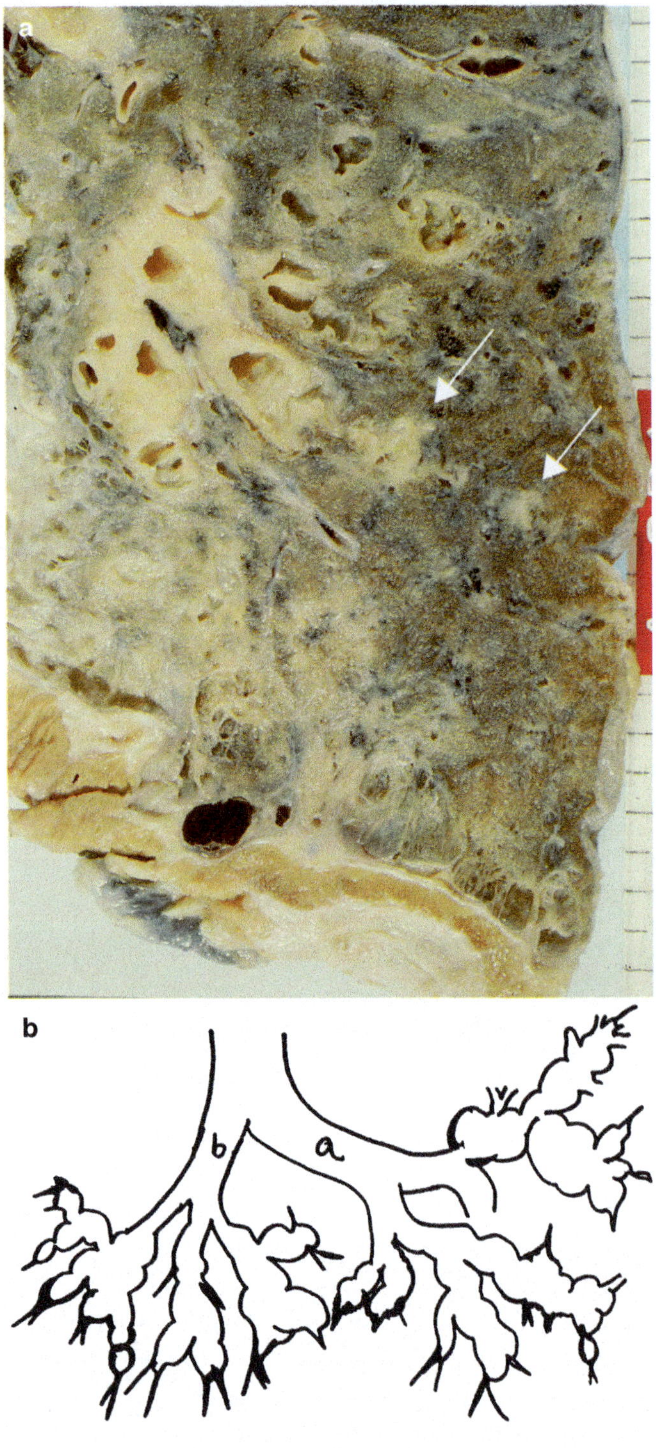

Fig. 3.15 Macroscopic view of an autopsy patient with CDB (a, left lower lobe) and macroscopic reconstruction of a segmental bronchus (b, B9). Tubular or cystic bronchiectasis is evident, and airway occlusion (CDB) (a, arrow) is visible at the edges of the bronchiectasis

Both bronchiectasis and CDB are lesions that cause severe destruction of tissues, and it is difficult to identify the primary lesion based on their morphological features alone. However, recently, a number of studies have reported that the bronchi

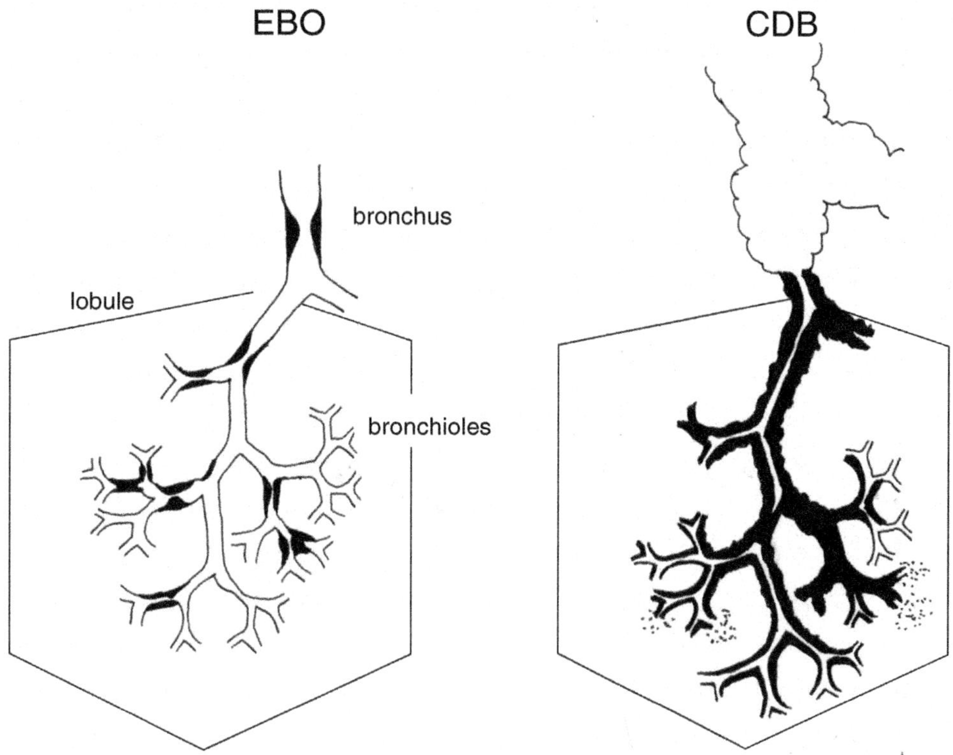

Fig. 3.16 Schema of EBO and CDB

become dilated after the onset of CDB [10–12], and we suggest that bronchiectasis may develop as a secondary lesion in patients with CDB. Bronchiectasis may be due to the destruction and weakening of the bronchial wall proximal to the CDB lesion as a result of the inflammation spreading from CDB to the bronchi or to a secondary airway infection.

CDB can easily be seen with the naked eye at the edge of the dilated part of the bronchus. Parts of the airway replaced with fibrosis appear as grayish-white fibrotic scarring, and granulation tissue with aggregations of foamy macrophages can be seen as yellow granulation (Fig. 3.15).

3.3 Summary (Fig. 3.16 and Table 3.1)

1. RA-associated bronchiolitis obliterans can be categorized as follows: (1) EBO, in which airway obstruction is due to lesions in the airway lumen and there is little destruction of the airway wall, and (2) CDB, in which transmural inflammation results in destruction of the airway wall.
2. EBO and CDB not only differ in their pathologies but also have markedly different clinical presentations and should be regarded as separate conditions.
3. At least some cases of RA-associated bronchiectasis are probably secondary to bronchiolitis obliterans, and to CDB, in particular.

Table 3.1 Summary of clinical and pathological characteristics of EBO and CDB

	EBO	CDB
Clinical course	Acute–subacute	Chronic
Chronic sinusitis	Rare	Common
Bacterial infection	Rare	Common
Distribution of lesions	Focal, multiple	Continual
Destruction of bronchiolar wall	Rare	Severe
Involvement of respiratory bronchioles	Rare	Common
Bronchiectasis	Rare	Very common

References

1. Cohen M, Shan SA. Bronchiectasis in systemic disease. Chest. 1999;116:1063–74.
2. White ES, Tazalaar HD, Lynchi JP III. Bronchiolar complications of connective tissue diseases. Semin Respir Crit Care Med. 2003;24:543–66.
3. Lange W. Ueber eine eigenthuemliche Erkrankung der kleinen Bronchien und Bronchiolen. Dtsch Arch Klin Med. 1901;70:342–64.
4. Colby TV, Myers JL. Clinical and histologic spectrum of bronchiolitis obliterans, including bronchiolitis obliterans organizing pneumonia. Semin Respir Med. 1992;13:119–33.
5. Colby TV. Bronchiolar pathology. In: Epler GR, editor. Diseases of the bronchioles. New York: Raven Press; 1994. p. 77–100.

6. Geddes DM, Corrin B, Brewerton DA, Davies RJ, Turner-Warwick M. Progressive airway obliteration in adults and its association with rheumatoid arthritis. Q J Med. 1977;184:427–44.
7. Hayakawa H, Sato A, Imokawa S, Toyoshima M, Chida K, Iwata M. Bronchiolar diseases in rheumatoid arthritis. Am J Crit Care Med. 1996;154:1531–6.
8. Yousem SA, Colby TV, Carrington CB. Follicular bronchitis/bronchiolitis. Hum Pathol. 1985;16:700–6.
9. Homma S, Sakamoto S, Kawabata M, Kishi K, Tsuboi E, Motoi N, et al. Comparative clinicopathology of obliterative bronchiolitis and diffuse panbronchiolitis. Respiration. 2006;73:481–7.
10. Sugino K, Hebisawa A, Uekusa T, Hatanaka K, Abe H, Homma S. Histopathological bronchial reconstruction of human bronchiolitis obliterans. Path Int. 2011;61:192–201.
11. Morita S, Sato A, Hayakawa H, Chida K, Tsukamoto K, Toyoshima M, et al. Follicular bronchiolitis associated with rheumatoid arthritis. Nihon Kyobu Shikkan Gakkai Zasshi. 1996;34:921–5. (in Japanese; abstract in English).
12. Ishiguro T, Takayanagi N, Tokunaga D, Yanagisawa T, Sugita Y, Kawabata Y. A case of follicular bronchiolitis in which progressive bronchiectasis developed over 7 years. Nihon Kokyuki Gakkai Zasshi. 2011;49:827–32. (in Japanese; abstract in English).

4 Imaging of Airway Diseases of Rheumatoid Arthritis

Fumikazu Sakai

Abstract

Varying kinds of airway disease are frequently seen in rheumatoid arthritis (RA) patients. It is mandatory to know immunologic and pathologic features of RA in order to explain frequent occurrence of airway diseases in RA patients. Causes of airway diseases encompass infectious and noninfectious process. Noninfectious process may be related to hyperreactive state to endogenous/exogenous agents in RA patients. This noninfectious destructive disease of airway may become one of predisposing factors of respiratory tract infection. Respiratory tract infection can accelerate autoimmune inflammatory process in airway and vice versa.

Phenotype of airway disease includes bronchitis and bronchiectasis in large airways and cellular bronchiolitis, follicular bronchiolitis, bronchiolitis obliterans, and cellular and destructive bronchiolitis in small peripheral airway. Existence of airway disease may be a predisposing factor of infection and may lead to poor prognosis of patients. CXR and CT features of these airway diseases are well correlated with pathologic features and one of very useful tools to recognize airway disease in RA patients.

Keywords

Rheumatoid arthritis • Bronchiectasis • Airway disease • Bronchiolitis obliterans • Cellular and destructive bronchiolitis

4.1 Introduction

It is well known that patients with rheumatoid arthritis (RA) have often airway disease. High incidence of airway disease may be related to RA itself or infection and sometimes related to immunocompromised state induced by antirheumatic drugs and both of them.

Airway lesion is classified into disease of large- and middle-sized bronchi and peripheral small airway (less than 1 mm in diameter) disease based on the level of bronchi. Large to intermediate airway disease includes bronchiectasis and bronchitis. Peripheral airway diseases include bronchiolitis of varying etiologies and subtypes [1].

F. Sakai, M.D.
Department of Diagnostic Radiology, Saitama International Medical Center, Saitama Medical University, Saitama, Japan
e-mail: fmksakai@yahoo.co.jp

4.2 X-Ray Diagnosis of Airway Disease

Chest X-ray (CXR) and computed tomography (CT) are most frequently used diagnostic modalities for lung disease complicated in RA patients. High-resolution CT (HRCT) is one of the most valuable modalities in examining lung diseases including airway lesion.

On CXR, bronchitis and bronchiectasis can be identified as linear opacity and/or increased vascular markings corresponding to thickened bronchial wall, sometimes described as "tram line" (Figs. 4.1 and 4.2). Tram line is seen as paralleling linear opacities representing bronchial wall thickening of relatively large bronchi. In advanced case of cystic bronchiectasis, the bronchiectatic wall forms curvilinear opacities.

T. Gono et al. (eds.), *Lung Disease Associated with Rheumatoid Arthritis*, https://doi.org/10.1007/978-981-10-6750-1_4

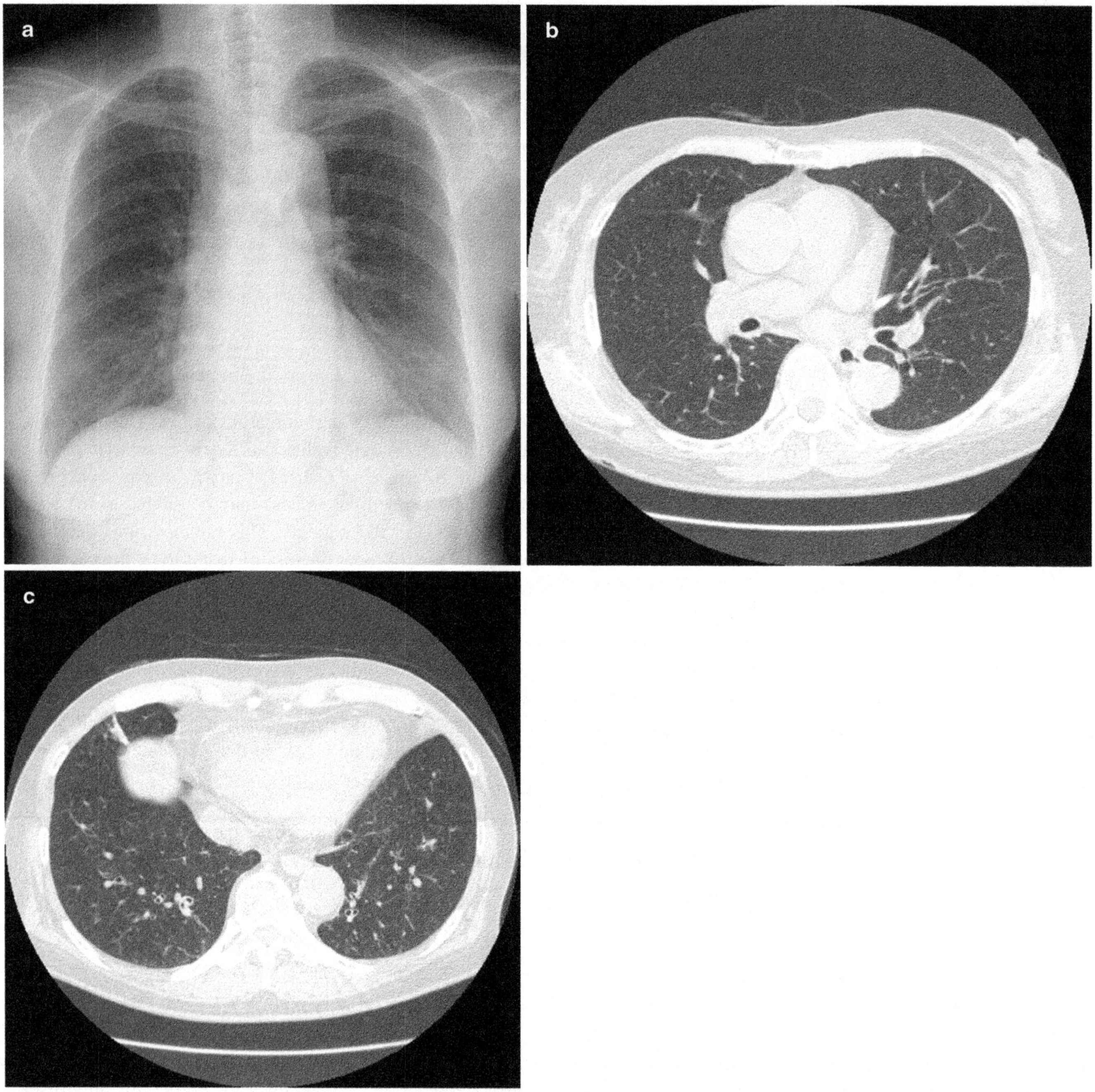

Fig. 4.1 Bronchiectasis in a RA patient (by the courtesy of Dr. H. Tokuda). (**a**) CXR. Bronchial wall thickening is identified as linear shadow, sometimes paralleling line, so-called tram line. (**b**) HRCT at the middle lung shows bronchiectasis with bronchial wall thickening, corresponding to linear opacities and tram lines. (**c**) HRCT. Minimal dilatation of bronchi with wall thickening is noted. A few small centrilobular nodules are identified

Bronchiolitis shows ill-defined small nodular opacities on CXR (Fig. 4.2). Bronchiolitis is often complicated with air trapping and overinflation of the lung, which evokes small heart shadow and flat shape, lower position of diaphragm on frontal projection (Fig. 4.3), and increased retrosternal clear space on lateral projection. In patients with air trapping, CXR at expiration shows less movement of diaphragm and decrease of lung volume.

4.3 CT Findings of Airway Disease

4.3.1 Bronchitis and Bronchiectasis

CT findings of airway lesion of large to intermediate bronchi include bronchial wall thickening and bronchiectasis. Bronchial wall at CT corresponds to bronchial

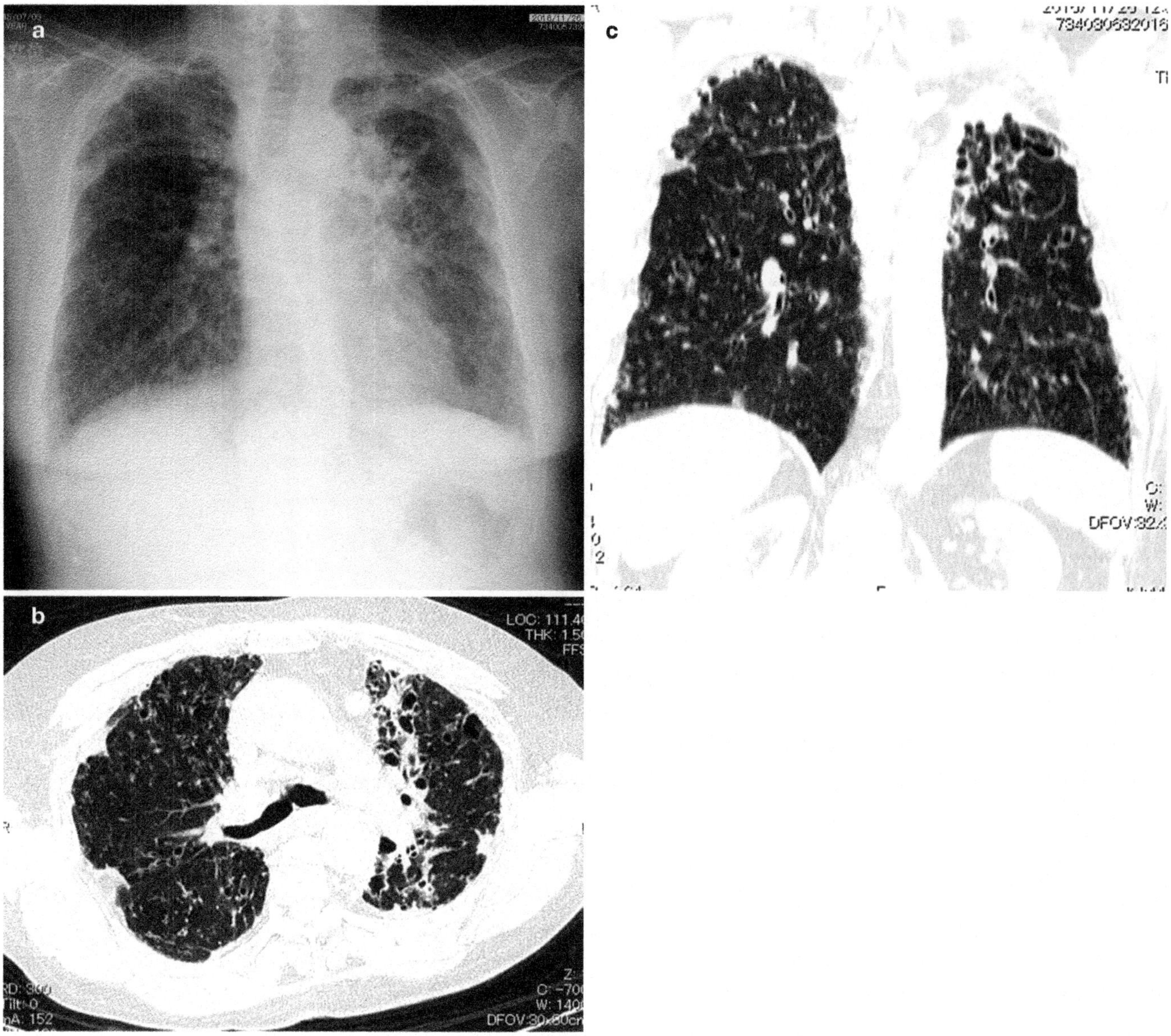

Fig. 4.2 Bronchobronchiolitis with bronchiectasis in RA. (**a**) CXR. CXR shows bronchial wall thickening (tram line) and small ill-defined nodular opacities. (**b**) HRCT. HRCT at the upper lung shows multiple centrilobular nodules and branching opacities. Bronchial wall thickening and bronchiectasis are noted predominantly in the medial aspect of the left lung. (**c**) Coronal CT. Coronal reformatted image shows bronchiectasis predominantly in the left upper lung. Bronchial wall thickening and centrilobular nodular opacities are shown in bilateral lungs

mucosa, submucosal tissue, cartilages if present, smooth muscles of the airway, and peribronchial connective tissues surrounding bronchus. These tissues cannot be discriminated on CT images except calcified cartilages of large central airways. Pathologic process of peribronchial lung parenchyma may not be differentiated from bronchial disease on CT.

Thickening of bronchial wall is related to inflammatory process caused by infectious, noninfectious, or both of them. Pathologically edematous change of mucosa and submucosal tissue, cellular infiltration and intramural organization in acute phase, and proliferation of mucous gland and fibrotic change may be related to bronchial wall thickening.

Thickness of airway has been investigated mainly in patients with COPD, correlating with pulmonary function tests and degree of obstructive impairment [2]. Destructive changes of bronchial wall ultimately result in bronchiectasis. Shape of bronchiectasis is classified as cylindrical, cystic, and varicose regardless of causes of bronchial wall destruction.

According to Naidich and coworkers [3], inner diameter of normal bronchial lumen is narrower than outer diameter

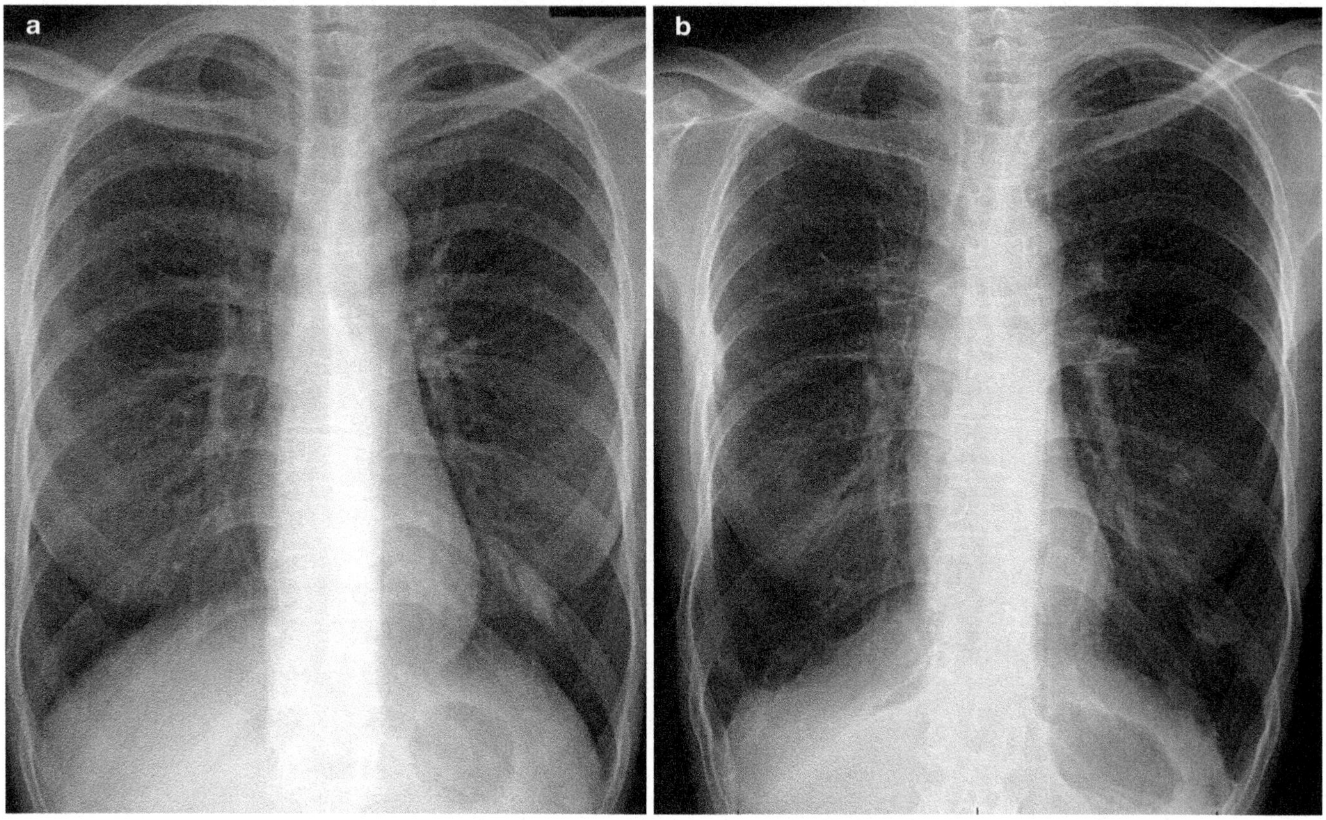

Fig. 4.3 Bronchiolitis obliterans in a RA patient (by the courtesy of Dr. H. Tokuda). (**a**) CXR. CXR showed overinflation of lungs and increased lung volume. Lower position and flat shape of bilateral diaphragm are also noted. (**b**) CXR 4 years later. Four years later, overinflation of bilateral lungs and flattering of the diaphragm were found

of accompanying pulmonary artery (usually intraluminal diameter of bronchus is approximately 70% of diameter of accompanying pulmonary artery). Thus, if bronchial lumen is larger than the diameter of accompanying pulmonary artery, it should be considered as dilated (bronchiectasis) (Figs. 4.1 and 4.2). However, these criteria have some limitations in determining bronchiectasis because pulmonary artery caliber may change according to pulmonary perfusion state and is not an absolute standard (Fig. 4.4).

Other diagnostic criteria of bronchiectasis include non-tapering bronchus, because normal bronchial lumen shows gradual narrowing of lumen along perihilar to peripheral regions. Also bronchiectasis should be considered when HRCT demonstrates packing of mucus in lumen of bronchi, that is, cylindrical shadow (mucoid impaction) (Fig. 4.5).

4.3.2 Bronchiolitis

Lumen of normal peripheral small airway cannot be recognized in the areas as far as 1 cm apart from the chest wall by HRCT. Smaller bronchi whose lumen is narrower than 1 mm in inner diameter cannot be discriminated as bronchioles even at HRCT.

HRCT manifestations of peripheral airway lesion (bronchiolitis) include varieties of findings: centrilobular nodules, branching opacities (Fig. 4.6), and mosaic appearance (Fig. 4.7).

Centrilobular nodular and branching opacities are caused by bronchiolar wall thickening and peribronchiolar pathologic process that is mainly composed of cellular infiltration. These findings are most prominently seen in cellular bronchiolitis.

Centrilobular nodules and branching opacities are not identified in constrictive bronchiolitis (e.g., bronchiolitis obliterans) because the main pathologic feature of restrictive bronchiolitis is fibrosis and lack of prominent cellular infiltration in bronchial walls (Fig. 4.8) [4–12].

Mosaic appearance is defined as intermingled white (radiopaque) and black (radiolucent) areas at CT. Sometimes decreased opacity areas are observed as lobular/multilobular pattern, and their borders of increased opacity areas are linear [13]. Mosaic appearance is usually seen in airway disease or pulmonary vascular disease. Radiolucent areas may represent as increased aeration (air trap) in airway disease and decreased perfusion (blood volume) in vascular disease (Figs. 4.5 and 4.8) [6–12].

Pulmonary vasculature is attenuated in air-trapped (black) areas in airway disease, because reactive vaso-

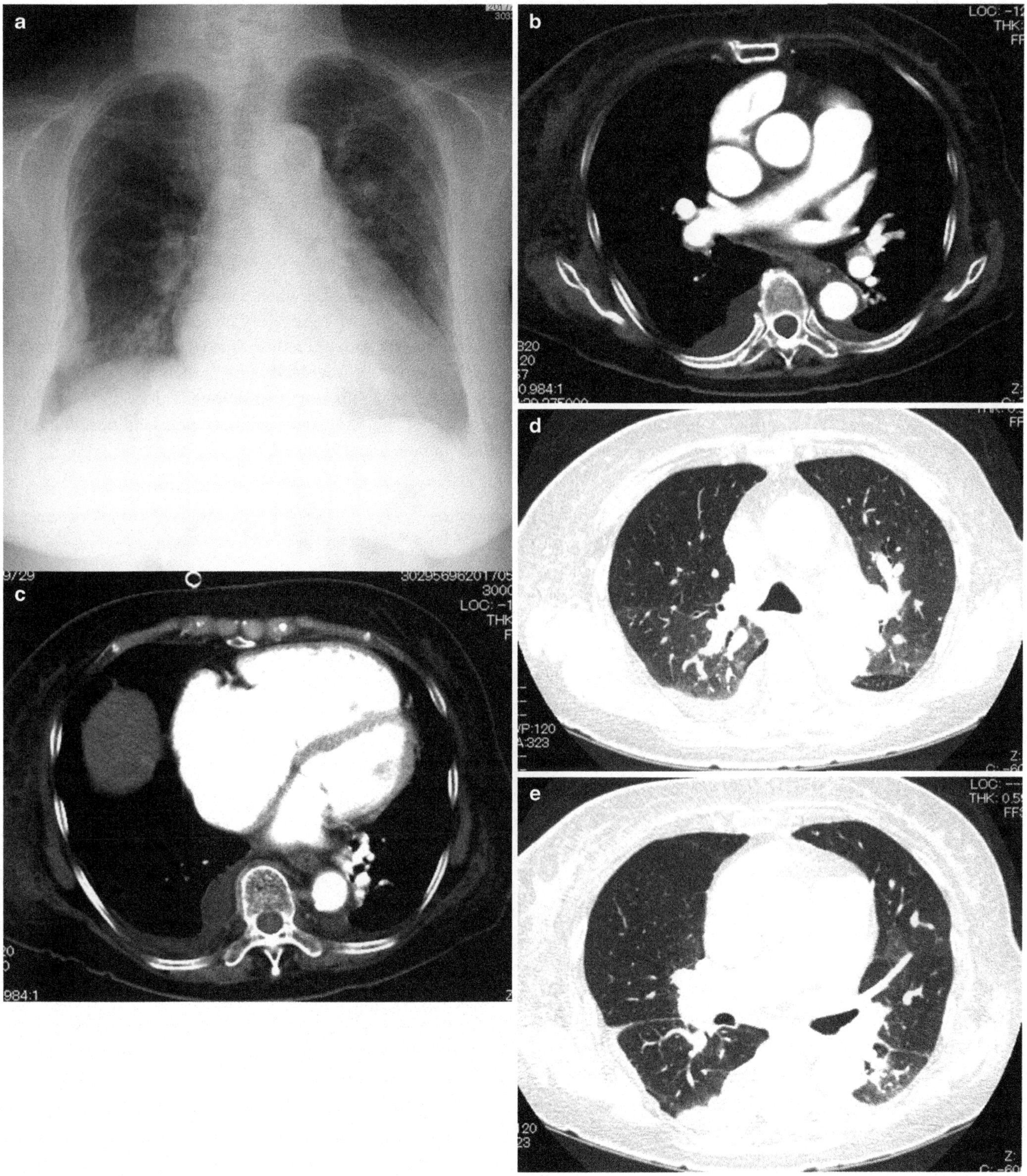

Fig. 4.4 Pulmonary hypertension. (**a**) CXR. Chest X-ray shows cardiomegaly with central pulmonary artery dilation. Diameter of main pulmonary artery is measured 32 mm, larger than the ascending aorta. (**b**) CECT. CECT shows dilatation of the central pulmonary artery, suggesting pulmonary hypertension. (**c**) CECT. CECT shows dilation of the right ventricle, suggesting right heart overload. (**d**) HRCT. In a case where diameter of pulmonary arteries is increased, ratio of bronchial lumen and pulmonary artery caliber are unreliable. Mosaic appearance of lung fields is noted. Intermingled radiopaque (white) and radiolucent (black) areas are shown; the borders of these two different areas are sometimes straight apparently. Vessels within radiolucent areas are attenuated. (**e**) HRCT. Mosaic appearance is also noted in more caudal section

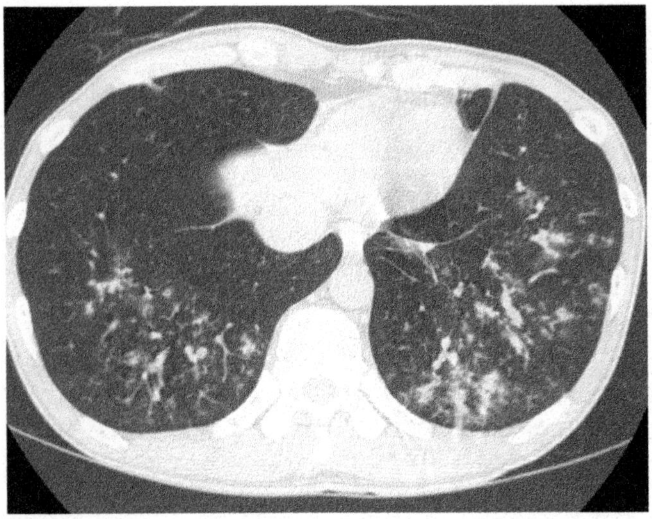

Fig. 4.5 Bronchobronchiolitis with mucoid impaction in RA. HRCT images show thick bronchial walls. Mucoid impaction is identified as tubular opacities

constriction causes decreased blood circulation in areas with hypoventilation by regulatory process to reduce ventilation perfusion mismatch. CT at expiration shows exaggeration of mosaic appearance in airway disease (Figs. 4.7 and 4.9) [11]. While normal or nearly normal areas (white areas) show decreased attenuation at expiration CT, air-trapped areas (black areas) remain aeration as at inspiration CT. Sometimes shape of air-trapped areas is almost same shape or size in expiratory CT as that in inspiration CT.

Even in pulmonary parenchymal disease, spurious mosaic appearance is observed when degrees of disease severity are inhomogeneous. More severely involved areas which are less aerated show relatively radiopaque (white) when surrounded by less severely involved area which are more aerated (black). In such situation, expiration CT does not show exaggeration of inhomogeneous appearance, and vasculature in black area is not attenuated.

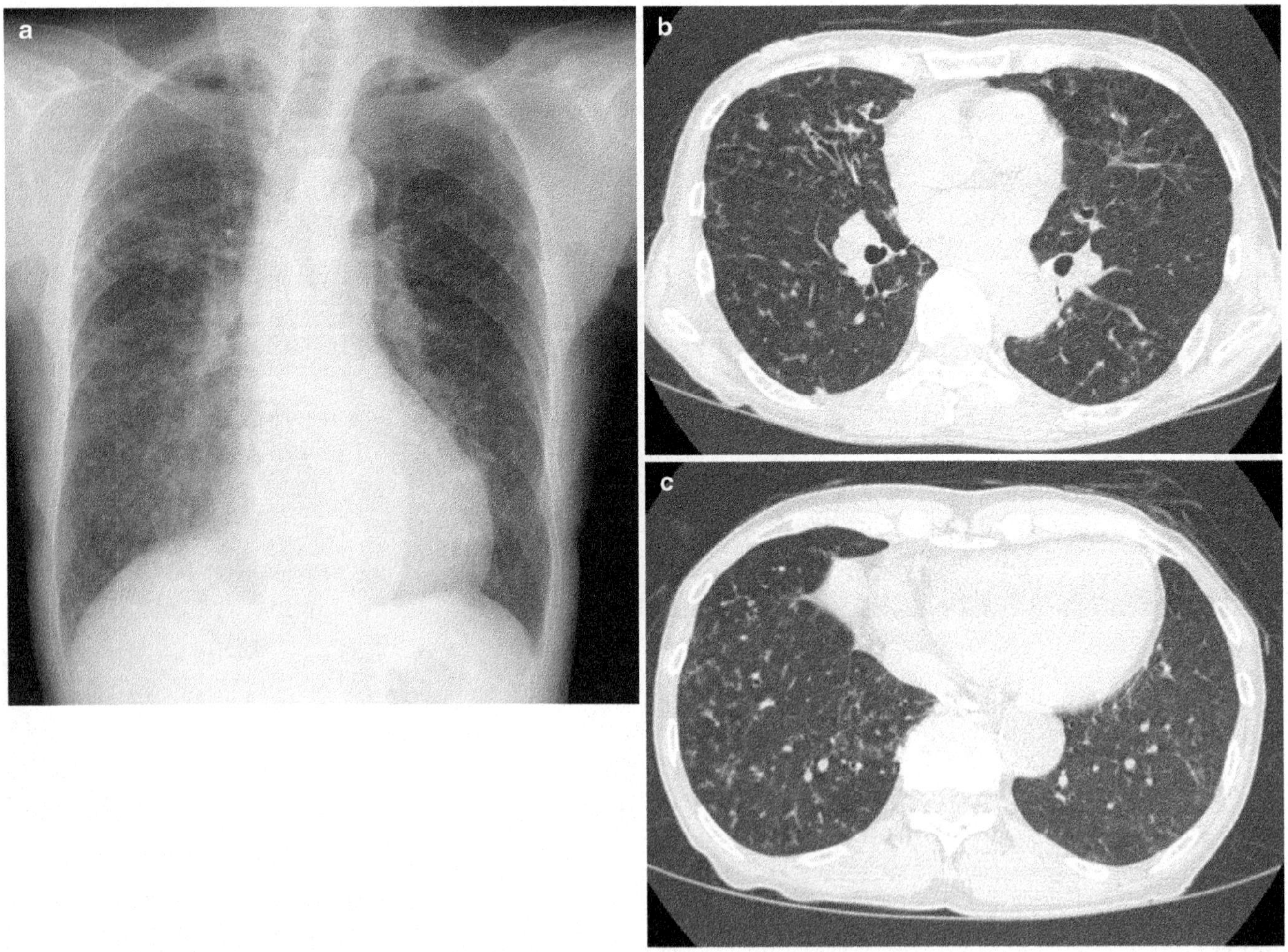

Fig. 4.6 Bronchiolitis in RA. (**a**) CXR. CXR shows overinflation of bilateral lungs. CXR shows bronchial wall thickening and small centrilobular nodular opacities, suggesting bronchiolitis. (**b**) HRCT. HRCT images show bronchiectasis with bronchial wall thickening and small centrilobular nodular or branching opacities. (**c**) HRCT. HRCT at more caudal level shows definite centrilobular nodules and branching opacities, suggesting bronchiolitis

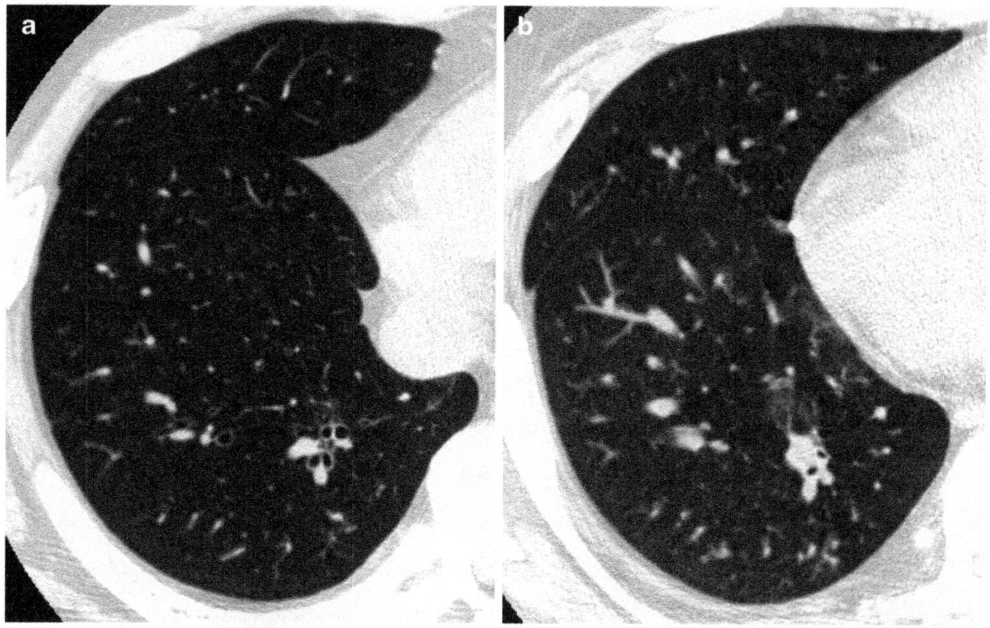

Fig. 4.7 Bronchiolitis obliterans in RA. (**a**) HRCT at full inspiration. HRCT images at full inspiration show scanty small centrilobular nodules. Panlobular or multilobular radiolucent areas are obtained, surrounded by normal lung. (**b**) HRCT at full expiration. HRCT at expiration shows exaggeration of mosaic appearance

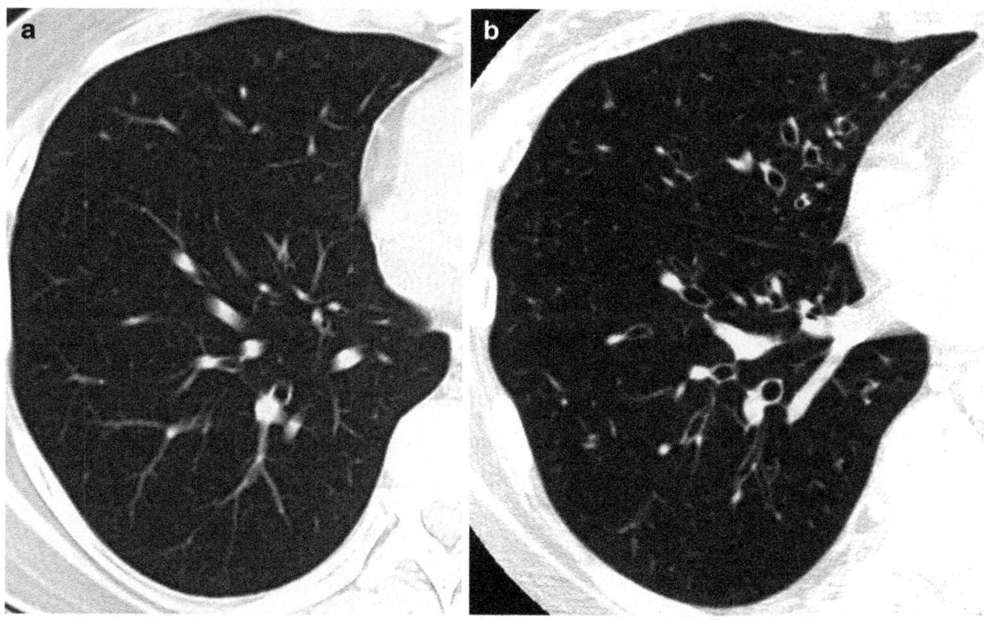

Fig. 4.8 Bronchiolitis obliterans in post-bone marrow transplantation. (**a**) Early stage. HRCT shows almost normal appearance. (**b**) Advanced stage. In advanced stage, the lumen of bronchi is larger than the accompanying pulmonary arteries. There are slight centrilobular/branching opacities, suggesting bronchiolitis. It requires great caution to compare calibers of bronchi because calibers of bronchi may change, depending on the degree of inspiration

4.4 Airway Disease in RA Patients

Many previous papers described high incidence of airway lesion (bronchial wall thickening and/or bronchiectasis) in RA patients. The incidence of airway lesion is reported to be approximately 20–40% [12, 14–22]. The incidence of bronchitis and bronchiectasis in RA patients seems to be ten times as frequent as in general population. Obstructive impairment of pulmonary function tests and pathologic analysis show more frequent bronchiolitis/small airway disease in RA patients.

Frequency of respiratory tract infection is higher than general population [23–26], and the overall survival is shorter in RA patients with airway lesion [27, 28]. The use of antirheumatic drugs including biologic agents is one of the risk factors of respiratory tract infection [25, 26, 29–32]. Airway lesion seems to be a very important problem in management of RA patients [26].

4.4.1 Diseases of Large to Intermediate Airway

4.4.1.1 Noninfectious Airway Disease

Destructive change of bronchial wall leads to bronchiectasis [33]. Etiologies of bronchiectasis are varying, infectious and noninfectious. Bronchiectasis is one of the most important

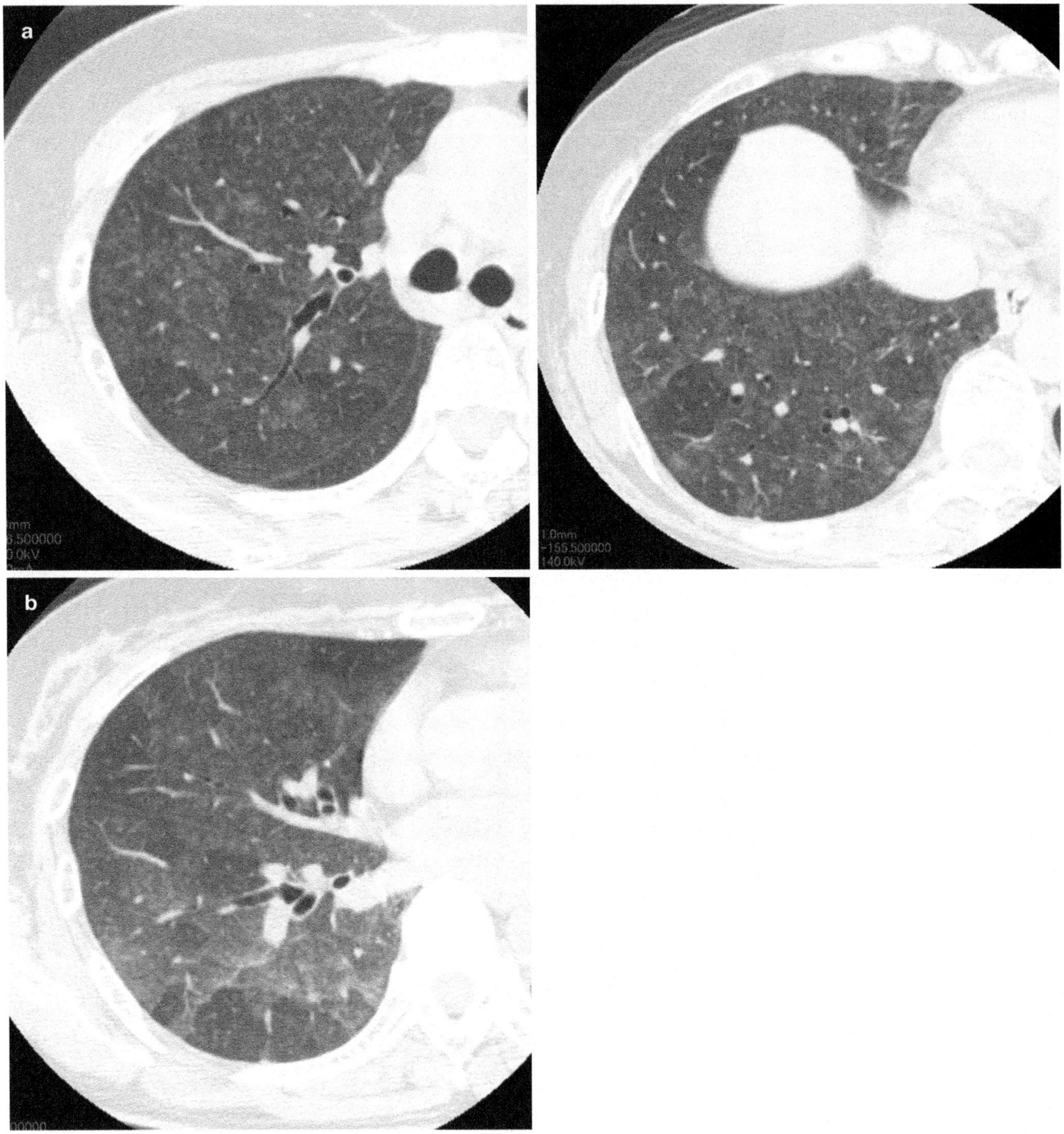

Fig. 4.9 Air trap proved at expiration CT in hypersensitivity pneumonia. (**a**) HRCT at full inspiration. Centrilobular faint ground-glass opacities are evident. Rectangular radiolucent areas are intermingled (mosaic appearance). (**b**) HRCT at full expiration. At full expiration, mosaic appearance is exaggerated

sequelae of severe lower respiratory infection. Conversely, existence of bronchiectasis itself also becomes one of the risk factors of infection. This circulus vitiosus results in progression of bronchial wall destruction [34–36].

According to previous reports [12, 14–17], RA patients show airway lesion including bronchiectasis very frequently at HRCT; the frequency is reported to be approximately 20–40% (Figs. 4.2, 4.5, and 4.6).

In RA patients, immunologic process may play important roles in the formation of destructive change of bronchi. Noninfectious immunologic process can cause destructive change of the bronchial wall. Recent studies disclosed the existence of normal bacterial flora of the lower respiratory tract. Exaggerated reaction to this bacterial flora may be related to autoimmune inflammation of airway in RA patients [37]. RA patients show hyperreactive change to endogenous or exogenous agents including the normal endobronchial flora. Rich bronchus-associated lymphoid tissues (BALT) play important roles in autoimmune inflammatory process and production of autoantibodies.

4.4.1.2 Infectious Airway Disease

In addition to airway disease due to noninfectious autoimmune mechanism, infectious airway disease is frequently seen in RA patients. Destructive change of airway by noninfectious immunologic mechanism becomes one of the predisposing factors of airway infection. Immunosuppressive state induced by antirheumatic drugs is also another predisposing factor of infectious airway disease.

Varying kinds of organism including bacterial, mycobacterial, fungal, and viral infection may sometimes occur in RA patients [24, 26, 27]. Bacterial infection is the most frequent complication in RA patients practically, and *Pseudomonas aeruginosa* and *Haemophilus influenzae* are the most frequent causative bacteria [26].

Nontuberculous mycobacteriosis (Fig. 4.10) is one of the most important differential diagnoses of airway disease.

Under biologics therapy, increased incidence of mycobacterial infection is reported [25, 29, 38, 39]. Clinicians should be alert for complications of nontuberculous mycobacteriosis, particularly when airway disease is preexisting before initiation of biologic agents in RA patients.

Nontuberculous mycobacteriosis is divided into two forms: nodular bronchiectatic form and fibrocavitary form. Nodular bronchiectatic form shows bronchiectasis, small nodular opacities, and patchy consolidation/ground-glass opacity, predominantly in the right middle lobe and left lin-

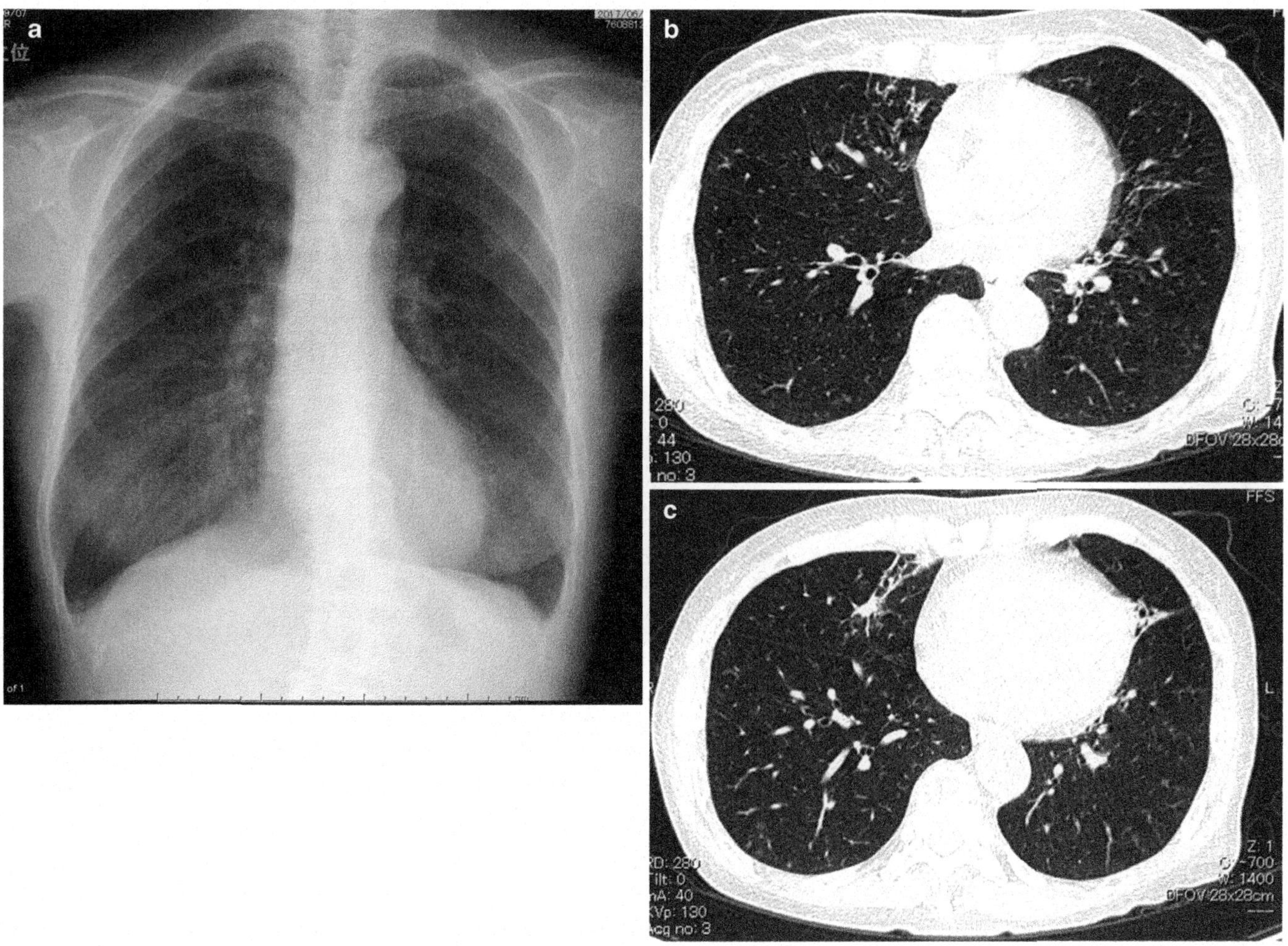

Fig. 4.10 *Mycobacterium avium-intracellulare* complex in RA. (**a**) CXR. CXR shows overinflation of bilateral lungs. Patchy abnormal opacities are evident in the medial aspect of right lower lung field. (**b**) HRCT. HRCT shows bronchiectasis and centrilobular nodular opacities in the right middle lobe. Less severe same lesion is noted in the lingual division of the left upper lobe. (**c**) HRCT. Small centrilobular nodular opacities are noted in S9 of the right lower lobe

gual segment. Small centrilobular opacities may be seen in other segments.

Differential diagnosis between nodular bronchiectatic form of nontuberculous mycobacteriosis and airway lesion caused by RA itself seems to be difficult based on imaging features alone (Fig. 4.11). Actually mycobacterial organism cannot be detected despite repeated bacteriologic study utilizing bronchoscopy in many cases presenting nodular bronchiectatic form of nontuberculous mycobacteriosis.

Nontuberculous mycobacteriosis had generally been thought to be contraindication for the use of biologic agents [39–41]. In Japan, possibility of biologics therapy has been sought because of high effectiveness of biologic agents for rain condition of treatment success of once deteriorated nontuberculous mycobacteriosis [40, 41]. The indication of biologic agents for patients with nontuberculous mycobacteriosis remains under debate at the present. Most of RA patients with worsened *mycobacterium avium-intracellulare* complex infection after treatment of biologic agents have good responses to medical treatment, and their prognosis was relatively good. On the other hand, in patients with *Mycobacterium abscessus* infection, anti-mycobacterium therapies have been poorly responded in our study [30].

Easy and groundless diagnosis of nontuberculous mycobacteriosis without bacteriological proof could deprive RA patients of a chance of treatment with effective biologic agents.

4.4.2 Diseases of Small Airway

4.4.2.1 Noninfectious Disease

RA patients frequently show bronchiolitis of infectious and noninfectious causes. Varying kinds of noninfectious small airway disease are noted in RA patients [42–45]. Follicular bronchiolitis, cellular bronchiolitis mimicking diffuse pan-

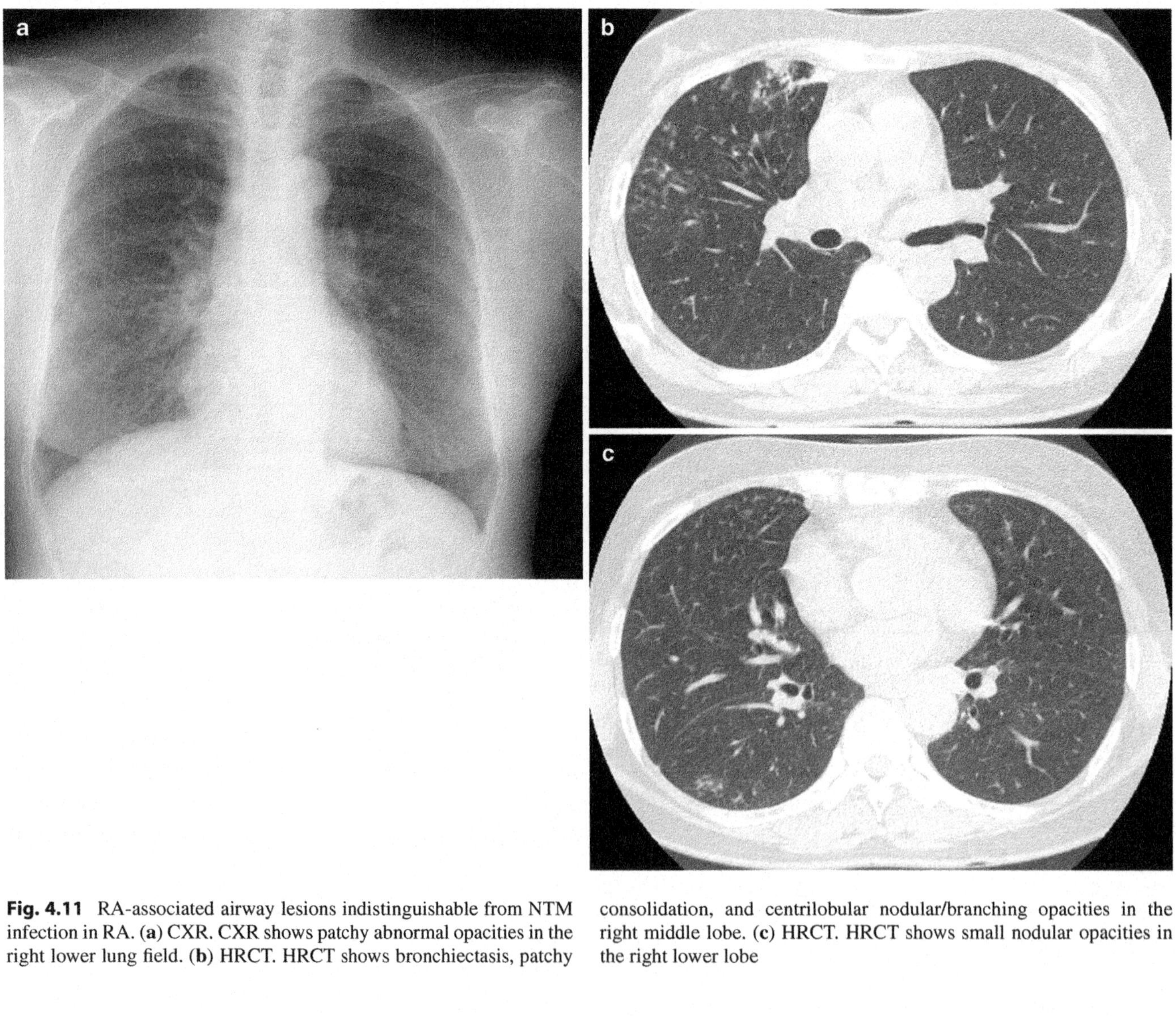

Fig. 4.11 RA-associated airway lesions indistinguishable from NTM infection in RA. (**a**) CXR. CXR shows patchy abnormal opacities in the right lower lung field. (**b**) HRCT. HRCT shows bronchiectasis, patchy consolidation, and centrilobular nodular/branching opacities in the right middle lobe. (**c**) HRCT. HRCT shows small nodular opacities in the right lower lobe

bronchiolitis (DPB) [46], and bronchiolitis obliterans (BO) have been described so far. At HRCT images, cellular and destructive bronchiolitis may show prominent centrilobular nodules/branching opacity mimicking diffuse panbronchiolitis because of prominent cellular infiltration, different from bronchiolitis obliterans.

Follicular bronchiolitis (FB) is most frequently seen in RA and Sjogren syndrome; histologically abundant lymph follicles with germinal center are evident in the bronchiolar wall and pulmonary parenchyma with infiltration of mononuclear cells [43]. Active inflammatory process and varying kinds of cytokine and autoantibody are produced in the bronchus-associated lymphoid tissues (BALT) in FB and related to inflammatory reaction in other organs such as in articular cartilages [47].

FB shows centrilobular nodular and/or bronchial opacity on HR images. Bronchial wall thickening and peribronchial cellular infiltration correspond to those image findings [48, 49]. Sometimes thickening of bronchovascular bundle and interlobular septa can be noted, corresponding to proliferation of lymphatic tissue.

Bronchiolitis obliterans (endobronchiolitis obliterans) is also called as constrictive bronchiolitis [50]. In RA patients, RA itself and drugs for treatment of RA may cause this state.

Bronchiolitis obliterans (BO) is caused by continuous injury of bronchioles. Pathologically reactions to bronchiolar epithelial injury induce exudation of fibrin and infiltration of inflammatory cell into bronchiolar lumen. In progression of disease process, granuloma formation and fibrosis occur. Scanty cellular infiltration is observed in advanced fibrotic cases. This disease process results in stenosis or obstruction of bronchial lumen [51]. Usually disease process is observed diffusely in bilateral lungs, but sometimes involvement is focal or patchy. And between involved areas, normal bronchioles are seen; thus, degree of severity is inhomogeneous.

BO is seen in varying conditions: after bone marrow transplantation, lung transplantation, and the use of drugs for treatment of connective tissue diseases including RA. It has not been fully clarified concerning differences of pathology and imaging features of BO between post-plantation BO and BO of RA.

On CT images, BO often shows scanty centrilobular nodular or branching opacities because fibrotic stage of BO lacks abundant cellular infiltration in bronchial wall (restrictive bronchiolitis) [52, 53]. Overinflation of the lung may obscure centrilobular nodular or branching opacities (Fig. 4.12).

More proximal bronchi usually show bronchial wall thickening and dilatation on CT images. Bronchial wall thickening of central airway may be related to concomitant infection or noninfectious autoimmune mechanism.

According to Sugino and coworkers [54], bronchiolitis obliterans in RA patients is subdivided into two types: endobronchiolitis obliterans (EBO) and cellular and destructive bronchiolitis (CDB). CDB is frequently seen in RA, Sjogren syndrome, and other autoimmune diseases, while EBO is typically seen as a manifestation of GVHD following bone marrow transplantation.

CDB, a subtype of bronchiolitis obliterans, is formed through destructive change and fibrosis of bronchial wall, which is caused by inflammation of whole bronchial wall, resulting in stenosis or obstruction of bronchial lumen.

Homma and coworkers have reported significant overlap of diffuse panbronchiolitis and bronchiolitis in RA patients in clinical features, CT, and pulmonary function tests [51]. CDB may put over clinical and CT features of DPB like bronchiolitis in RA patients (Fig. 4.13).

Major radiological differential diagnosis of noninfectious airway lesion includes infectious bronchiolitis, inhalational airway disease, and so on. Infectious bronchiolitis is a common complication of RA patient.

4.4.2.2 Infectious Process

As infectious lesion of large to intermediate airway diseases, causative organisms include bacterial and mycobacterial, viral, mycoplasma, and so on. As for the infection of small airway, drug-induced hypoimmunity and autoimmune process is one of the predisposing factors. Bronchiolitis by nontuberculous mycobacteriosis and tuberculosis is the most important infection.

4.5 Relationship Between Airway Disease and Interstitial Pneumonia

Although interstitial pneumonia in RA patient (RA-IP) often shows UIP pattern (RA-UIP), peribronchovascular reticular opacities are often observed in addition to subpleural regions. Honeycombing in RA-UIP is sometimes composed of thin-walled and large-sized cysts as compared to IPF/UIP and shows peribronchovascular distribution.

These findings could suggest that RA-UIP is closely related to airway disease.

Detailed investigation of CT images and pathologic findings conducted recently showed airway-centered nature of interstitial pneumonia in RA patients. They implied novel theory on histogenesis of those large cystic changes not documented before. Those cysts may be caused by constellation of bronchiectasis, mimicking cystic lesions associated with UIP. These issues are well discussed in other chapters (please refer to Sects. 2.4, 5.4, and 7.6) of this book.

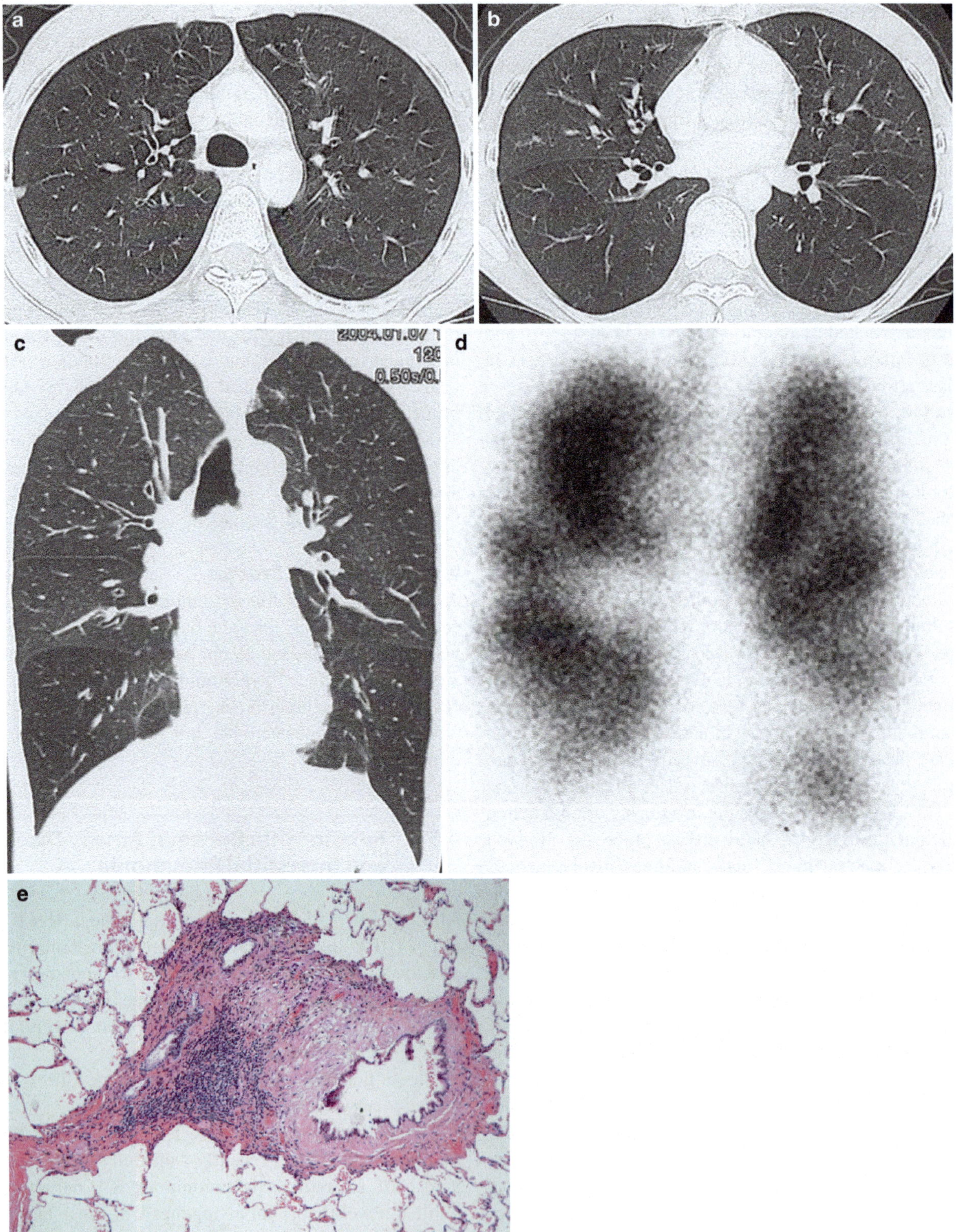

Fig. 4.12 BO in RA treated with penicillamine (by the courtesy of Dr. H. Tokuda). Five months after the administration of D-penicillamine for RA. (**a**) HRCT at initial presentation. HRCT image shows dilatation and bronchial wall thickening of relatively proximal bronchi. There are scanty centrilobular nodules/branching opacities. Mosaic perfusion is also not evident. (**b**) HRCT at initial presentation (at more caudal level). HRCT shows mosaic appearance in bilateral lower lobes. (**c**) Coronal reformatted CT images. Reformatted coronal CT shows enlargement of lung volume and lower position of the diaphragm. Mosaic appearance and bronchial wall thickening are also noted. (**d**) Ventilation scintigraphy. Radioisotope is inhomogeneously uptaken in the lungs. (**e**) Pathologic specimen obtained by VATS. Lymphocytic infiltration and granuloma formation were found in the bronchial wall, resulting in fibrosis and luminal stenosis of the bronchiolar wall

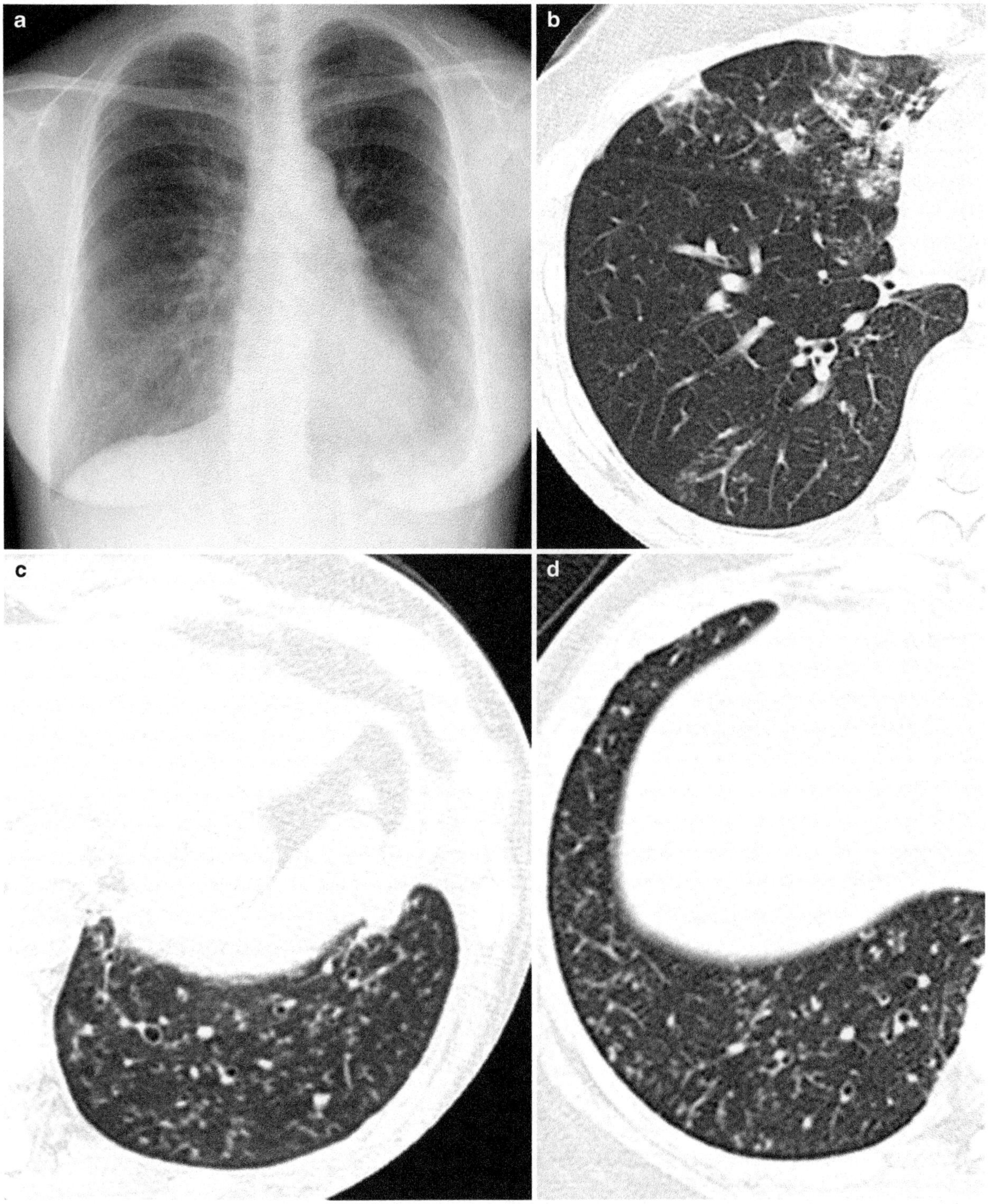

Fig. 4.13 CDB in RA (by the courtesy of Dr. H. Tokuda). Progressive dyspnea in RA patient. BAL fluid shows TCC 1.2×10^5 (neutrophil 41%, lymphocyte 8%, macrophage 46%). Progressive decrease of FEV 1.0% is also noted. Culture of the sputum showed *Pseudomonas aeruginosa*. (**a**) CXR. CXR shows consolidation in the medial aspect of the right lower lung. (**b**) HRCT. HRCT shows patchy consolidation and small centrilobular nodular on the right middle lobe. (**c**) HRCT 3 years after (**a**) and (**b**), just before VATS. HRCT shows small centrilobular nodular opacities in bilateral lower lobes. (**d**) HRCT of the right lung (VATS). (**e**) Pathologic specimen by VATS. Cellular infiltration in and around small bronchi and bronchioles was identified in microscopic specimen. Destructive change of small bronchi was also noted. (**f**) Pathologic specimen. Destructive change of bronchial wall resulted in the disappearance of elastic membrane and smooth muscles of the bronchial wall. (**g**) Pathologic specimen. Abundant lymphocytes and polymorphonuclear leukocyte infiltrate into the bronchial wall. Final pathological diagnosis was decided as cellular and destructive bronchitis

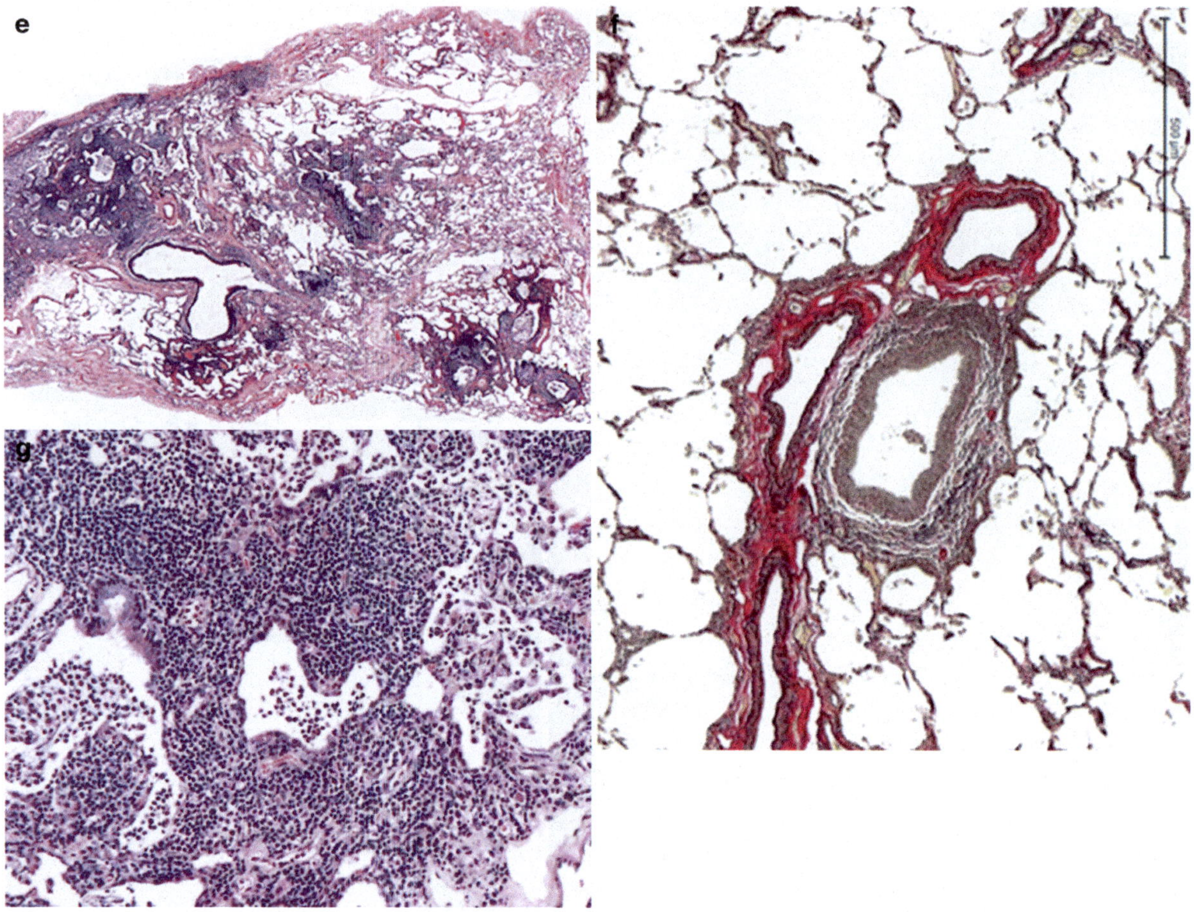

Fig. 4.13 (continued)

References

1. Colby TV, Travis WD. Bronchiolar disorders. In: Travis WD, Colby TV, et al., editors. Non-neoplastic disorders of the lower respiratory tract. Washington, DC: American Registry of Pathology and AFIP; 2002. p. 351–80.
2. Hasegawa M, Makita H, Nasuhara Y, Odajima N, Nagai K, Ito Y, Betsuyaku T, Nishimura M. Relationship between improved airflow limitation and changes in airway calibre induced by inhaled anticholinergic agents in COPD. Thorax. 2009;64:332–8.
3. Naidich DP. Bronchiectasis. In: Naidich DP, Webb WR, Grenier PA, et al., editors. Imaging of the airways. Philadelphia: Lippincott Williams & Wilkins; 2005. p. 107–45.
4. Ng YL, Paul N, Patosis D, et al. Imaging of lung transplantation: review. AJR Am J Roentogenol. 2009;192:S1–S13.
5. Gunn ML, Godwin JD, Kanne JP, et al. High resolution CT findings of bronchiolitis obliterans syndrome after hematopoietic transplantation. J Thorac Imaging. 2008;23:244–50.
6. Waitches GM, Syern EJ. High resolution CT of peripheral airway disease. Radiol Clin N Am. 2002;40:21–9.
7. Worthy SA, Mueller NL. Small airway diseases. Radiol Clin N Am. 1998;36:163–73.
8. Choi YW, Rossi SE, Palmer SM, et al. Bronchiolitis obliterans syndrome in lung transplant recipient: correlation of computed tomography findings with bronchiolitis obliterans syndrome stage. J Thorac Imaging. 2003;18:72–9.
9. Miller WT Jr, Kotloff RM, Bllumenthal NP, et al. Utility of high resolution computed tomography in predicting bronchiolitis obliterans syndrome following lung transplantation. J Thorac Imaging. 2001;16:76–80.
10. Ng CS, Desai SR, Rubens MB. Visual quantification and observer variation of signs of small airway disease at inspiratory and expiratory CT. J Thorac Imaging. 1999;14:279–85.
11. Kim HG, Shin HJ, Kim YH, et al. Quantitative computed tomography assessment of graft versus host disease related bronchiolitis obliterans in children. Eur Radiol. 2015;25:2931–6.
12. Remy-Jardin M, Remy J, Cortet B, et al. Lung changes in rheumatoid arthritis: CT findings. Radiology. 1994;193:375–82.
13. Meyer CA, Pina JS, Taillon D, Godwin JD. Inspiratory and expiratory high-resolution CT findings in a patient with Sjögren's syndrome and cystic lung disease. Am J Roentgenol. 1997;168(1):101–3.
14. Despaux J, Manzoni P, Toussirot E, et al. Prospective study of the prevalence of bronchiectasis in rheumatoid arthritis using high-resolution computed tomography. Rev Rhum Engl Ed. 1998;65:453–61.
15. Wilsher M, Voight L, Milne D, et al. Prevalence of airway and parenchymal abnormalities in newly diagnosed rheumatoid arthritis. Respir Med. 2012;106:1441–6.
16. Mori S, Koga Y, Sugimoto M, et al. Comparison of pulmonary abnormalities on high-resolution computed tomography in patients with early versus longstanding rheumatoid arthritis. J Rheumatol. 2008;35:1513–21.

17. Izumiyama T, Hama H, Miura M, et al. Frequency of broncho-bronchiolar disease in rheumatoid arthritis: an examination by high-resolution computed tomography. Mod Rheumatol. 2002;12: 311–7.
18. Tsuchiya Y, Takayanagi N, Sugiura H, et al. Lung diseases directly associated with rheumatoid arthritis and their relationship to outcome. Eur Respir J. 2011;37:1411–7.
19. Wilczynska MM, Condliffe AM, McKeon DJ. Coexistence of bronchiectasis and rheumatoid arthritis: revisited. Respir Care. 2013;58:694–701.
20. Tanaka N, Kim JS, Newell JD, et al. Rheumatoid arthritis-related lung diseases: CT findings. Radiology. 2004;232:81–91.
21. Tokuda H. Lung complication of RA Airway lesion and its imaging diagnosis. Rinsho Hoshasenn. 2015;60:1085–96. In Japanese.
22. Lieberman-Maran L, Orzano IM, Passero MA, et al. Bronchiectasis in rheumatoid arthritis: report of four cases and a review of the literature——implications for management with biologic response modifiers. Semin Arthritis Rheum. 2006;35:379–87.
23. Nannini C, Medina-Velasquez YF, Achenbach SJ, et al. Incidence and mortality of obstructive lung disease in rheumatoid arthritis: a population-based study. Arthritis Care Res. 2013;65:1243–50.
24. Doran MF, Crowson CS, Pond GR, et al. Frequency of infection in patients with rheumatoid arthritis compared with controls: a population-based study. Arthritis Rheum. 2002;46:2287–93.
25. Terasaki H, Fujimoto K, Hayabuchi N, et al. Respiratory symptoms in rheumatoid arthritis: relation between high resolution CT findings and functional impairment. Radiat Med. 2004;22:179–85.
26. Takayanagi N. Biological agents and respiratory infections: causative mechanisms and practice management. Respir Investig. 2015;53:185–200.
27. Wolfe F, Caplan L, Michaud K. Treatment for rheumatoid arthritis and the risk of hospitalization for pneumonia: associations with prednisone, disease modifying antirheumatic drugs, and anti-tumor necrosis factor therapy. Arthritis Rheum. 2006;54:628–34.
28. Swinson DR, Symmons D, Suresh U, et al. Decreased survival in patients with co-existent rheumatoid arthritis and bronchiectasis. Br J Rheumatol. 1997;36:689–91.
29. Komazaki Y, Miyazaki Y, Fujie T. Serodiagnosis of Mycobacterium avium complex pulmonary disease in rheumatoid arthritis. Respiration. 2014;87:129–35.
30. Takayanagi N, Tsuchya H, Tokunaga D. Respiratory tract infection complicated in RA patients. Nihon Kokyuki Gakkai Zasshi. 2007;45:465–73. (In Japanese).
31. Galloway JB, Hyrich KL, Mercer LK, et al. Anti-TNF therapy is associated with an increased risk of serious infections in patients with rheumatoid arthritis especially in the first 6 months of treatment: updated results from the British Society for Rheumatology Biologics Register with special emphasis on risks in the elderly. Rheumatology. 2011;50:124–31.
32. Mori S, Yoshitama T, Hidaka T, Sakai F, Hasegawa M, Hashiba Y, Suematsu E, Tatsukawa H, Mizokami A, Yoshizawa S, Hirakata N, Ueki Y. Comparative risk of hospitalized infection between biological agents in rheumatoid arthritis patients: a multicenter retrospective cohort study in Japan. PLoS One. 2017;12(6):e0179179.
33. Takemura T. Pathologic feature of lung lesion complicated in RA. Nihon Kyoubu Rinsho. 2007;66:470–84. In Japanese.
34. Whitwell F. A study of the pathology and pathogenesis of bronchiectasis. Thorax. 1952;7:213–39.
35. Fuschillo S, De Felice A, Balzano G. Mucosal inflammation in idiopathic bronchiectasis: cellular and molecular mechanisms. Eur Respir J. 2008;31:396–406.
36. Morrissey BM. Pathogenesis of bronchiectasis. Clin Chest Med. 2007;28:289–96.
37. Boyton RJ, Reynolds CJ, Quigley KJ, et al. Immune mechanisms and the impact of the disrupted lung microbiome in chronic bacterial lung infection and bronchiectasis. Clin Exp Immunol. 2013;171:117–23.
38. Mori S, Tokuda H, Sakai F, Johkoh T, Mimori A, Nishimoto N, Tasaka S, Hatta K, Matsushima H, Kaise S, Kaneko A, Makino S, Minota S, Yamada T, Akagawa S, Kurashima A, NTM-BIORA (NTM infection in Biologic-treated RA patients) Study Investigators. Radiological features and therapeutic responses of pulmonary nontuberculous mycobacterial disease in rheumatoid arthritis patients receiving biological agents: a retrospective multicenter study in Japan. Mod Rheumatol. 2012;22:727–37.
39. Winthrop KL, Baxter R, Liu L, et al. Mycobacterial diseases and antitumour necrosis factor therapy in USA. Ann Rheum Dis. 2013;72:37–42.
40. Tokuda H. Non tuberculous mycobacterosis. Japanese Respiratory Society Guideline for therapy for biologic agent; Biologic agent and respiratory disease. Tokyo: Japanese Society of Respiratory Medicine; 2014. p. 59–70. In Japanese.
41. Japanese Society of Tuberculosis. Guideline for the diagnosis of nontuberculous mycobacteriosis. Kekkaku. 2008;83:525–6. In Japanese.
42. Hayakawa H, Sato A, Chida K, et al. Bronchiolar disease in rheumatoid arthritis. Am J Respir Crit Care Med. 1996;154:1531–6.
43. Yousem SA, Colby TV, Carrington CB. Follicular bronchitis/bronchiolitis. Hum Pathol. 1985;16:700–6.
44. Mori S, Koga Y, Sugimoto M. Different risk factors between interstitial lung disease and airway disease in rheumatoid arthritis. Respir Med. 2012;106:1591–9.
45. Mori S, Koga Y, Sugimoto M. Small airway obstruction in patients with rheumatoid arthritis. Mod Rheumatol. 2011;21:164–73.
46. Homma S, Kawabata M, Kishi K, Tsuboi E, Narui K, Nakatani T, Uekusa T, Saiki S, Nakata K. Diffuse panbronchiolitis in rheumatoid arthritis. Eur Respir J. 1998;12:444–52.
47. Rangel-Moreno J, Hartson L, Navarro C, et al. Inducible bronchus-associated lymphoid tissue(iBALT)in patients with pulmonary complications of rheumatoid arthritis. J Clin Invest. 2006;116:3183–94.
48. Howling SJ, Hansell DM, Wells AU, Nicholson AG, Flint JD, Müller NL. Follicular bronchiolitis: thin-section CT and histologic findings. Radiology. 1999;212:637–42.
49. WY O, Effmann EL, Redding GJ, Godwin JD. Follicular hyperplasia of bronchus-associated lymphoid tissue causing severe air trapping. AJR Am J Roentgenol. 1999;172:745–7.
50. Devouassoux G, Cottin V, Lioté H, et al. Characterisation of severe obliterative bronchiolitis in rheumatoid arthritis. Eur Respir J. 2009;33:1053–61.
51. Homma S, Sakamoto S, Kawabata M, Kishi K, Tsuboi E, Motoi N, Hebisawa A, Yoshimura K. Comparative clinicopathology of obliterative bronchiolitis and diffuse panbronchiolitis. Respiration. 2006;73:481–7.
52. Konen E, Gutierrez C, Chaparro C, Murray CP, Chung T, Crossin J, et al. Bronchiolitis obliterans syndrome in lung transplant recipients: can thin-section CT findings predict disease before its clinical appearance? Radiology. 2004;231:467–73.
53. Aquino SL, Webb WR, Golden J. Bronchiolitis obliterans associated with rheumatoid arthritis: findings on HRCT and dynamic expiratory CT. J Comput Assist Tomogr. 1994;18:555–8.
54. Sugino K, Hebisawa A, Uekusa T, et al. Histopathological bronchial reconstruction of human bronchiolitis obliterans. Pathol Int. 2011;61:192–201.

5 Therapeutic Strategy for Airway Disease in Rheumatoid Arthritis

Hitoshi Tokuda

Abstract

Despite the high prevalence of airway disease in patients with rheumatoid arthritis (RA), its significance in the clinical practice of RA has not been well discussed. The significance of airway disease can be summarized as follows. (1) It can predispose patients to infectious diseases such as pneumonia and nontuberculous mycobacterial disease. (2) It may cause progressive impairment of lung function, leading to obstructive malfunction and ultimate respiratory failure. (3) In some cases, airway inflammation can result in the destruction of bronchioles and surrounding lung parenchyma, leading to the formation of cysts mimicking a honeycomb lung. In this chapter, we discuss these problems by presenting typical clinical cases and consider the pathogenesis of those processes and finally show the treatment strategy for each problem, based on the limited available literature and the author's opinion. The most important point is that airway disease is an extra-articular manifestation of RA, and if left untreated, it may exacerbate the patients' medical condition and cause deterioration with serious consequences. These problems should be addressed from the viewpoint of how to control the inflammation caused by the excessive immune response of RA.

Keywords

Rheumatoid arthritis • Airway disease • Bronchiectasis • Bronchiolitis • Respiratory infection

5.1 Introduction

Although the high prevalence of airway disease in patients with rheumatoid arthritis (RA) (30–40%; see Chap. 2) has been recognized for decades, little has been discussed about its significance in the clinical setting of RA or its effects on the clinical course and implications for patient prognosis. So far, only a few studies have indicated the harmful effects, that it can predispose patients to bacterial infection or nontuberculous mycobacteriosis (NTM) [1, 2] or that it may cause obstructive lung disease with poor prognosis [3].

H. Tokuda, M.D., Ph.D.
Department of Respiratory Medicine, Tokyo Yamate Medical Center, Japan Community Health Care Organization (JCHO), Tokyo, Japan
e-mail: tokuda@car.ocn.ne.jp

In the author's opinion, the clinical significance of airway disease in RA patients can be summarized as follows:

1. It can predispose patients to infectious diseases including bacterial pneumonia and NTM disease.
2. It may cause progressive obstructive impairment of lung function, leading to chronic respiratory failure and eventual cor pulmonale.
3. In some cases, airway inflammation can result in the destruction of the peripheral airway and lung parenchyma, leading to the formation of cysts mimicking a honeycomb lung.

These problems are important not only because they may impair the medical condition of RA patients but also they may be major obstacles to the use of potent disease-modifying antirheumatic drugs (DMARDs), methotrexate (MTX),

T. Gono et al. (eds.), *Lung Disease Associated with Rheumatoid Arthritis*, https://doi.org/10.1007/978-981-10-6750-1_5

and biological agents. However, the proper management of these problems has scarcely been discussed, except to stress their potential risk.

In the following sections, these issues are considered in detail item by item with presentation of typical clinical cases. The treatment strategy for each problem is discussed based on the limited available literature and the author's personal experience.

5.2 Airway Disease Can Predispose to Infectious Diseases and Cause Poor Prognosis

5.2.1 Bacterial Infections

Many previous observational studies have reported a high frequency of pulmonary infections, especially bacterial pneumonia, in RA patients [4, 5]. However, the reason why has not been well elucidated. Three possible mechanisms are assumed [1]:

1. The possibility that immune dysfunction of RA patients may disturb proper activation of protective immunity.
2. The possibility that tissue impairment and structural distortion of the lung caused by excessive immune response may form a niche for infectious microorganisms.
3. The immunosuppressive effects of drugs used for RA treatment.

Until recently, the third factor has been stressed. Surely corticosteroid therapy as the most important risk factor of infection is widely recognized. However, no consensus has been reached on whether MTX and biological agents are risk factors [5–7]. As for biological agents, Galloway and colleagues reported that under anti-TNF (tumor necrosis factor) therapy, infections tend to occur within 6 months after the initiation of treatment [7, 8].

The second factor mentioned above has emerged as a factor of no less importance in recent studies [9]. Takayanagi reported that among RA patients with bacterial pneumonia, bronchiectasis (BE) or interstitial lung disease (ILD) was found as an underlying disease in 87% of them (Fig. 5.1) [1].

BE is regarded as a poor prognostic factor in RA patients in observational studies. In a study in the USA, the reported 5-year survival of RA patients complicated with BE was 69%, and the causes of death were respiratory infection and cor pulmonale [10]. In Japan, Tsuchiya and colleagues reported that the 10-year survival for RA patients complicated with BE was 82%, better than that of the US study, but similarly, the final causes of death were respiratory infection and cardiac failure [11]. Also in a prospective longitudinal study conducted in France in which 55 RA patients and 82 non-RA patients were followed up for 10 years, RA patients with diffuse BE had a significantly poorer prognosis than the subjects in the other groups, and the causes of death were likewise lung disease or heart disease [12]. Thus, in patients complicated with BE, it is

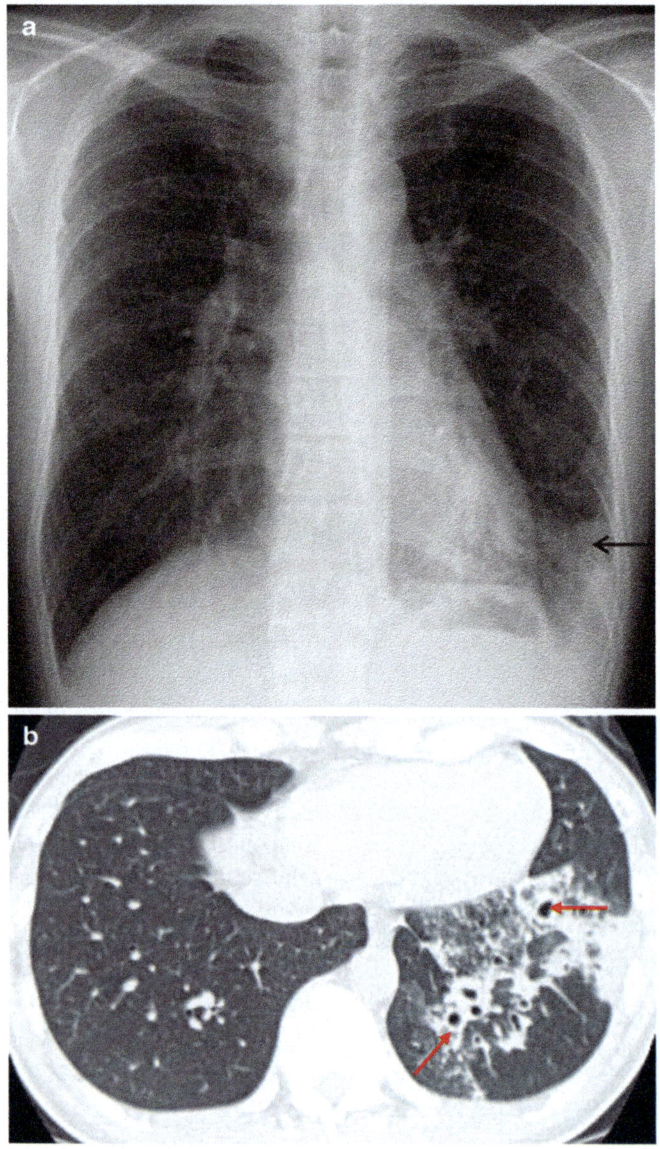

Fig. 5.1 Pneumonia in RA patients often develops at the base of preexisting lung disease, such as bronchiectasis or interstitial lung disease. (**a**) A 42-year-old male with RA for 15 years. He presented with high fever for 2 days. Chest radiograph shows patchy opacities in the left lung base, suggesting pneumonia (*arrow*). (**b**) HRCT reveals dilated bronchi in the area of consolidation in the left lower lobe (*red arrows*). Preexisting bronchiectasis was assumed to be the predisposing factor for pneumonia in this case

possible that recurrent lung infections and eventual respiratory and cardiac failure result in their poor prognosis. Therefore, the control of infection is currently the most important issue in the treatment of RA patients.

5.2.1.1 Recurrent Infection and Progressive Deterioration of Medical Condition

As mentioned above, even with the recent advances of antimicrobial chemotherapy, infection may recur based on underlying lung disease in the clinical practice of RA treatment, ultimately leading to fatality in some cases. Why cannot we control such deterioration? The mechanism of these disease courses has scarcely been discussed or clarified so far.

These problems are considered here by discussing three clinical cases of RA with BE.

Case 1 Early stage. Lung shrinkage develops insidiously through recurrent pneumonia and successive organization.

In Fig. 5.2, we present a 67-year-old woman with RA for 18 years. Her disease activity of RA began to increase 3 years before admission to the respiratory division of our hospital, and MTX therapy was begun. Chest radiography at that time (Fig. 5.2a) showed no remarkable abnormalities except for apical scars. However, high-resolution computed tomography (HRCT) on the same occasion revealed BE in the middle lobe and lingular division (Fig. 5.2b).

During the following 3 years, she complained of slight symptoms of respiratory tract infection including cough, sputum, and low-grade fever, and CT done at one of those episodes revealed pneumonia at the base of the BE (Fig. 5.2c). Her chest radiograph on admission (Fig. 5.2d) showed elevation of the bilateral hilum and diaphragm, indicating shrinkage of the upper and middle lung, and lingular division. Despite proper antimicrobial treatment for each infectious episode (presumably pneumonia), organizing pneumonia (OP) in the affected area had occurred successively that had caused lung shrinkage (Fig. 5.2e).

To understand this process, refer to the surgical lung biopsy specimen from another patient with RA (Fig. 5.2f, g). In Fig. 5.2f, consolidation localized at the subpleural area is seen with shrinkage. In the magnified view (Fig. 5.2g), this area shows OP. We can see from this pathological specimen that organization occurring after pneumonia can cause lung shrinkage when left untreated.

In the present patient, frequent chest X-rays and CT scans revealed these changes. However, if such examinations had not been performed due to an absence of symptoms (a common pattern in the clinical settings of RA!), her lung shrinkage would not have been detected until it had reached an advanced stage.

Case 2 Early to late stage. Deterioration occurs through recurrent infection.

In the daily practice of RA treatment, chest imaging is not conducted so often. Thus, one day we may notice that marked structural distortion has taken place in the patient's lungs without any corresponding history. The explanation is as follows: recurrent lung infections had occurred insidiously, with only minimal symptoms such as a "common cold," and destruction of the lung progressed without being noticed, finally leading to a marked degree of structural distortion. With such structural change, the patient would suffer more and more infection until the final catastrophe.

In Fig. 5.3, we present such a case of a 77-year-old woman with RA for 18 years. Chest radiography 10 years ago showed slight change of a moderate degree in the middle lobe and lingular division, a common finding in RA patients (Fig. 5.3a, b). She complained of cough and sputum from that time and was treated with medications with no effect. Soon, the disease activity of RA increased, and therapy with MTX and prednisolone was started. She suffered a compression fracture of her thoracic vertebrae 4 years later that caused kyphosis, thus reducing her daily activities. The chest radiograph on that occasion revealed the collapse of the right S6 and marked volume loss in the lower lobes (Fig. 5.3c, d). On HRCT (Fig. 5.3e, f), not only the middle lobe and lingular division but also all segments of the bilateral lower lobe had shrunk, which was assumed to be brought about by recurrent infections and their incomplete cure, that is, organization leading to the collapse of lung parenchyma—the same mechanism as in Case 1. At this point, her vital capacity was 49%, indicating the marked reduction in lung volume. From 5 months ago, her cough worsened, and she was referred to our institution, where fluoroquinolone was prescribed with satisfactory effect. However, after several months, she suffered from severe pneumonia that was barely conquered through the use of every therapeutic effort including intense antimicrobial therapy and other supportive therapies (Fig. 5.3g–j).

We can draw an important lesson from these two cases. In RA patients, recurrent infection may occur with minimal symptoms and may insidiously progress to devastation of the lung. Without chest imaging, we are unaware of this progression and deterioration. Rheumatologists must be alert to these possibilities and appropriately address the respiratory signs and symptoms of patients at each visit, and if a subtle sign is recognized, must not hesitate to conduct chest imaging and appropriate treatment if necessary.

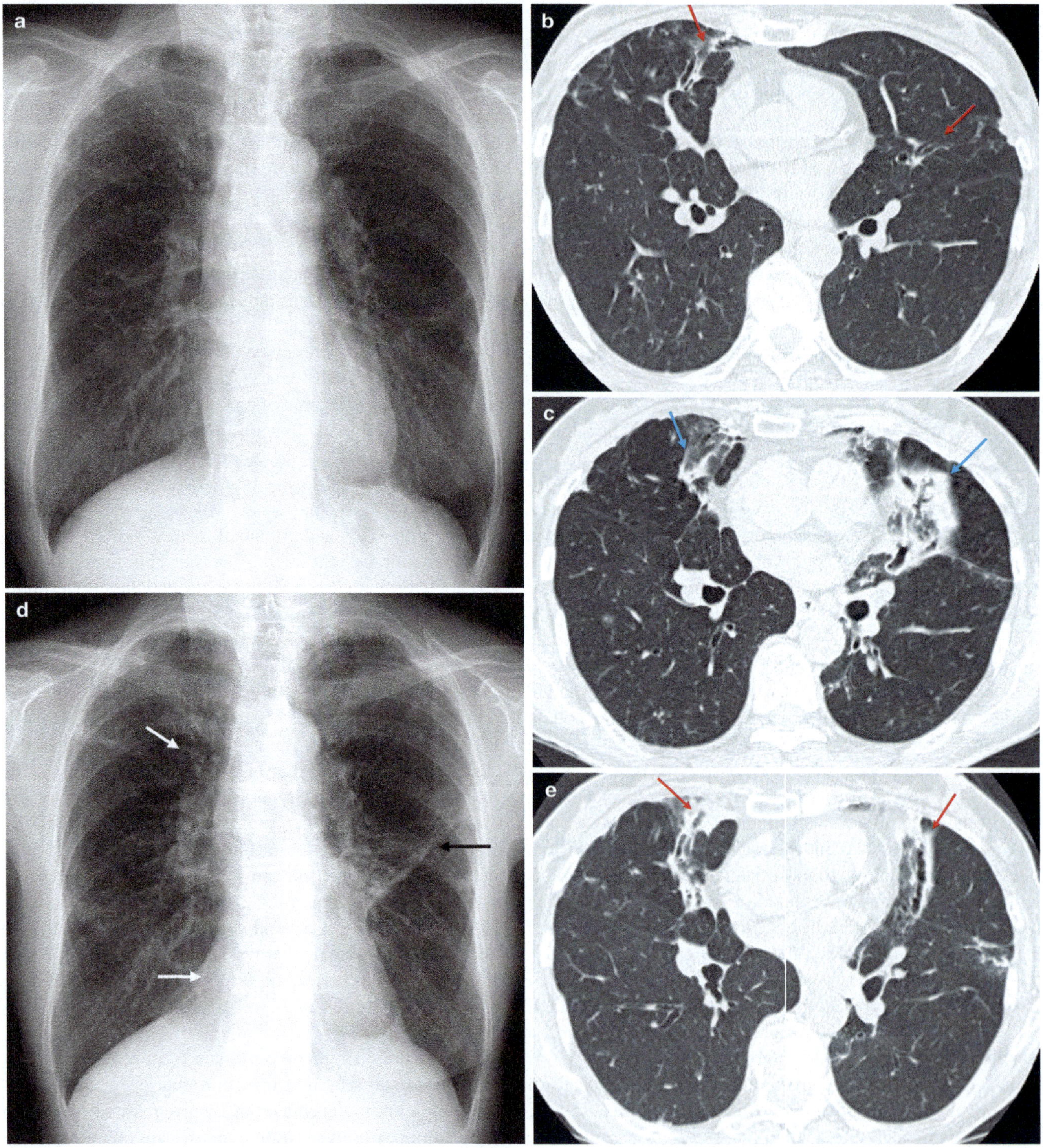

Fig. 5.2 (**a**) A 67-year-old woman in whom recurrent pneumonia based on bronchiectasis resulted in shrinkage of the lung during 2 years' clinical course. (**a**) Chest radiograph 2 years ago shows no abnormality except for apical scar. (**b**) HRCT scan conducted at the same time with (**a**), that is, 2 years ago, revealed bronchiectasis of slight degree in the middle lobe and lingular division (*red arrows*). (**c**) During these 2 years, she suffered from recurrent pneumonia. HRCT scan at one of those episodes shows pneumonia occurring at the base of those bronchiectases (*blue arrows*). She was treated with antibiotics with improvement of symptoms each time. (**d**) However, chest radiograph taken on the referral to the respiratory department demonstrates cicatrized shadow in the left middle lung field (*black arrow*) and also lifting up of the bilateral hilum and diaphragm (*white arrows*), suggesting shrinkage of the upper and middle lung. (**e**) In HRCT, consolidated areas around the segmental bronchi of the right middle lobe and left lingular division demonstrate collapse of those areas (*red arrows*), probably due to organization of pneumonia. The shrinkage of the lung seen in (**d**) is caused by such a process. (**f**, **g**) Organization causes collapse and shrinkage of the lung in RA patients. Surgical lung biopsy (SLB) specimen of another case. A 67-year-old woman in whom RA-related organizing pneumonia (OP) was suspected clinically. (**f**) Consolidated area with shrinkage is seen in subpleural area. Panoramic view. (**g**) Magnified view of the circle in f shows remnant alveolar structure in the dense collagen deposition, indicating that this lesion is OP. Photomicrographs courtesy of Dr. T. Takemura

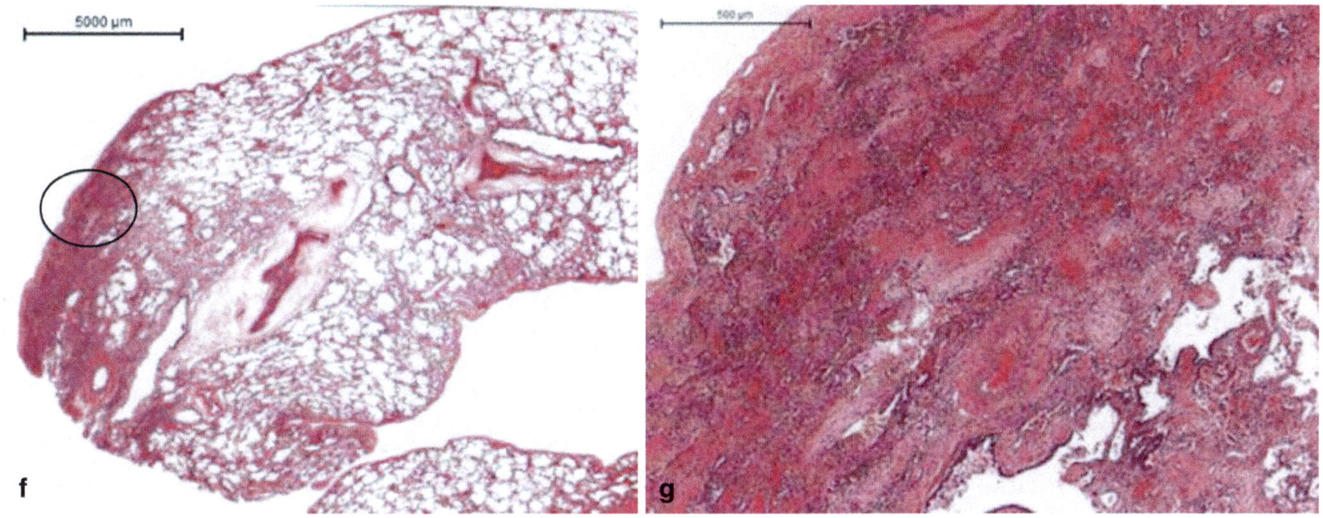

Fig. 5.2 (continued)

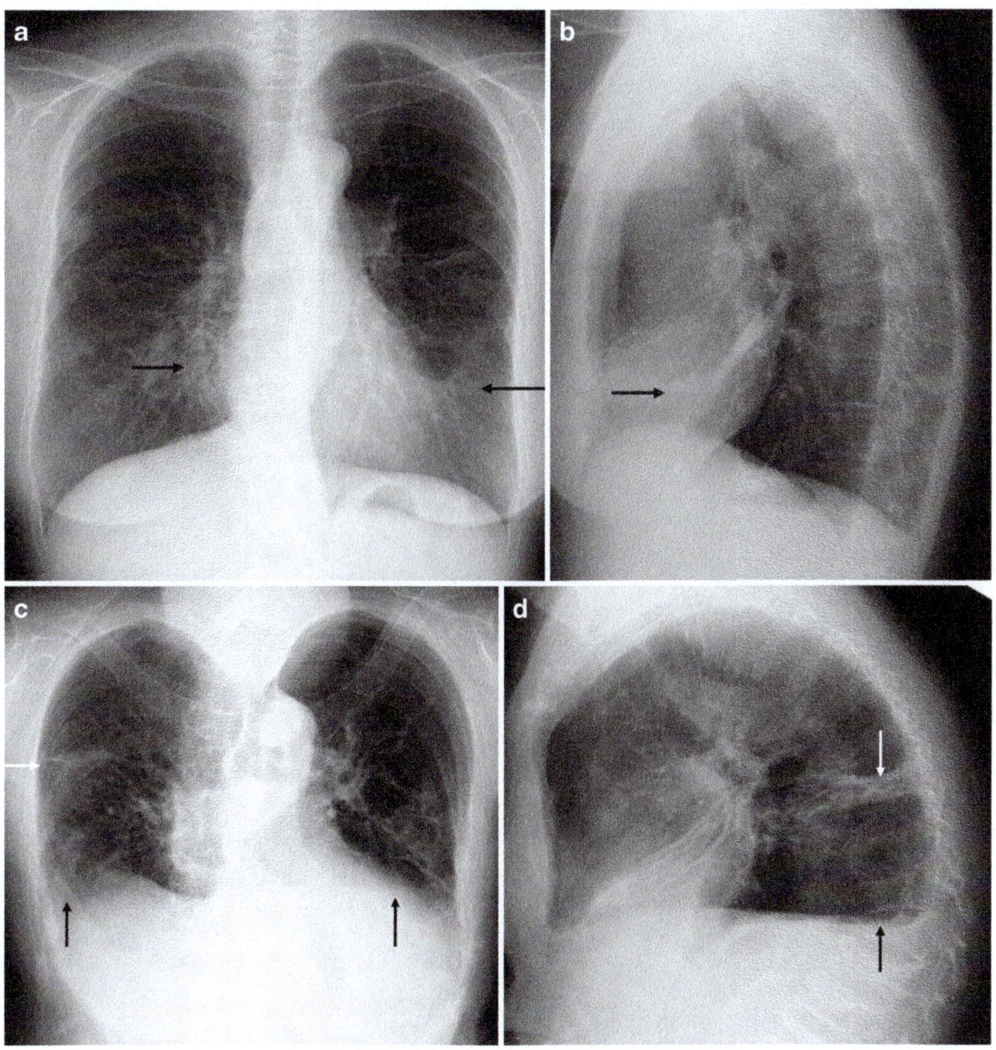

Fig. 5.3 (**a**, **b**) A case of recurrent pneumonia following lung shrinkage and deterioration. A 77-year-old woman of RA for 18 years. (**a**, **b**) Chest radiograph 10 years ago shows only collapse of the right middle lobe and left lingular division of slight degree (*arrows*), suggesting bronchiectasis of these regions. (**c**, **d**) Four years later, compression fracture of thoracic vertebrae occurred and caused severe kyphosis. (**c**, **d**) Chest radiograph shows collapse of right S6 (*white arrow*) in addition to middle lobe and lingular division, along with marked shrinkage of lower lobe (*black arrows*). (**e**, **f**) HRCT demonstrates diffuse bronchiectasis in bilateral lower lobes and the collapse of the adjacent lung parenchyma (presumably through organization) (*red arrows*). These findings and scarce pulmonary vasculature in the lung fields indicate loss of normal lung parenchyma. Recurrent infection and incomplete cure in each episode resulted in these conditions. (**g**, **h**) Serious pneumonia, nearly fatal, occurred in bilateral lower lung, which was barely conquered with every effort. (**i**, **j**) HRCT demonstrates widespread pneumonia at the base of these bronchiectases (*red arrows*)

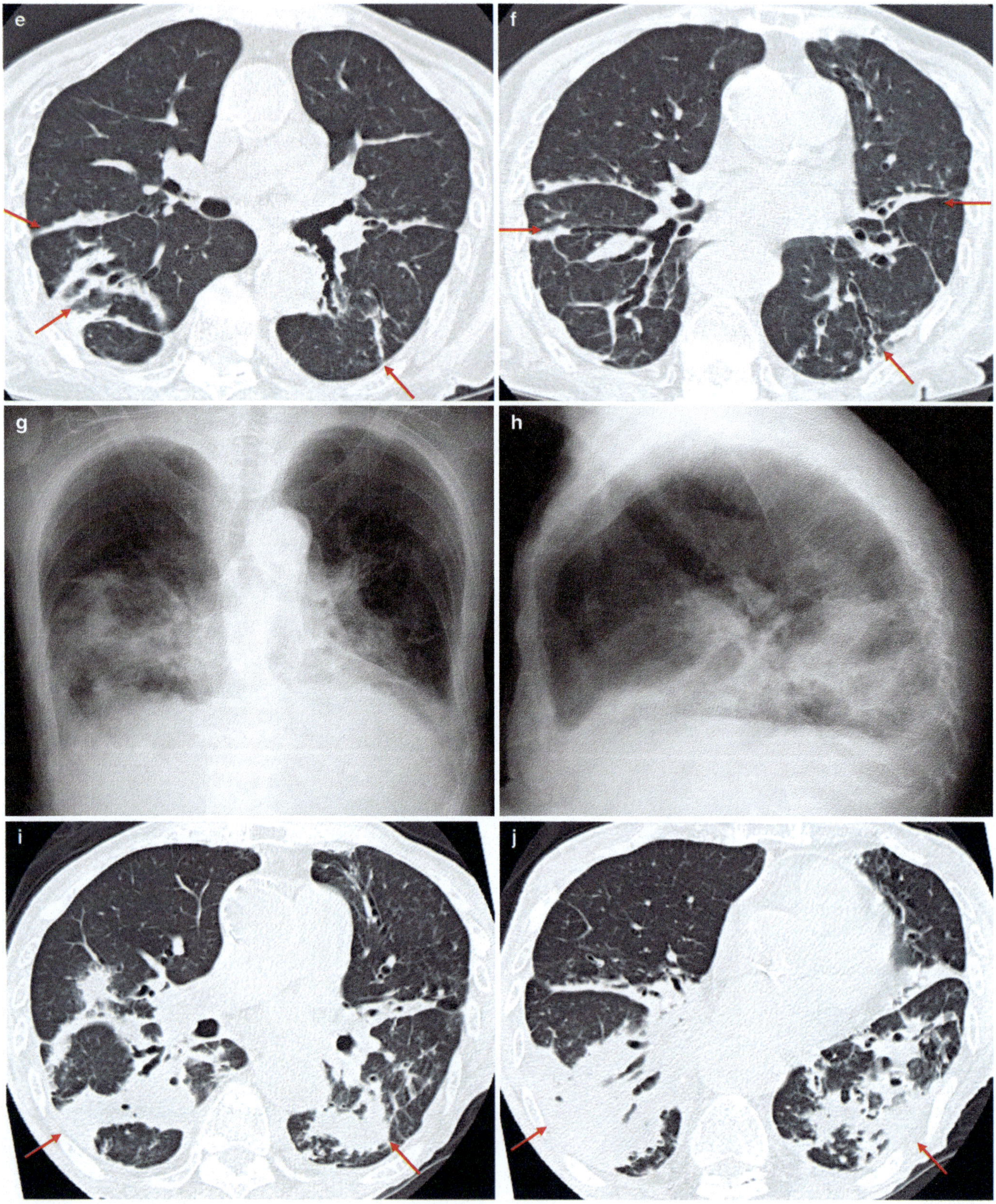

Fig. 5.3 (continued)

Case 3 Late stage. Recurrent pneumonia in advanced-stage BE is fatal.

In Fig. 5.4, we present a case of repeated pneumonia based on advanced BE that follow a fatal course. A 66-year-old man with a past history of smoking one pack/day for 10 years was diagnosed as RA 6 years ago. One year before admission to the respiratory division of our hospital, he developed dyspnea on exertion. Chest radiography on his first visit (Fig. 5.4a) showed a severe degree of apical scarring and shrinkage of the bilateral upper lungs. Reticular shadows were seen bilaterally in the lower lung field that resembled that of ILD, but differed from usual ILD in that the lung base showed hyperinflation rather than shrinkage. On HRCT (Fig. 5.4b–d), extensive BE was visible, with coexisting emphysematous change. A wedge-shaped consolidation were seen in the dorsal area of the lung base, within which dilated bronchi were visible. Although mimicking honeycombing at first glance, it is not difficult to identify this as bronchodilation due to the continuity to bronchial structures in the central area. These bronchial dilatations were assumed to be caused by inflammatory destruction (see Sect. 2.3). These dilated bronchi can provide a niche for pathogenic bacteria such as *Pseudomonas* and thus a favorable environment for persistent infection, which was the case in this patient. Over the following 2 years, he suffered several occurrences of severe pneumonia, each of which required hospitalization.

In a chest radiograph taken in the final stage of the disease (Fig. 5.4e), lung destruction had progressed, and reticular shadows were spread through the lung base. These changes were shown in detail in a HRCT image (Fig. 5.4f). At this stage, his lung function deteriorated step by step, and he deceased during his seventh hospitalization due to severe pneumonia and cor pulmonale (Fig. 5.4g).

This case shows the typical course of a RA patient complicated with recurrent bacterial infection based on advanced BE and ultimate death due to respiratory and cardiac failure. Once a patient progresses to this stage, current antimicrobial therapy is insufficient. Thus, we must intervene in the disease course before the patient reaches this late stage.

Here, another viewpoint may be proposed. The severe inflammation occurring at such a late stage may be difficult to control with antibiotics alone. In such a condition, an exuberant immune response is assumed, and if so, the additive use of a proper immunosuppressive agent might be attempted. Many reports have affirmed the efficacy of corticosteroid therapy in addition to antibiotics to control severe pneumonia [13], hence such a trial should be considered in these severe cases as well.

How this process of deterioration can be checked blocked will be described in the next section.

5.2.1.2 How to Control Bacterial Infection

For a detailed description, see Chap. 10. Importantly, it is crucial to choose appropriate antibiotics, taking the specific characteristics of RA patients into account [1, 14]. The pathogenic bacterial profile of RA patients is different from that of non-RA subjects. A high frequency of *Pseudomonas* as a causative agent is reported. It is well known that *Pseudomonas* is common in general subjects with underlying lung diseases such as BE, and, as previously stated, RA patients are often complicated with BE. The choice of antibiotics should be made considering these profiles. Therefore, in RA patients with underlying lung diseases, the use of fluoroquinolones is justified as one of the best choices because of their wide-spectrum activity and coverage of *Pseudomonas*. The efficacy and safety of a short, 5-day course of fluoroquinolones have been validated by many studies [15].

Of note, rather than being an exogenous infection, the bacterial pneumonia of RA patients is an endogenous one caused by bacteria colonizing in existing lung lesions. Thus, before beginning treatment for RA, it is mandatory to perform HRCT scanning to determine the presence or absence of underlying lung disease, and once such disease is found in a patient, the physician should be very alert to the possibility of the patient developing pneumonia after a slight upper respiratory infection (such as a common cold) and should not hesitate to perform chest imaging and give adequate antibiotics when necessary.

Pneumococcal vaccination has also been validated as a preventive measure to reduce the burden of pneumococcal colonization [1]. Most importantly, however, controlling the activity of RA itself leads to a good result in controlling the infection in the end. For details, refer to Sect. 2.1.4.

5.2.1.3 How to Treat OP That Follows Pneumonia

As shown by Cases 1 and 2 (Figs. 5.2 and 5.3), it is often difficult to control the pulmonary infection of RA patients with antibiotic therapy alone. The problem is OP. In cases of persistent symptoms, a remnant radiographic shadow, and suspended C-reactive protein (CRP) despite appropriate antibiotic therapy, the possibility of OP should be considered. Treatment is sometimes easy with the proper use of corticosteroids [16]. The OP of RA is described in detail in Chap. 12.

Not infrequently, however, subsequent OP in RA patients shows no symptoms, and when it is unrecognized and left untreated, the affected area of the lung collapses, generating permanent fibrosis and reducing the lung volume, as described above. Thus, physicians must be very cautious to perform a chest X-ray examination even with the slightest suspicion of OP.

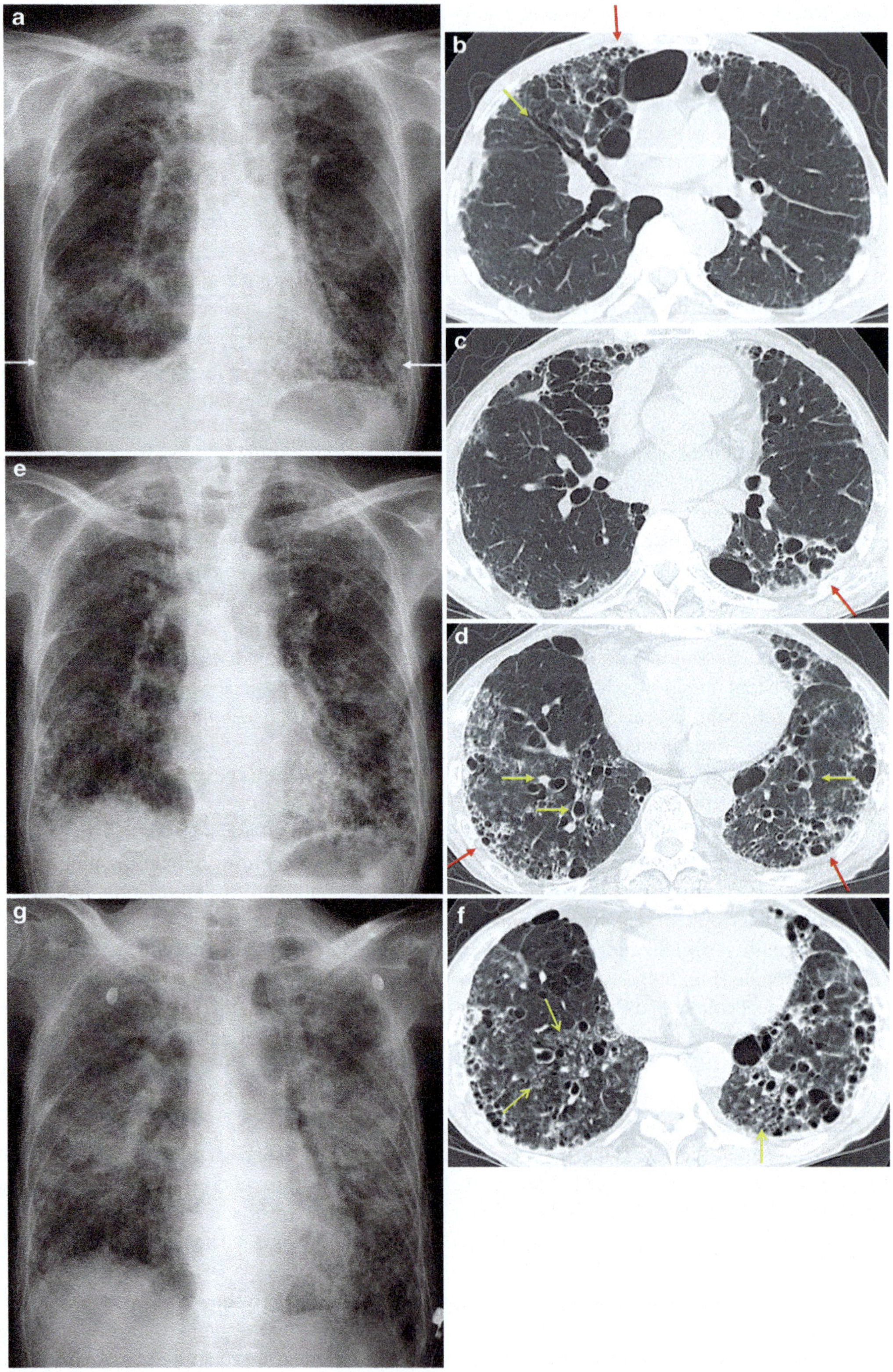

Fig. 5.4 (**a**) A 66-year-old man with RA for 6 years, in whom repeated bouts of pneumonia based on advanced BE lead to a fatal course. (**a**) A chest radiograph taken at his first visit to our respiratory department. In addition to extensive scarring at the apex and shrinkage of bilateral upper lung, reticulonodular shadows at bilateral lung base are noted (*arrows*). These findings are not compatible with ILD, which is usually accompanied by lung shrinkage at the lung base. (**b–d**) HRCT reveals diffuse bronchiectasis in middle and lower lobes (*yellow arrows*) and cluster of cysts mimicking honeycombing in bilateral lung base (*red arrows*), which are contiguous to dilated bronchi, suggesting that these cysts are bronchial in origin. (**e**) Chest radiograph taken 1 year later, near his death. Reticulonodular shadow and patchy opacities are prominent in bilateral lower lung fields. (**f**) HRCT reveals extensive ground glass opacity and centrilobular nodules (*yellow arrows*) around dilated bronchi, showing expansion of infection. (**g**) Chest radiograph on his last admission for severe pneumonia

5.2.1.4 Choice of DMARDs in Cases of Recurrent Respiratory Infection

Among RA patients, there are many in whom bacterial infection occurs repeatedly at the base of airway disease. Now it has become a serious problem whether such RA patients should be or should not be treated with potent DMARDs such as MTX or biologics, when they are necessary to control the disease activity of RA. Many physicians think that their use should be restrained in such cases [8]. However, as has been stressed so far, airway disease is an extra-articular manifestation of RA brought about by the dysregulated inflammatory response of the RA itself. Thus, when necessary treatment of RA is abandoned on the reason of repeated infection, not only the joint disease but also the airway disease will deteriorate also. Therefore, to improve the prognosis of RA patients, tireless administration of potent antirheumatic drugs is mandatory to control such infections as well as the disease activity of the RA [17]. Also, by adding biological agents, the required dosage of corticosteroid can be decreased, thus reducing the risk of infection, which is the desirable course [18].

Nevertheless, when the biologics therapy is initiated, respiratory infections tend to occur particularly during the first 6 months [8]. To overcome this stage, the early recognition of infection and prompt and adequate treatment are essential. To accomplish this goal, the short-term use of fluoroquinolone should be considered as the first option.

A successful case is presented in Fig. 5.5, in which sufficient control of RA disease activity and respiratory infection was achieved in parallel. A 75-year-old woman had RA for 20 years. MTX therapy was initiated 7 years ago, and sequential dose escalation of MTX was required. At the same period, cough, sputum production, and weight loss developed, diagnosed as respiratory infection (Fig. 5.5a), and MTX was withheld temporarily. We treated her with fluoroquinolone and obtained good control of the infection. The HRCT scan showed pneumonia in the left lung (Fig. 5.5c) and BE in the opposite side, which was supposed to be the site of origin of this infection (Fig. 5.5b). Immediately after the infection was resolved, MTX was resumed at a dose of 15 mg. However, for a while after that, pneumonia occurred frequently and was treated by

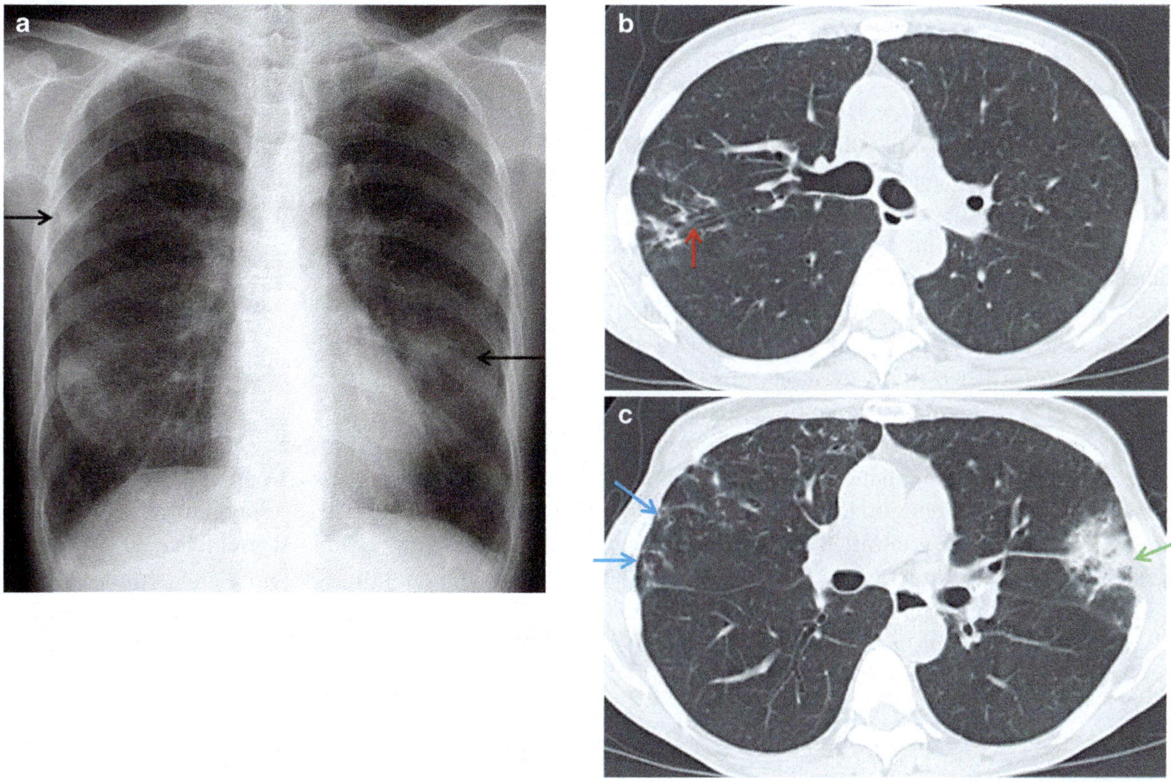

Fig. 5.5 (**a**) A case in whom disease control of RA with persistent use of potent DMARD resulted in conquering recurrent respiratory infection. (**a**) Chest radiograph taken during the unstable period shows patchy opacities in bilateral lung fields (*arrows*), indicating pneumonia. (**b**) HRCT shows bronchiectasis (*red arrow*) and bronchiolitis (*blue arrow*) in S2 of the right upper lobe. (**c**) A focal consolidated area indicating bacterial pneumonia (*green arrow*). She expectorated *Pseudomonas aeruginosa*, which was assumed to colonize the deformed airway and be the causative organism of this pneumonia. (**d**) Chest radiograph taken 5 years later from (**a**). Her condition had become stable, without any bouts of infection. Linear shadows are seen in right upper lung field (*arrow*), suggesting remnant bronchiectasis. There are no other pathological shadows. (**e, f**) HRCT reveals remnant bronchiectasis in the right upper and middle lobe with scanty micronodules (*red arrows*). Despite successful control of RA, anatomical change of bronchi remained. But as the fact, pneumonia does not occur for these several years. Effective control of RA also resulted in good control of respiratory infection

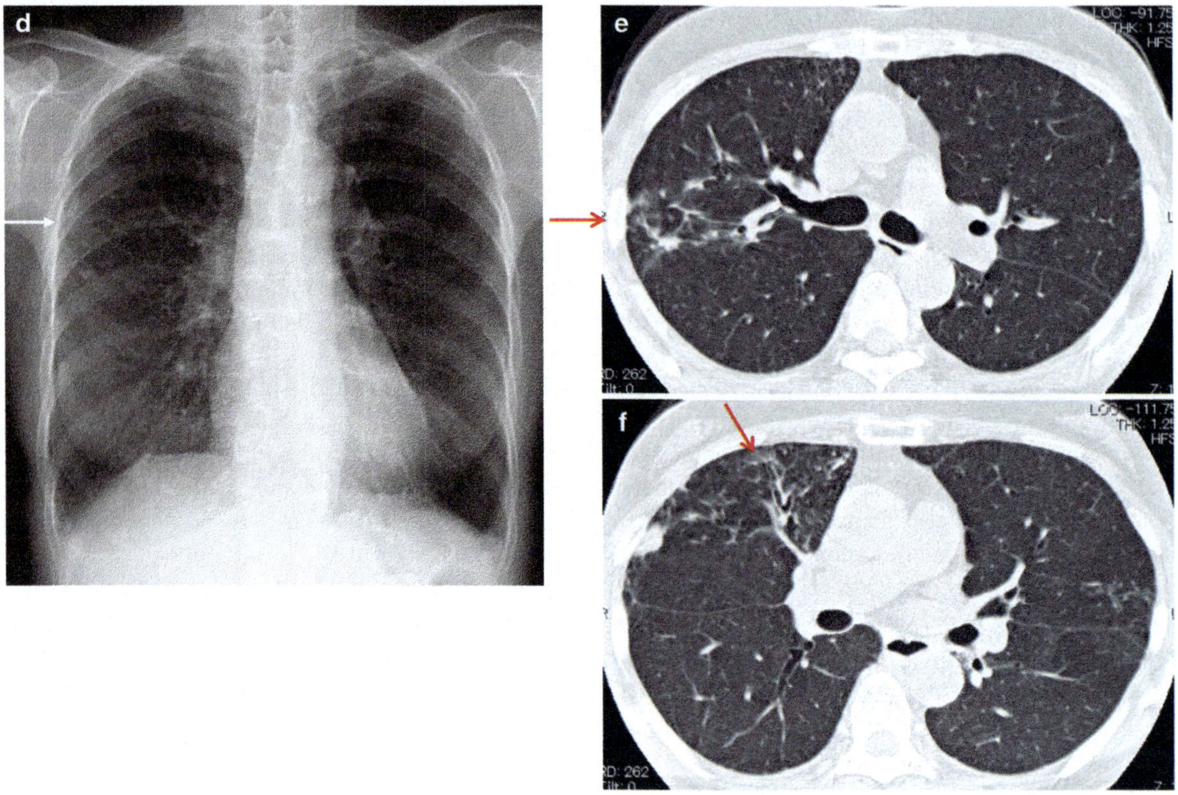

Fig. 5.5 (continued)

hospitalization or in the outpatient clinic. During the year, a total of six episodes of pneumonia occurred, but they all were conquered with proper treatment, that is, by the prompt use of fluoroquinolone. During this period, MTX was withheld only at the time of infection and was resumed immediately after control of the infection was obtained, ultimately leading to final success in the control of the RA. Thereafter, no further respiratory infections occurred (Fig. 5.5d), and the patient has been infection-free for 6 years. Note that on a recent HRCT, BE has not disappeared (Fig. 5.5e, f), indicating that although the structural changes in the airway may remain, infectious episodes do not occur when the RA is controlled. This fact clearly shows that the pulmonary infection of RA patients is not exogenous but is often endogenous, caused by the immunological conflict between colonizing bacteria and the host immune system.

5.2.2 NTM Disease

Since the introduction of biologics therapy for RA patients, NTM disease has been reported frequently as a serious complication and has become a worldwide problem. In Japan, according to post-marketing surveillance (PMS) and subsequent notification to the Pharmaceuticals and Medical Devices Agency (PMDA), 109 patients under biologics treatment were confirmed to be suffering from this disease in early 2013. This figure is not directly comparable with the estimated incidence of NTM disease in the general population in Japan, but certainly, it is extraordinarily high. An epidemiological study conducted in the USA reported the incidence of NTM disease of RA patients to be twice as high as that of the general population (over 50 years of age) and five times higher still in the case of biologics use, resulting in an overall incidence ten times higher (Table 5.1) [18]. The high morbidity in cases of biologics treatment could be understood, but how should we understand the high morbidity in RA patients receiving no biologics therapy at all?

Mori and colleagues reviewed 13 patients with NTM disease developed during biologics therapy and found that in most cases, airway diseases such as BE and bronchiolitis

Table 5.1 Incidence rate of NTM disease in the USA, observed in general population and in patients with RA with and without anti-TNF therapy (2000–2008) (cited and modified from ref. 18)

Population	Crude incidence rate (95% CI)
General population >50 years old	11.8 (11.1–12.6)
RA patients without anti-TNF therapy	19.2 (14.2–25.0)
RA patients with anti-TNF therapy	105 (59–173)

preceded NTM disease, affirmed by comparing CT findings (Fig. 5.6a, b) [2]. Generally speaking, nontuberculous mycobacteria are ubiquitous in the environment, and they could colonize in structural derangements of the lung such as BE and ILD, leading to the later onset of disease. Airway diseases of RA provide just such an environment, and the high incidence of NTM disease in RA patients can be explained from this viewpoint. Thus, preexisting airway disease in RA patients may be the largest predisposing factor for NTM disease. Therefore it is strongly advocated HRCT scanning to be performed to check for the presence of airway disease before the introduction of biologics therapy.

Of note, there is some difficulty in the use HRCT as a diagnostic tool of NTM disease in RA patients. The differential diagnosis on CT between the airway disease of RA and NTM disease is confusing. The findings of both diseases on CT imaging resemble so much (Fig. 5.6c, d). Both show extensive BE and centrilobular micronodular and branching opacities distributed segmentally. To the best of the author's knowledge, there has been no report to date in which these two diseases were reviewed and compared to determine the possibility of differential diagnosis. However, from the author's experience, differential diagnosis is absolutely impossible [19]. After all, when NTM disease is suspected, physicians have no choice but to perform repeated sputum examinations or bronchoscopy, if necessary. Also, as the serum anti-GPL antibody testing developed in Japan in recent years has high specificity in *Mycobacterium avium* complex disease despite its insufficient sensitivity in RA patients, this should be combined for use as well [20]. The diagnosis and treatment of NTM disease are described in detail in Chap. 11.

One point to be emphasized is that even if NTM disease develops during biologics treatment, the prognosis is not poor. Winthrop and colleagues reported that among 18 cases of NTM disease that developed during biologics treatment, seven patients died, indicating a mortality of 38%, a

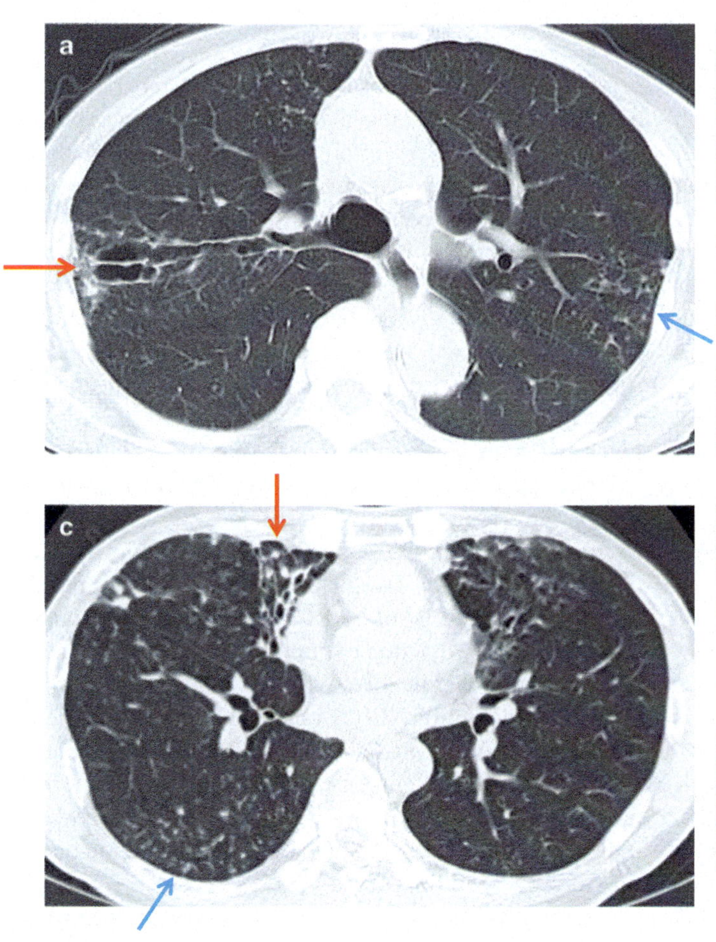

Fig. 5.6 (**a**, **b**) Nontuberculous mycobacterial disease in RA patients develops on RA-specific airway disease. (**a**) HRCT 1 year before onset of NTM disease. Bronchiectasis of the right upper lobe (*red arrow*) and bronchiolitis in left upper lobe (*blue arrow*) are visible (airway disease of RA). (**b**) HRCT at the onset of NTM disease shows infiltrative shadows that appear (*yellow arrows*) at the same place of the preexisting airway diseases. (**c**, **d**) NTM disease and RA airway disease are indistinguishable on HRCT image. Both resemble so closely with each other. (**c**) Airway disease of RA, (**d**) NTM disease. Bronchiectasis (*red arrows*) and centrilobular micronodules (*blue arrows*) are seen in both

miserable prognosis. Based on this fact, they warn against the easy use of biologic agents [18]. In Japan, however, no deaths have been reported in more than 100 cases of NTM disease, according to PMS of biologic agents. Also, Mori and colleagues, who reviewed the case series of 13 patients in Japan, reported no deaths and stated that all patients responded well to the antimicrobial therapy [2]. Of interest, the period from the start of biologics therapy to the onset of NTM disease in Japan is 8 months on average, whereas it is 3 years on average in the US study [18], which suggests that the discovery of NTM disease may be earlier in Japan than in the USA. If the lung destruction has progressed, NTM disease become difficult to control, but if it is treated early when the lung destruction is less, it is not a difficult disease to control. During biologics treatment, a miserable prognosis can be avoided by periodic chest radiography to check for the occurrence of NTM disease and any other lung complications.

5.3 Airway Diseases May Cause Obstructive Lung Disease

5.3.1 Airway Obstruction in RA Patients

Many authors who used HRCT to assess the prevalence of airway diseases in RA patients also reported a high frequency of airway obstruction on pulmonary function testing [21, 22]. As a criterion of airway obstruction, FEF_{25-75} is used more than FEV_1, and the reported prevalence ranges from 8 to 65%. Such obstruction is attributed to bronchiolitis, which is often accompanied with BE, or COPD in smoking patients. As stated above, the disorder of the peripheral airways is often relevant to that of the central airway in RA patients.

Despite the recognition of obstructive airway disease, it has not been well discussed in relation to the clinical course and prognosis of RA, except for the rare disorder called bronchiolitis obliterans (BO).

Nannini and colleagues focused on this problem in a longitudinal cohort study [3], which is a part of the famous Rochester Epidemiology Project with its high confidence as a population-based study. With an FEV_1 of 70% or less in lung function testing and the physician's clinical diagnosis being set as the criteria for obstructive lung disease (OLD), comprising of COPD, BE, and bronchiolitis, long-term follow-up results were compared and analyzed in RA and non-RA cohorts. The lifetime risk of developing OLD was 9.6% for RA patients (hazard ratio [HR] 1.54) compared with non-RA patients. Survival of RA patients diagnosed as having OLD was worse compared to those without OLD (HR 2.09). They concluded that patients with RA are at higher risk of developing OLD, which is significantly associated with premature death. They discussed the reason for this increased risk and postulated that RA-related immune dysfunction may predispose to excessive inflammatory responses in small airway. This study is valuable because of its population-based nature and long observational period in that it minimized the risk of referral bias. It should be regarded as the fundamental study for future research.

In clinical settings of RA, however, such an obstructive disorder is not necessarily evident. This is probably due to the low level of daily activity of RA patients, who rarely complain of dyspnea on exertion until the end stage. Without the complain of dyspnea, lung function testing would not generally be performed in routine practice.

5.3.2 Bronchiolitis Obliterans

BO (bronchiolitis obliterans) is a rare disorder clinically characterized by progressive dyspnea and impairment of lung function and characteristic pathological changes in the bronchioles. Prognosis is poor in patients with RA and several systemic disorders.

Devouassoux and colleagues investigated a 25-case series of obliterative bronchiolitis in RA [23]. They reported that BE coexisted in many cases, and airway obstruction was progressive, resistant to every effort including corticosteroids and other immunosuppressive drugs, and only one exceptional case was treated successfully with etanercept, a TNF blocker.

A typical case is presented here, a 39-year-old woman with recurrent respiratory infections in whom lung function deteriorated over a short period (Fig. 5.7). RA was diagnosed 14 years ago and treated with MTX and corticosteroid. She complained of cough, sputum, and sinusitis from 10 years ago for which macrolide and inhaled steroids were given but with no effect. From 1 year before dyspnea on exertion appeared, with progressive obstructive changes shown in lung function testing. She expectorated *Pseudomonas aeruginosa*, and neutrophils predominated in her bronchoalveolar lavage fluid analysis. Her anti-CCP antibody was 92.9 U/mL. HRCT 4 years before admission to the respiratory division of our hospital (Fig. 5.7b) showed BE in the right middle lobe, with surrounding patchy opacities and bronchiolitis. HRCT conducted just before the surgical lung biopsy (SLB) (Fig. 5.7d) revealed increased bronchiolitis in the right lower lobe. However, a micronodular shadow in the left lower lobe disappeared, which was not indicative of improvement but rather of completion of scarring of bronchiolitis.

Pathological findings of the SLB specimen revealed intense infiltration of lymphocytes and neutrophils in the bronchiolar walls and surrounding lung tissue (Fig. 5.7f). In the magnified view (Fig. 5.7g), disruption of elastin and marked narrowing of the lumen are observed, which are typical findings of cellular and destructive bronchiolitis. Two courses of steroid pulse therapy were administered with no

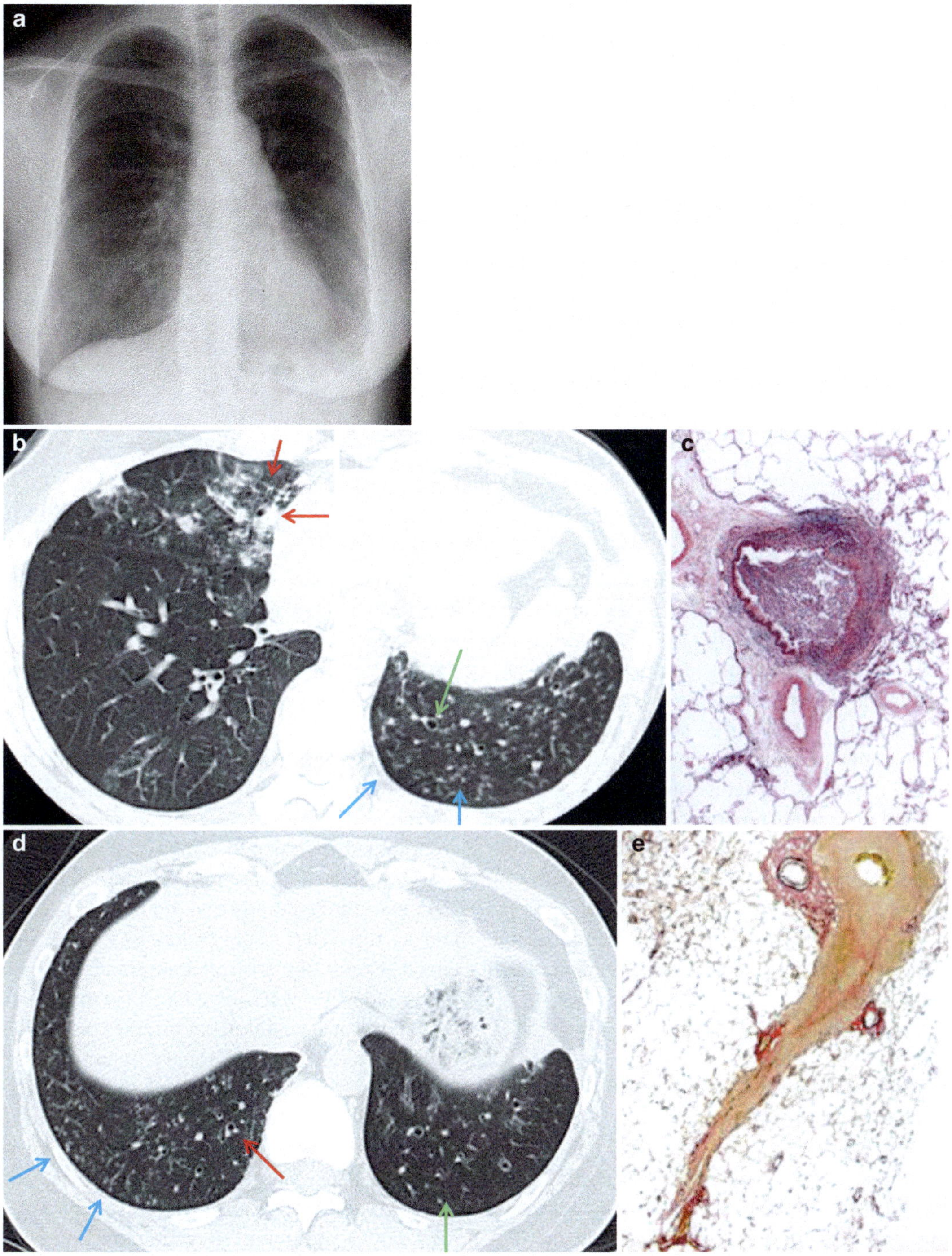

Fig. 5.7 (**a**) A case of obliterative bronchiolitis (cellular and destructive type, histologically). A 39-year-old female with RA for 14 years. She had complained cough and sputum for 10 years, which exacerbated 1 year ago. Also she complained exertional dyspnea recently. (**a**) Chest radiograph shows pleural adhesion in left side of the thorax, suggesting preceding inflammatory episodes. (**b**) HRCT scan done 4 years ago. Bronchiectases with surrounding opacities are seen in the right middle lobe (*red arrows*). In the left lower lobe, many centrilobular micronodules (*blue arrows*) are seen as well as bronchiectasis (*green arrow*), the former of which indicates active stage of bronchiolitis. (**c**) Photomicrograph of an active phase of cellular and destructive bronchiolitis of another case, which could correspond to the micronodules seen in CT image (**b**). Photomicrograph courtesy of Dr. A. Hebisawa. (**d**) HRCT scan done before the SLB. Micronodules have increased in number in the right lower lobe (*blue arrows*) along with bronchiectasis (*red arrow*). In the left lower lobe, micronodules have disappeared (*green arrow*) suggesting complete cicatrization, not the improvement, of bronchiolitis. (**e**) Photomicrograph of cicatrized stage of cellular and destructive bronchiolitis of another case. HRCT cannot demonstrate such a tiny cicatrized focus. Photomicrograph courtesy of Dr. A. Hebisawa. (**f**) SLB specimen, panoramic view. (**f**) Several bronchioles are seen. The wall of the bronchioles and surrounding lung tissue are infiltrated with inflammatory cells (*red arrows*). A dilated bronchus is also visible (*blue arrows*). Photomicrograph courtesy of Dr. T. Takemura. (**g**) The wall and surrounding lung tissue are infiltrated with lymphocyte and neutrophils. Epithelia are eroded and lined with regenerative cells, with marked narrowing of the lumen (*arrows*). A typical finding of cellular and destructive bronchiolitis. ×15 HE. Photomicrograph courtesy of Dr. T. Takemura

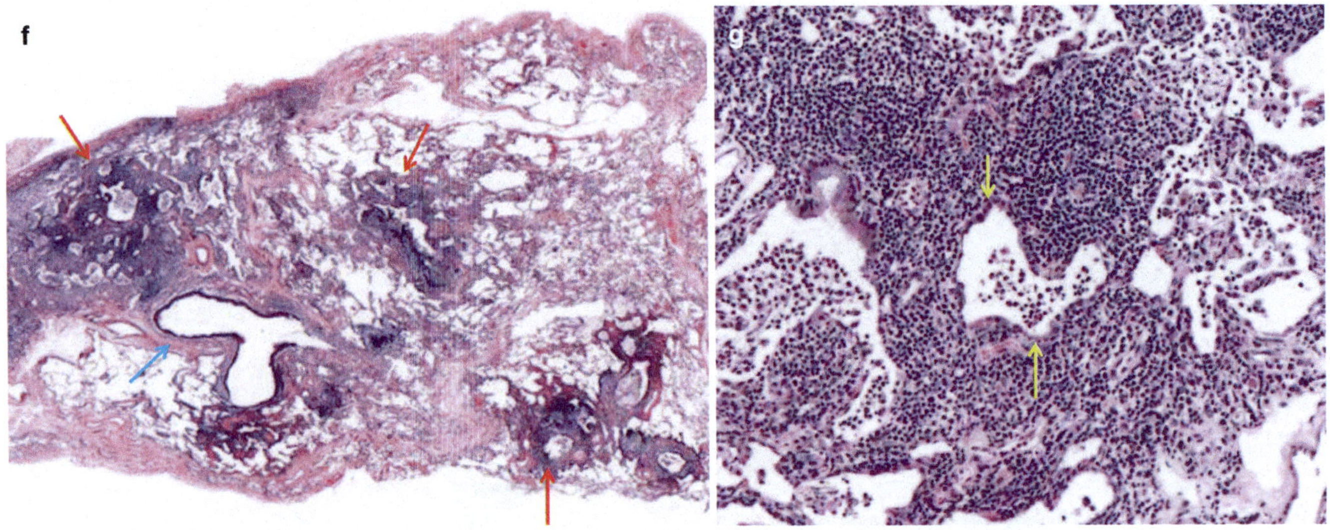

Fig. 5.7 (continued)

effect. Only biologics therapy (certolizumab pegol) could control her cough, sputum production, and deterioration of respiratory function, which not only ceased to worsen but even improved after several months' treatment. This case clearly shows that the airway disease of RA is an extra-articular manifestation of RA, and in severe cases, neither corticosteroid nor other immunosuppressants but only biologics can control the disease progression.

As Nannini and colleagues reported [3], and as this case shows, patients suffering from progressive airway obstruction do exist and might be more frequent than is currently estimated. Because RA patients rarely complain of dyspnea because of restricted daily activities, it is challenge for the physician to recognize the presence and development of airway obstruction.

5.3.3 How to Control the Progression of Airway Obstruction

Long-term macrolide administration has been evaluated as an effective therapy for chronic respiratory tract infection such as BE or diffuse panbronchiolitis (DPB) in non-RA patients. Conversely, Hayakawa and colleagues studied 12 cases of bronchiolitis in RA and reported that in the majority of the cases, no improvement of lung function was obtained with macrolide therapy, in contrast with DPB in non-RA subjects [24].

As airway disease is assumed to be the result of an excessive immunological response of RA patients, it is natural to think that treatment of the RA itself with potent DMARDs, such as MTX and biologics, can be effective in controlling the persistent airway inflammation. The BO mentioned above is one example. Treatments toward this direction should be attempted in the future.

Another case in which treatment of the RA itself improved airway disease refractory to macrolide therapy is presented here. A 65-year-old woman with a diagnosis of RA for 2 years (Fig. 5.8a). Her MMP-3 was 392 ng/mL, anti-CCP antibody 391 U/mL, PaO_2 67.5 Torr, %VC 69.5%, and FEV_1 54.6%. She was initially treated for RA with prednisolone and salazosulfapyridine. On HRCT, diffuse BE was found throughout the entire lung, with micronodules surrounding the areas of BE (Fig. 5.8b). She complained of chronic cough and sputum. She was initially diagnosed as having DPB, and was prescribed long-term macrolide therapy that did not improve her symptoms. During the first 2 years of RA treatment, she also experienced several bouts of pneumonia. Two years later, tacrolimus and MTX were introduced for disease control of RA, which was successful. Concurrently, her respiratory symptoms decreased, her pulmonary function improved, and the episodes of pneumonia ceased to occur. These improvements were also confirmed on HRCT, which showed that the bronchodilation and bronchial wall thickening had disappeared (Fig. 5.8c). The airway diseases are caused by the RA itself. Long-term macrolide therapy was ineffective, and only potent RA therapy resolved her airway disorder.

5.3.4 How to Control Persistent Cough and the Role of Antibiotics: A Hint for Controlling Chronic Inflammation of the Airway in RA Patients

In general, RA patients with airway disease would not complain of respiratory symptoms such as cough or sputum production despite their severity. Meanwhile, patients who suffer persistent cough or sputum production do exist not

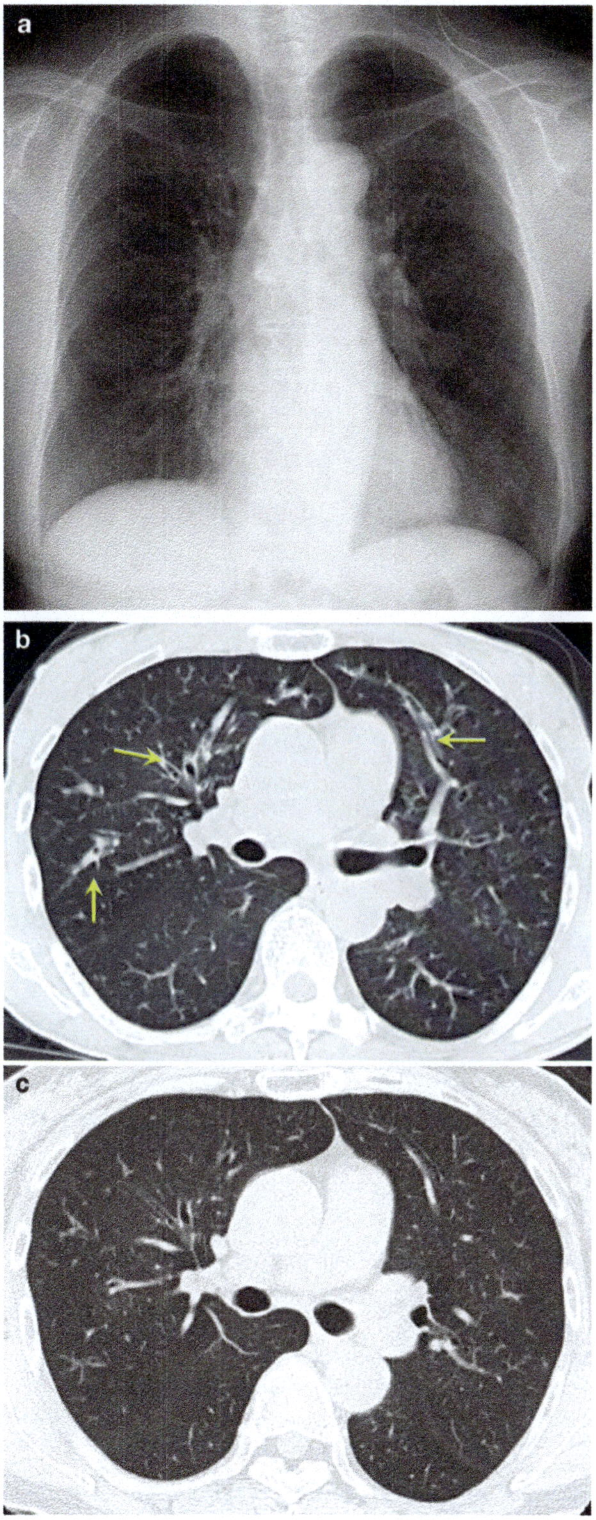

Fig. 5.8 (**a**) Diffuse bronchiectasis could be controlled with treatment of RA itself, not with macrolide therapy. (**a**) Chest radiograph in a 65-year-old woman with RA for 2 years. She complained of cough and sputum for several years. Macrolides were prescribed, but with no effect. Also she suffered from recurrent pneumonia. (**b**) CT scan shows diffuse bronchiectasis with wall thickening in the entire lung (*yellow arrows*). (**c**) CT scan done 5 years later shows diminished bronchial dilatation and wall thickening. During this period, treatment of RA with DMARDs have been done, with success. No treatment for respiratory infection per se, such as long-term macrolide

infrequently. Although they lack constitutional symptoms such as fever, and their serum CRP or erythrocyte sedimentation rate is usually not elevated, these obstinate symptoms bother patients greatly, decrease their quality of life, and discourage the physician from treating them with the potent DMARDs necessary to control the RA. The cause of these symptoms is assumed to be derived from chronic inflammation of the airways. Then how can we control these obstinate symptoms resulting from airway inflammation?

As mentioned above, there are a few proposed therapeutic strategies, including long-term macrolide or inhaled corticosteroid (ICS) therapy. Although the effects of long-term macrolide therapy are established for symptom reduction in non-RA subjects, its efficacy in RA subjects has not been investigated. In the author's clinical experience, the effect of macrolide therapy against the chronic cough and sputum production of RA patients is limited.

ICS is also used in non-RA subjects with BE to control chronic symptoms and has received a favorable appraisal [25], but no such study exists for patients with RA. In the author's experience, ICS was effective in some anecdotal cases, but the conditions of the responders were not clear. Dosage is an important factor for efficacy, and ciclesonide at a high dose of 800–1600 μg per day is preferred. With this treatment, concerns about the risk for infection may be raised, but in large-scale meta-analyses of the use of ICS for COPD and asthma, only a slightly increased risk of upper respiratory infection or mild pneumonia was observed [26]. To date, no studies of ICS for RA patients have been performed.

The author has found that short-term antimicrobial therapy is effective for this purpose. For RA patients who suffer from chronic cough for more than 1 month, after the evaluation of lung status with HRCT and confirmation of the presence of airway disease such as BE, 7 days of fluoroquinolone is prescribed, not necessitating the presence of apparent respiratory infection as a condition. This therapy has been prescribed for over 30 patients, and in 80% of them, a good or very good response was obtained without the relapse of symptoms within several weeks. Moreover, more than half of the patients did not relapse and required no additional treatment for the next several months or years (unpublished data).

A typical case is presented below. A 72-year-old woman with a history of RA for 10 years had suffered a dry cough for 10 months and weight loss of 6 kg (Fig. 5.9a, b). HRCT (Fig. 5.9c) showed BE and severe inflammation in the surrounding lung. She did not produce sputum, which may be a wonder, but in reality, this is common in RA practice. Fluoroquinolone of 7 days without any other drugs completely cured the obstinate cough, and it has not recurred over a 2-year follow-up period. Her weight steadily increased as well.

Only 1 week of quinolone therapy was effective, with almost a permanent effect for a symptom derived from

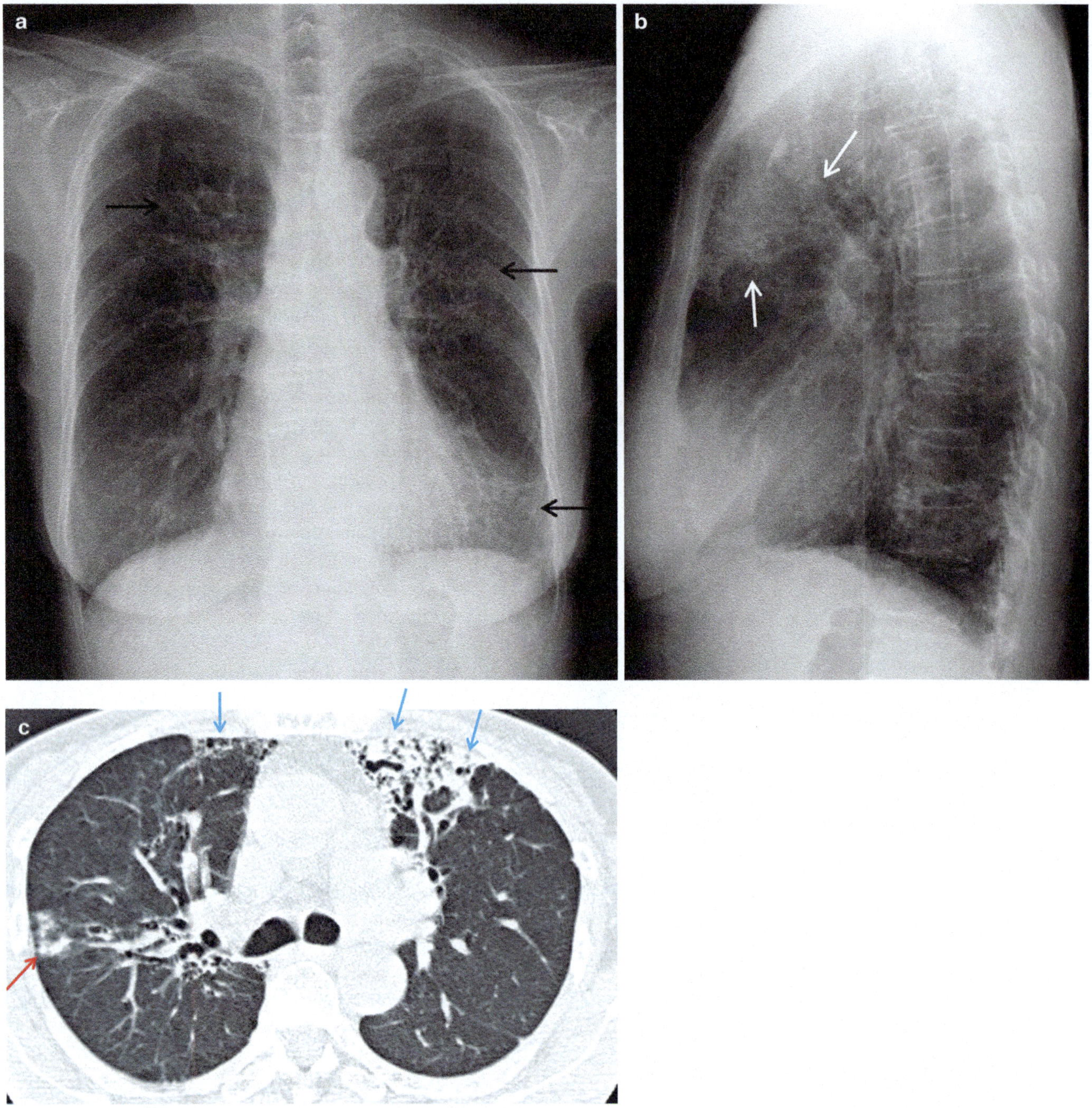

Fig. 5.9 (**a**, **b**) A 72-year-old female with RA for 10 years. She complained of nonproductive cough since 10 months ago, with weight loss of 6 kg. (**a**) Posteroanterior chest radiograph shows reticular opacities in bilateral hilar regions and in left lower lung field (*black arrows*). She had been diagnosed as having ILD. (**b**) However, lateral radiograph clearly shows that opacities have segmental distribution, suggesting airway origin (*white arrows*). (**c**) HRCT reveals bronchiectasis with surrounding lung consolidation (*blue arrows*). Patchy consolidation is also seen in the right lung field, suggesting focal pneumonia (*red arrow*)

chronic inflammation over a long period. This fact is peculiar and incomprehensible in the context of conventional medical theory, but an interpretation might be possible when we introduce the new concept of the microbiome. With the recent advances in genome analysis technology, it is clarified that microbiome is found also in the lower respiratory tract, which only a decade ago was considered to be sterile. Researches have disclosed that the change in the composition of the microbiome (dysbiosis) may result in host immune modulation (dysregulation), thus evoking chronic inflammation in the respiratory tract.

M. Blaser, a prestigious investigator for his contribution to the early days of microbiome research, reported the results of a study on the effects of antibiotics on the gut microbiome of mice in his famous monograph, *Missing Microbes* [27]. According to his theory, the gut microbiome of a mouse is unique and stable individually, and even when confounding factors are introduced externally, the constitution of the microbiome is rapidly restored. In the mice given three pulse of amoxicillin, the biodiversity of gut microbiome would bounce back to normal in a short period, whereas in mice given tylosin (potent macrolide antibiotic), the biodiversity was lost and would not go back to normal even several months after. Such a phenomenon has been verified also in humans with Ciprofloxacin. We are tempted to interpret our clinical experience along such a hypothesis. One week of quinolone therapy changed the microbiome of the lower respiratory tract and corrected the dysbiosis for a long period, thus leading to modulation of the dysregulated immunity, thereby calming the airway inflammation for the next few months to years in these patients.

5.4 Airway Disease Can Cause Honeycomb-Like Change Through Inflammatory Destruction of Bronchioles and Lung Parenchyma

As mentioned in Chap. 2, persistent inflammation that destroys the bronchiolar wall and surrounding alveolar tissue can eventually form clustered cysts at the peripheral airways in the subpleural area that mimics honeycombing. This change is not infrequently observed and has been erroneously recognized as ILD of the usual interstitial pneumonia (UIP) pattern on the HRCT image and even on pathology (as shown in Fig. 5.10). Revision of these pathological mechanisms is discussed in detail in Chap. 7.

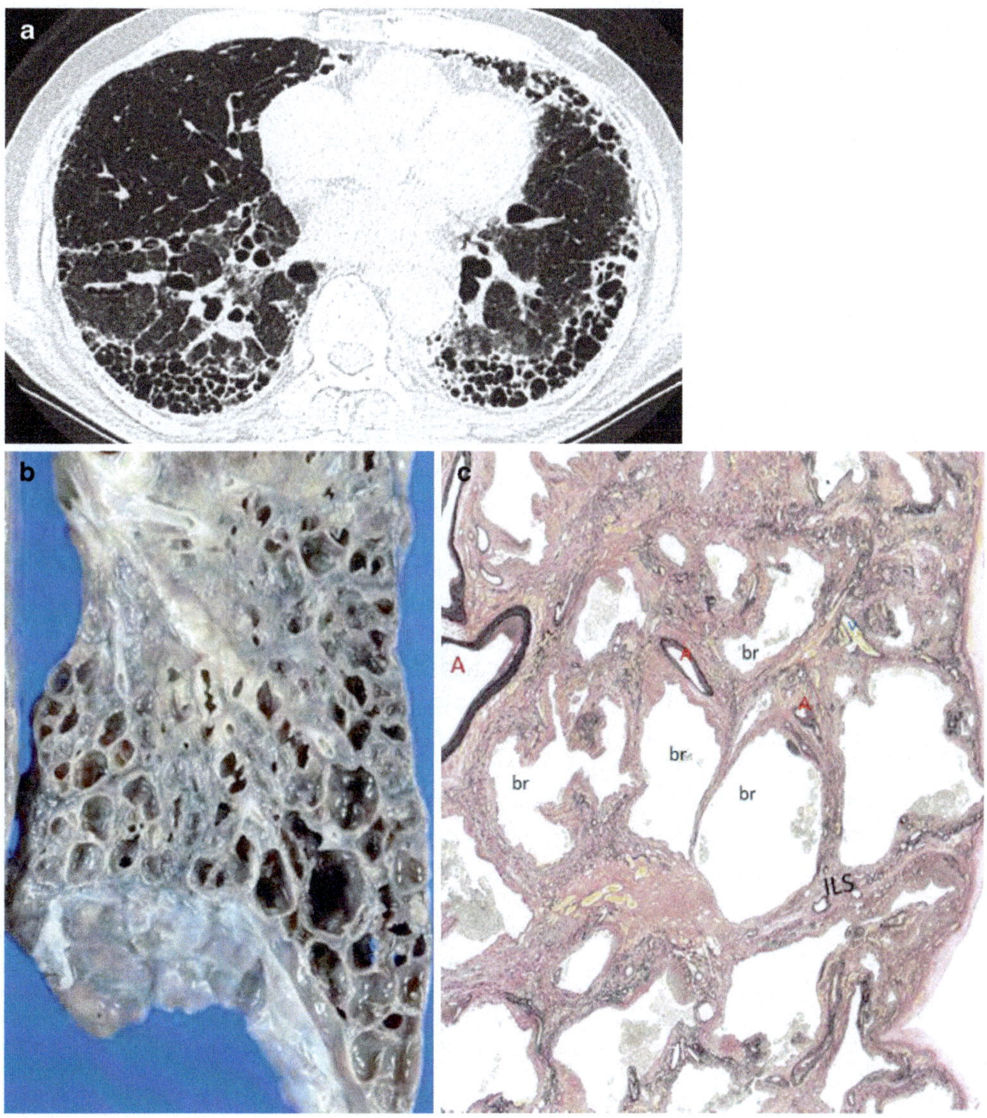

Fig. 5.10 (**a**) In RA patients, persistent inflammation may destruct peripheral airway and cause honeycomb-like change. A 65-year-old male. (**a**) HRCT shows multiple cysts clustered in subpleural area of bilateral lower lobe, mimicking ILD of UIP pattern. CT image courtesy of Dr. S. Izumi. (**b**, **c**) Autopsy specimen of the patient who deceased due to severe pneumonia with respiratory failure. (**c**) Multiple cysts are visible, resembling honeycombing usually seen in chronic fibrosing ILD, especially UIP pattern. Macroscopic view. (**d**) Pathological examination revealed that all those cysts are dilated bronchi or bronchiole formed through the inflammatory destruction. *A* artery, *br* bronchus, *ILS* interlobular septum. ×4, EVG. Photomicrograph courtesy of Drs. T. Takemura and S. Izumi

Generally, the prognosis of RA-ILD is good compared with that of idiopathic ILD, but among them, those judged as UIP pattern on pathological or radiological images are reported to have a poor prognosis, although agreement has not been reached among researchers [28–31]. Even if this is so, the reason for the poor prognosis remains to be clarified. In the author's opinion, some UIP patterns in RA-ILD are, in fact, caused by cyst formation through the airway inflammation, and therefore, they should be considered as airway disease, not ILD. In such cases, control of the airway inflammation may contribute to an improvement of prognosis. Potent DMARDs may be effective for the systemic control of inflammation, and for local control, additional ICS and/or other attempts should be tried. Needless to say, caution must be taken against possible infection when such immunosuppressive therapy is administered.

Conclusion

Now, with the advances in the management of RA and the therapeutic goal focused on remission coming into sight, lung complications have emerged as the most important obstacle against this new therapeutic strategy. In this chapter we have shown that preexisting lung diseases, especially airway disease, are the most important risk factor for lung complications, and we offered modest proposals for how to conquer them. The author has also pointed out the possibility of long-standing inflammation causing a honeycomb-like structural change at the distal airway that mimics ILD.

Chest HRCT is the most competent tool to grasp these underlying lung diseases and their progression in RA patients, but, unfortunately, it had not been popular in the clinical practice of RA, restricting comprehension of the exact situation. Recently, however, chest HRCT is being frequently performed in RA clinics in Japan and in other countries before initiating and also during the disease-modifying treatment of RA. Accompanying this trend over the past few years, enormous amounts of new knowledge are being accumulated regarding the development and progression of lung diseases of RA. In the not-so-distant future, active studies and discussion will be undertaken on this issue based on the accumulated evidence. Thus, the pathogenesis of airway disease and a part of ILD in RA will be elucidated, and therapeutic strategies can be established on the basis of such scientific evidence.

References

1. Takayanagi N. Biological agents and respiratory infections: causative mechanisms and practice management. Respir Investig. 2015;53:185–200.
2. Mori S, Tokuda H, Sakai F, Johkoh T, Mimori A, Nishimoto N, et al. Radiological features and therapeutic responses of pulmonary nontuberculous mycobacterial disease in rheumatoid arthritis patients receiving biological agents: a retrospective multicenter study in Japan. Mod Rheumatol. 2012;22:727–37.
3. Nannini C, Medina-Velasquez YF, Achenbach SJ, Crowson CS, Ryu JH, Vassallo R, et al. Incidence and mortality of obstructive lung disease in rheumatoid arthritis: a population-based study. Arthritis Care Res (Hoboken). 2013;65:1243–50.
4. Wolfe F, Caplan L, Michaud K. Treatment for rheumatoid arthritis and the risk of hospitalization for pneumonia: associations with prednisone, disease-modifying antirheumatic drugs, and anti-tumor necrosis factor therapy. Arthritis Rheum. 2006;54:628–34.
5. Doran MF, Crowson CS, Pond GR, O'Fallon WM, Gabriel SE. Frequency of infection in patients with rheumatoid arthritis compared with controls: a population-based study. Arthritis Rheum. 2002;46:2287–93.
6. Listing J, Strangfeld A, Kary S, Rau R, von Hinueber U, Stoyanova-Scholz M, et al. Infections in patients with rheumatoid arthritis treated with biologic agents. Arthritis Rheum. 2005;52:3403–12.
7. Galloway JB, Hyrich KL, Mercer LK, Dixon WG, Fu B, Ustianowski AP, et al. Anti-TNF therapy is associated with an increased risk of serious infections in patients with rheumatoid arthritis especially in the first 6 months of treatment: updated results from the British Society for Rheumatology Biologics Register with special emphasis on risks in the elderly. Rheumatology (Oxford). 2011;50:124–31.
8. Strangfeld A, Eveslage M, Schneider M, Bergerhausen HJ, Klopsch T, Zink A, et al. Treatment benefit or survival of the fittest: what drives the time-dependent decrease in serious infection rates under TNF inhibition and what does this imply for the individual patient? Ann Rheum Dis. 2011;70:1914–20.
9. Lieberman-Maran L, Orzano IM, Passero MA, Lally EV. Bronchiectasis in rheumatoid arthritis: report of four cases and a review of the literature—implications for management with biologic response modifiers. Semin Arthritis Rheum. 2006;35:379–87.
10. Swinson DR, Symmons D, Suresh U, Jones M, Booth J. Decreased survival in patients with co-existent rheumatoid arthritis and bronchiectasis. Br J Rheumatol. 1997;36:689–91.
11. Tsuchiya Y, Takayanagi N, Sugita Y, Miyahara Y, Tokunaga D, Kawabata Y, et al. Lung diseases directly associated with rheumatoid arthritis and their relationship to outcome. Eur Respir J. 2011;37:1411–7.
12. Puéchal X, Génin E, Bienvenu T, Le Jeunne C, Dusser DJ. Poor survival in rheumatoid arthritis associated with bronchiectasis: a family-based cohort study. PLoS One. 2014;9:e110066.
13. Siemieniuk R, Meade M, Alonso-Coello P, Briel M, Evaniew N, Prasad M, et al. Corticosteroid therapy for patients hospitalized with community-acquired pneumonia: a systematic review and meta-analysis. Ann Intern Med. 2015;163:519–28.
14. Tokuda H, Harigai M, Watanabe A, Hideto Kameda H, Tomono K, Takayanagi N, et al. Consensus statements for medical practice: biological agents and lung disease. Abridged English translation by the Japanese Respiratory Society. Respir Investig. 2017;55:229–51.
15. Gotfried MH, Grossman RF. Short-course fluoroquinolones in acute exacerbations of chronic bronchitis. Expert Rev Resp Med. 2010;4:661–72.
16. Kawasumi H, Gono T, Tanaka E, Kaneko H, Kawaguchi Y, Yamanaka H. Clinical characteristics and cytokine profiles of organizing pneumonia in patients with rheumatoid arthritis treated with or without biologics. J Rheumatol. 2016;43:738–44.
17. Banno S, Nobata H, Kitagawa W, et al. Safety and efficacy of biological therapy with rheumatoid arthritis associated pulmonary disease as interstitial lung disease or airway disease. Mod Rheumatol. 2015;163(25 Suppl):W66–5. http://www.ryumachi-jp.com/publication/pdf/mr_supple_all_2015.pdf. Accessed 30 Jan 2017.

18. Winthrop KL, Baxter R, Liu L, Varley CD, Curtis JR, Baddley JW, et al. Mycobacterial diseases and anti-tumor necrosis factor therapy in USA. Ann Rheum Dis. 2013;72:37–42.
19. Tokuda H. Broncho-bronchial disorders in patients with rheumatoid arthritis [in Japanese]. Rinsho Hoshasen. 2015;60:1085–96.
20. Komazaki Y, Miyazaki Y, Fujie T, Sakashita H, Tsuchiya K, Tamaoka M, et al. Serodiagnosis of Mycobacterium avium complex pulmonary disease in rheumatoid arthritis. Respiration. 2014;87:129–35.
21. Mori S, Koga Y, Sugimoto M. Small airway obstruction in patients with rheumatoid arthritis. Mod Rheumatol. 2011;21:164–73.
22. Wilsher M, Voight L, Milne D, Teh M, Good N, Kolbe J, et al. Prevalence of airway and parenchymal abnormalities in newly diagnosed rheumatoid arthritis. Respir Med. 2012;106:1441–6.
23. Devouassoux G, Cottin V, Lioté H, Marchand E, Frachon I, Schuller A, et al. Characterization of severe obliterative bronchiolitis in rheumatoid arthritis. Eur Respir J. 2009;33:1053–61.
24. Hayakawa H, Sato A, Chida K, Toyoshima M, Chida K, Iwata M. Bronchiolar disease in rheumatoid arthritis. Am J Respir Crit Care Med. 1996;154:1531–6.
25. Tsang WT, Ho PL, Lam WK, Ip MS, Chan KN, Ho CS, et al. Inhaled fluticasone reduces sputum inflammatory indices in severe bronchiectasis. Am J Respir Crit Care Med. 1998;158:723–7.
26. Saag KG, Furst DE, Barnes PJ. Major side effects of inhaled glucocorticoids. UpToDate. https://www.uptodate.com/contents/major-side-effects-of-inhaled-glucocorticoids. Accessed 30 Jan 2017.
27. Blaser MJ. Missing microbes. New York: Henry Holt & Company; 2014. p. 164.
28. Assayag D, Elicker BM, Urbania TH, Colby TV, Kang BH, Ryu JH, et al. Rheumatoid arthritis-associated interstitial lung disease: radiologic identification of usual interstitial pneumonia pattern. Radiology. 2014;270:583–8.
29. Walsh S, Sverzellati N, Devaraj A, Keir GJ, Wells AU, Hansell DM. Connective tissue disease related fibrotic lung disease: high resolution computed tomographic and pulmonary function indices as prognostic determinants. Thorax. 2014;69:216–22.
30. Solomon J, Chung J, Cosgrove GP, Demoruelle MK, Fernandez-Perez ER, Fischer A, et al. Predictors of mortality in rheumatoid arthritis-associated interstitial lung disease. Eur Respir J. 2016;47:588–96.
31. Zamora-Legoff JA, Krause ML, Crowson CS, Ryu JH, Matteson EL. Patterns of interstitial lung disease and mortality in rheumatoid arthritis. Rheumatology (Oxford). 2017;56(3):344–50. pii: kew391.

Part III

Interstitial Lung Disease in Rheumatoid Arthritis

6 Comprehensive Understanding of Interstitial Lung Disease in Rheumatoid Arthritis

Takahisa Gono

Abstract

Rheumatoid arthritis-associated interstitial lung disease (RA-ILD) is complicated in approximately 10% of RA patients. High titers of rheumatoid factor or anti-citrullinated protein antibodies (ACPAs), smoking, male gender, older age, longer disease duration, and higher articular disease activity are factors associated with the development of RA-ILD. Genetic factors such as human leukocyte antigen and peptidyl-arginine deiminase (PADI) and environmental factors such as smoking and periodontal disease could be associated with the activation of autoimmunity against citrullinated proteins, the synthesis of ACPAs, and the development of RA or RA-ILD. Metalloproteinase 7 and interferon-r-inducible protein 10 are serum novel biomarkers for the identification of RA-ILD, although surfactant protein A (SP-A), SP-D, and KL-6 are useful conventional biomarkers for the evaluation of RA-ILD. Novel antibodies against the PADI enzyme isoforms 3 and 4 or citrullinated heat shock protein (Hsp) 90a and Hsp90b are associated with RA-ILD and could be useful for predicting the development of RA-ILD. ILD is one of the main causes of mortality in RA. Therefore, prompt management of ILD in RA is necessary. To provide a better prognosis for RA-ILD patients, more efforts need to be made to determine the pathophysiology and the biomarkers for RA-ILD and the causal relationship between the development of ILD and DMARDs.

Keywords

Rheumatoid arthritis • Interstitial lung disease • ACPA • Autoantibody • Biomarker

6.1 Introduction

Rheumatoid arthritis (RA) is an immune-mediated joint disease. Rheumatoid factor (RF) and/or antibodies against some types of citrullinated proteins, called anti-citrullinated protein antibodies (ACPAs), are found in most patients with RA. The treatment strategy for arthritis in RA has been organized and clarified by the American College of Rheumatology and the European League Against Rheumatism, which have proposed the guidelines or recommendations for the management of RA. Additionally, new agents for RA, such as biological disease-modifying antirheumatic drugs (bDMARDs) and targeted synthetic DMARDs (tsDMARDS), have been developed and have become available during the last 10 years. Progress in this area has led to better clinical outcomes for patients with RA. Accordingly, several critical issues have appeared. For example, pulmonary infection or interstitial lung disease (ILD) is occasionally complicated in RA patients during treatment with csDMARDs, including MTX and/or bDMARDs. These complications can lead to severe conditions and occasional fatal outcomes in RA patients. According to one previous study, half of the causes of death are respiratory complications in RA patients treated with bDMARDs, as shown in Fig. 6.1 [1]. Why are pulmonary lesions frequently complicated in patients with RA? The precise answer currently remains unknown. Therefore, we need to understand the

T. Gono, M.D., Ph.D.
Department of Allergy and Rheumatology, Nippon Medical School, Graduate School of Medicine, Tokyo, Japan
e-mail: t-gono@nms.ac.jp

T. Gono et al. (eds.), *Lung Disease Associated with Rheumatoid Arthritis*, https://doi.org/10.1007/978-981-10-6750-1_6

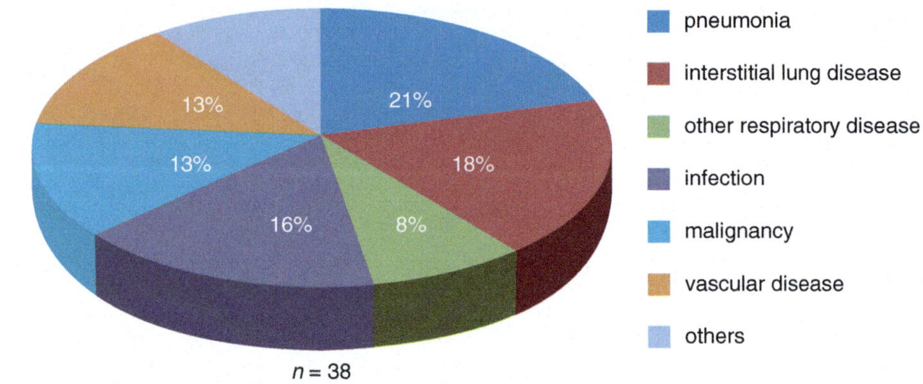

Fig. 6.1 Cause of death in RA patients treated with bDMARDs. *RA* rheumatoid arthritis, *bDMARDs* biological disease-modifying antirheumatic disease

present status and elucidate the pathophysiology and management of pulmonary complications in RA. These efforts will result in better outcomes and prognoses in RA patients.

In this section, we will focus on RA-associated ILD (RA-ILD) as a general discussion. Imaging, histopathology, and therapeutic strategy will later be separately described in more detail in each section.

6.2 What Is the Incidence and Prevalence Rate of RA-ILD?

According to a population-based study from the USA, the incidence rate of ILD was 7.9% in 582 RA patients who were followed up for a mean of 16.4 years [2]. Moreover, in 603 matched control patients without RA, the incidence of ILD was 1.2% [3]. In those RA patients, the 10-, 20-, and 30-year cumulative incidence rate of ILD was 3.5%, 6.3%, and 7.7%, respectively. In contrast, in the control subjects, the 10-, 20-, and 30-year cumulative incidence rates of ILD were 0.2%, 0.9%, and 0.9%, respectively. In other cohort studies from Japan, high-resolution computed tomography (HRCT) reveals ILD in 6.7–10.3% of RA patients [4, 5]. The prevalence of ILD is ~10% in RA patients, although respiratory symptoms are usually subclinical in RA patients with ILD.

6.3 What Symptoms Appear in RA-ILD?

As mentioned above, most patients with RA-ILD have clinically complained of few or no symptoms. The reasons may be because some patients with RA-ILD have limitations of exercise due to physical dysfunction in daily life, the extension of ILD is relatively limited, or the impairment of pulmonary function is mild. Symptoms could be missed or silent unless RA-ILD develops progressively and/or severely. In a previous study, HRCT revealed that ILD progressed in over one half of RA patients (12/21) with subclinical ILD for a mean follow-up of 1.5 years [6]. Clinicians should consider that no respiratory symptoms manifest until ILD progresses to some extent in RA and patients with RA-ILD need to receive follow-up chest radiography and pulmonary function tests regularly regardless of the presence or absence of symptoms.

As the severity of ILD progresses, patients with RA-ILD gradually suffer from a nonproductive cough and/or dyspnea on exercise. On the other hand, fever, dyspnea, cough, and malaise develop rapidly in acute exacerbation of chronic RA-ILD, drug-induced lung disease, or *pneumocystis* pneumonia. Secondary pulmonary hypertension is also a complication in the advanced stage of RA-ILD and can cause chronic respiratory failure and right heart failure. Related symptoms such as cyanosis, jugular venous distension, and edema will appear in advanced stages of ILD.

6.4 Clinical Factors and Characteristics of RA-ILD

As shown in Table 6.1, a presence of high titers of RF or ACPA, smoking, male gender, older age, longer disease duration, and higher articular disease activity are factors associated with the development of RA-ILD [3, 7, 8].

In a previous study, the clinical disease activity index (CDAI) in arthritis was positively correlated with ground-glass (GG) score in ILD in patients with RA. The fibrosis score was not correlated with CDAI. After treatment for arthritis, the GG score decreased along with a decline of the CDAI [9].

Therefore, prohibition of smoking and both early and appropriate treatment intervention for arthritis could be critical and preventive for the development of ILD in RA.

Table 6.1 Clinical factors associated with development of RA-ILD

Presence/high tiers of RF or ACPA
Smoking
Male
Older age
Longer disease duration
Higher articular disease activity

RA-ILD rheumatoid arthritis-associated interstitial lung disease, *RF* rheumatoid factor, *ACPA* anti-citrullinated protein antibody

6.5 What About the Prognosis for Patients with RA-ILD?

ILD is one of the major causes of death in patients with RA. In an inception cohort, 52 of 1460 RA patients developed RA-ILD [10]. Of these 52 patients, 39 patients died. The cause of death was attributed to RA-ILD in 28 patients. Median survival after diagnosis of RA-ILD was 3 years. Another recent study learned that the risk of mortality was three times higher in RA patients with ILD than in RA patients without ILD [2]. The median survival was 2.6 years in RA patients after a diagnosis of ILD, which was significantly lower than the expected median survival of 9.9 years in age- and gender-matched RA patients. The hazard ratio of mortality is 2.86 (95% CI 1.98–4.12) in RA-ILD patients compared to RA patients without ILD after adjusting for age, gender, and smoking.

The prognosis for RA-ILD patients depends on the extent of ILD and the degree of pulmonary dysfunction. The subtype of ILD is divided mainly into two forms, usual interstitial pneumonia (UIP) pattern and non-UIP pattern such as non-specific IP (NSIP), based on findings of HRCT in idiopathic pulmonary fibrosis (IPF) as shown in Table 6.2 [11]. As shown in Fig. 6.2, UIP-pattern ILD is characterized by honeycomb lesions and fibrotic changes predominantly in subpleural area and in the lung bases [11]. Moreover, NSIP has findings that are inconsistent with UIP (Fig. 6.3 and Table 6.2). The proportion of UIP ranged from 13% to 74% in RA-ILD [12]. In one study, UIP and NSIP were found in 103 (65%) and 39 (24%) subjects, respectively [13]. In other research, UIP and NSIP were found in 14 (27%) and 37 (73%) subjects, respectively [14]. The percentage of UIP and NSIP is different in each study. Results were dependent on the study design, such as methods used to recruit patients and screen for ILD. In clinical practice, it is occasionally difficult to classify UIP and NSIP clearly in RA-ILD. Findings that are a combination of UIP and NSIP are revealed in some RA-ILD patients.

Table 6.2 HRCT criteria for UIP pattern

UIP pattern (all four features)	Possibly UIP pattern (all three features)	Inconsistent with UIP pattern (any of the seven features)
Subpleural, basal predominance	Subpleural, basal predominance	Upper or mid-lung predominance
Reticular abnormality	Reticular abnormality	Peribronchovascular predominance
Honeycombing with or without traction bronchiectasis	Absence of features listed as inconsistent with UIP pattern	Extensive ground glass abnormality (extent > reticular abnormality)
Absence of features listed as inconsistent with UIP pattern		Profuse micronodules (bilateral, predominantly upper lobes)
		Discrete cysts (multiple, bilateral, away from areas of honeycombing)
		Diffuse mosaic attenuation/air-trapping (bilateral, in three or more lobes)
		Consolidation in bronchopulmonary segment(s)/lobe(s)

HRCT high-resolution computed tomography, *UIP* usual interstitial pneumonia; tomography

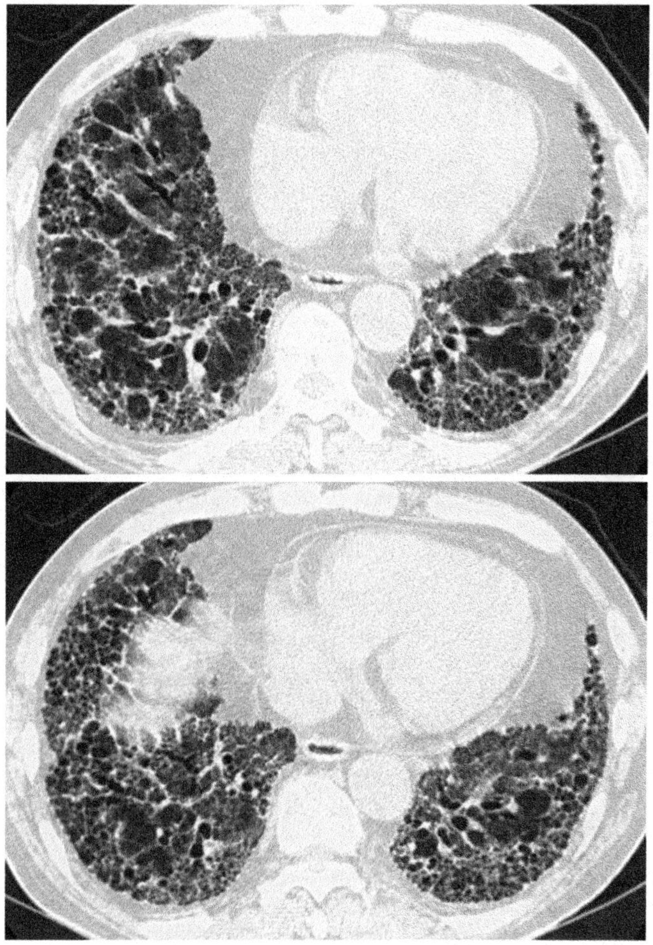

Fig. 6.2 Typical finding of UIP-pattern ILD in HRCT. *UIP* usual interstitial pneumonia, *ILD* interstitial lung disease, *HRCT* high-resolution computed tomography

6.6 What Are the Risk Factors Associated with Mortality in RA-ILD?

As shown in Table 6.3, male gender, smoking, older age, HRCT pattern such as extensive disease of ILD, fibrosis on histopathology, a lower baseline % predicted forced vital

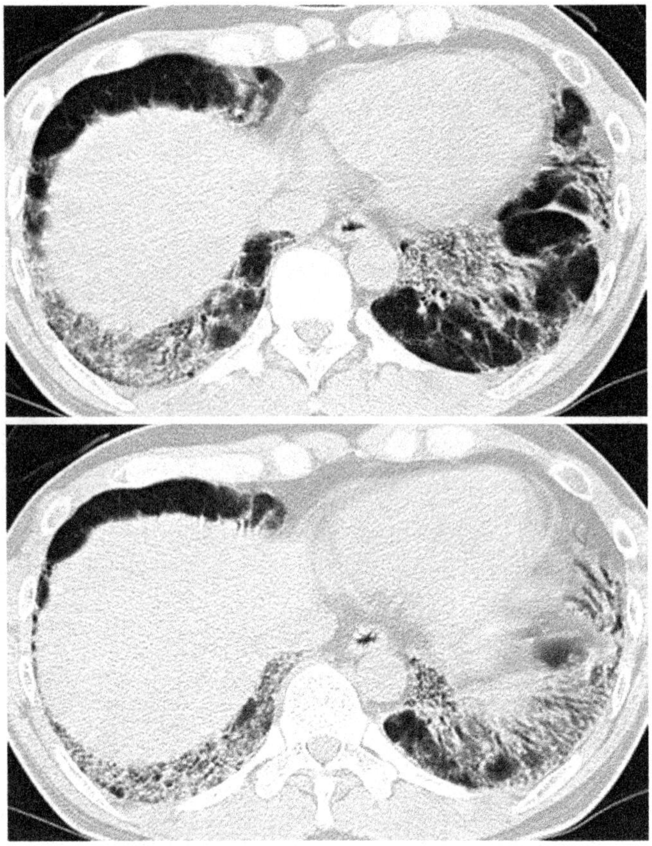

Fig. 6.3 Typical finding of NSIP pattern ILD in HRCT. *NSIP* nonspecific interstitial pneumonia, *ILD* interstitial lung disease, *HRCT* high-resolution computed tomography. These images are provided through the courtesy of H. Tokuda

Table 6.3 Risk factors for mortality in RA-ILD

Male
Smoking
Older age
HRCT pattern Presence of UIP, extensive disease of ILD
Fibrosis on lung histopathology
A lower baseline % predicted forced vital capacity
High articular disease activity

RA-ILD rheumatoid arthritis-associated interstitial lung disease, *HRCT* high-resolution computed tomography, *UIP* usual interstitial pneumonia

capacity (FVC), and higher articular disease activity are associated with increased mortality in RA-ILD [10, 13, 15–18]. Some of these factors are similar to the factors associated with complications of RA-ILD. Additionally, a 10% decline in % predicted FVC from baseline to anytime during follow-up is independently associated with mortality in RA-ILD [13]. Clinicians should carefully follow the FVC in RA-ILD patients.

Table 6.4 Risk factor for acute exacerbation of RA-ILD

Older age at diagnosis of ILD
UIP pattern on HRCT
Methotrexate usage

RA-ILD rheumatoid arthritis-associated interstitial lung disease, *HRCT* high-resolution computed tomography

6.7 Which Patients with RA-ILD Developed AE of ILD?

According to a previous report, 20% (11/51) of RA-ILD patients developed acute exacerbation with an overall 1-year incidence of 2.8%. Seven of these 11 RA-ILD patients with AE died as a result of the initial AE. As shown in Table 6.4, older age, UIP pattern on HRCT, and MTX usage are associated with the development of AE in RA-ILD [14].

6.8 Risk of Infections in RA-ILD

In Japanese postmarketing surveillance and reports regarding the usage of bDMARDs, such as TNF inhibitors (TNFi), a presence of pulmonary comorbidity and older age and corticosteroid use are risk factors for infection in RA patients [19]. One recent study assessed risk factors associated with infection in RA-ILD patients. In 181 RA-ILD patients, the mean age at diagnosis of ILD was 67 years, and the median follow-up period was 3 years [20]. The infection rate was higher during the first year after diagnosis of ILD (14.1 per 100 person-years (py)). The overall infection risk was higher in organizing pneumonia (OP) (27.1 per 100 py) than in UIP (7.7 per 100 py) or NSIP (5.5 per 100 py). With regard to antirheumatic therapy, the infection rates for RA-ILD patients treated with sulfasalazine or hydroxychloroquine alone and those treated with MTX or leflunomide alone were 2.9 and 7.4 per 100 py, respectively. On the other hand, prednisone use >10 mg/day resulted in the highest risk for serious infection as 15.4 per 100 py in RA-ILD [20]. Dose of corticosteroid for arthritis should be minimized as possible.

6.9 How to Differentiate the Diagnosis in RA-ILD?

RA-ILD is usually chronic ILD and presumed to be caused by RA itself autoimmunity. On the other hand, acute-onset ILD (acute ILD) is occasionally complicated in RA patients, but different from RA-ILD. The causes of acute ILD in RA include hypersensitivity to drugs such as MTX and bDMARDs, infections such as cytomegalovirus (CMV) and *Pneumocystis jirovecii,* and complications associated with other connective tissue diseases such as anti-aminoacyl-

Table 6.5 Differentiation diagnosis in ILD with RA

RA itself autoimmunity (RA-ILD)
Drugs (DMARDs)
Infection (cytomegalovirus, *Pneumocystis jirovecii*)
Other connective tissue disease (anti-ARS antibody syndrome, vasculitis)

ILD interstitial lung disease, *RA* rheumatoid arthritis, *DMARDs* disease-modifying antirheumatic drugs, *ARS* aminoacyl-tRNA synthetase

tRNA synthetase (ARS) antibody syndrome (Table 6.5). It is sometimes difficult to differentiate acute exacerbation of RA-ILD itself from acute ILD caused by other factors [21], particularly when chronic RA-ILD is already pre-existing. The most important way to differentiate the diagnosis of acute ILD in RA is to promptly conduct a microorganism test. Concretely, the CMV antigenemia assay and the measurement of β-D-glucan are useful for the detection of CMV and fungus such as *Pneumocystis jirovecii*. Additionally, sputum specimens are needed to isolate *Pneumocystis jirovecii* using staining measures and PCR methods. In regard to complications associated with other connective tissue diseases, a physical examination involving more than the joints should be conducted, and autoantibodies, including anti-ARS, anti-SS-A, and anti-neutrophil cytoplasmic antibodies, should be measured. If chronic RA-ILD and other connective tissue diseases are not pre-existing, the cause of acute ILD could be judged as hypersensitivity to drugs such as MTX or infections. When the described above microbial tests are all negative, drugs are considered to be the cause of ILD in RA patients without pre-existing ILD or connective tissue disease. Occasionally infections may induce acute exacerbation of RA-ILD. In this situation, RA-ILD develops progressively, even if infections are controlled with antibiotics. In such situation, treatment of ILD should be performed considering both of RA-ILD and infection.

6.10 Serum Biomarkers in RA-ILD

Surfactant protein A (SP-A), SP-D, and KL-6 have been found in idiopathic pulmonary fibrosis (IPF) and in connective tissue disease-associated ILD, including RA-ILD [22–24]. These markers reflect disruption of the blood-alveolar barrier and disease activity/severity of ILD but provide limited mechanistic insight [25].

Recent studies have found that metalloproteinase 7 (MMP-7) and interferon (IFN)-r-inducible protein 10 (IP-10)/CXCL10 are useful serum biomarkers for the identification of RA-ILD [26]. Serum levels of MMP-7 and IP-10/CXCL10 were higher in symptomatic RA-ILD than in subclinical RA-ILD. MMP-7 is a biomarker associated with survival in idiopathic pulmonary fibrosis (IPF) [27]. IPF patients with higher levels of plasma MMP-7 had a shorter survival time than those with lower levels of MMP-7. MMP-7 is overexpressed in alveolar epithelial cells in the IPF lung but not in the normal lung [27, 28]. MMP-7 is involved in wound healing [29]. MMP-7 is considered to be pathophysiologically associated with lung fibrosis. MMP-7 knockouts are protected from fibrosis [30]. Additionally, IP-10/CXCL10 is secreted by monocytes, endothelial cells, and fibroblasts in response to IFN-r and involved in recruitment of activated T cells. High levels of serum IP-10/CXCL10 were revealed in anti-Jo-1 antibody-associated ILD [25]. These fibrosis and inflammation processes could be associated with the pathophysiology of RA-ILD. In addition, tumor growth factor-beta, insulin-like growth factor-1, platelet-derived growth factors, IL-4, and IL-33 are associated with the development of RA-ILD [31–33].

Antibodies against the peptidyl-arginine deiminase (PAD) enzyme isoforms 3 and 4 (anti-PAD3/4) could be associated with RA-ILD [34]. The prevalence and extent of ILD was higher in RA patients with anti-PAD3/4 than in those without anti-PAD3/4. Immunoprecipitation and subsequent mass spectrum sequencing identified citrullinated heat shock protein (Hsp)90a and Hsp90b as candidate autoantigens in RA-ILD [35]. In enzyme-linked immunosorbent assay, sensitivity was 20–30%, and specificity was >95% relative to sera derived from patients with RA alone, those with MCTD or those with IPF. These autoantibodies might serve as useful biomarkers for predicting the development of ILD in RA.

6.11 Pathophysiology of RA-ILD

Minimal basic research regarding RA-ILD has been conducted. Among ever-smokers, the presence of interstitial lung lesions is associated with titers of RF or ACPA [36]. Moreover, these associations are not found among never-smokers. Therefore, smoking is linked to the production of RF/ACPA, which accelerates the development of ILD in RA. ILD occasionally precedes arthritis in RA. In one recent hypothesis, ACPA is initially produced in the lung. Additionally, ACPA is produced in articular sites, and it is known that arthritis develops in RA patients. The lung inflammation and autoimmune reactions are primarily associated with production of ACPA [37, 38]. Immunohistochemical studies showed increased expression of citrullinated proteins on the bronchial tissues in ACPA-positive early untreated RA patients compared to ACPA-negative RA patients. ACPA levels in bronchial alveolar fluid were higher than ACPA levels in the sera of ACPA-positive RA patients [38]. These findings suggested that ACPA is produced more commonly in the lung than in the joints of some RA patients. A broader ACPA repertoire in RA-ILD suggests a possible role for ACPA in the pathogenesis of ILD [39]. These greater numbers of ACPA are associated with an increase in the production of systemic inflammatory cytokines such as TNF-α and IL-6 [40]. This study suggests that more intensive inflammation and interactions between T cells and B cells occur more actively in RA-ILD patients. This hypothesis corresponds to some patients with RA. However, lung inflammation such as ILD is not always revealed in RA patients with ACPA. The development of ILD could be associated with articular disease activity in some RA patients in whom arthritis precedes ILD. There might be several different mechanisms for the development of ILD in RA. It remains unknown that the subtype of ILD such as UIP and NSIP is different in each RA-ILD patients.

Several HLA haplotype studies have been conducted in RA-ILD. In a Japanese study, DRB1*15 or *16 and DQB1*06 are associated with a high risk for the development of ILD in RA [4, 41]. Another study has demonstrated that high levels of ACPAs are associated with HLA-DRB1*15 in patients with RA [42]. Citrullination is a post-translational modification of proteins by PAD. The PAD type 4 (PADI4) gene is associated with a susceptible gene for RA [43]. Additionally, *Porphyromonas gingivalis* is associated with the development of periodontal disease and has the ability to carry PAD [44]. Recently, the complication of periodontal disease is associated with disease onset and disease severity in RA [45, 46]. Antibodies to *Porphyromonas gingivalis* are associated with ACPAs in RA patients [47]. In addition, smoking increases PADI2 in the lung [48]. Citrullinated proteins are found in the BAL of smokers but not in non-smokers [49]. Therefore, these genetic factors and environmental factors could be associated with the synthesis of ACPAs and the development of RA-ILD.

In the future, we need to conduct additional basic studies regarding RA-ILD and to determine the pathophysiology of RA-ILD more clearly. The presumptive pathophysiology is shown in Fig. 6.4.

6.12 A New Device for the Detection of ILD

Recently, it has been reported that transthoracic ultrasound (US) of the lung might be a useful noninvasive tool to detect ILD [50, 51]. US can detect the following findings: comet tail artifacts/B-pattern, subpleural nodes, and thickening of the pleural line. These findings were more frequently found in ILD patients than in patients without ILD. Certainly, CT is useful for the detection of minimal changes in the lung. However, the cost of this examination procedure and radiological risk are problems in CT. US can solve these issues. In a previous study, a B-line score > 10 was defined as the presence of ILD [51]. The B-line score was computed in 28 anterior and 44 posterior sites. In this study, 39 RA-ILD patients were enrolled. The sensitivity and specificity of lung US were 92% and 56%, respectively, as the gold standard of HRCT. The B-line score was significantly correlated with the HRCT score. In the future, lung US might be available for screening and follow-up of ILD, although many examiners of the lung US need to be educated to detect lung lesions accurately and in a reproducible manner with US.

6.13 Do Biologic DMARDs Improve Progressive RA-ILD or Prevent Acute Exacerbations of RA-ILD?

Whether biologic DMARDs can improve progressive RA-ILD or prevent exacerbations of RA-ILD has remained unknown and controversial. In some cases, ILD improved when treated with bDMARDs [52–54]. In other cases, bDMARDs such as TNFi exacerbated ILD [21, 55]. We need to conduct prospective studies or collect many cases of RA-ILD treated with bDMARDs to clarify the answers to these questions.

6.13.1 TNFi and RA-ILD

In a retrospective study regarding the association between TNFi use and the new development of ILD in RA patients with pre-existing RA-ILD, 58 patients had pre-existing RA-ILD out of 163 RA patients treated with bDMARDs [56]. A new ILD event occurred more frequently in RA patients who were being treated with TNFi than in patients who were not administered a drug from this class. Of 58 RA-ILD patients, 14 had new ILD events within 12 months after commencement of bDMARDs. All 14 patients were treated with TNFi. No new events of ILD occurred in patients treated with non-TNFi bDMARDs such as tocilizumab (TCZ) and abatacept (ABT).

With regard to the mortality rate in patients being treated with TNFi, one previous study provided evidence that the mortality rate was not increased in RA-ILD patients treated with TNFi compared to those treated with traditional DMARDs [17]. The adjusted mortality rate was 0.81 (95% CI 0.38–1.73) in RA-ILD patients treated with TNFi compared to those treated with traditional DMARDs. However, the presence of ILD is one of the risk factors associated with infection and mortality in RA. Clinicians should take precautions against infection and complications of pulmonary disease.

6.13.2 TCZ and RA-ILD

Regarding an association between TCZ use and the development of ILD, a study in which 395 patients treated with TCZ were enrolled found that 78 patients had pre-existing ILD

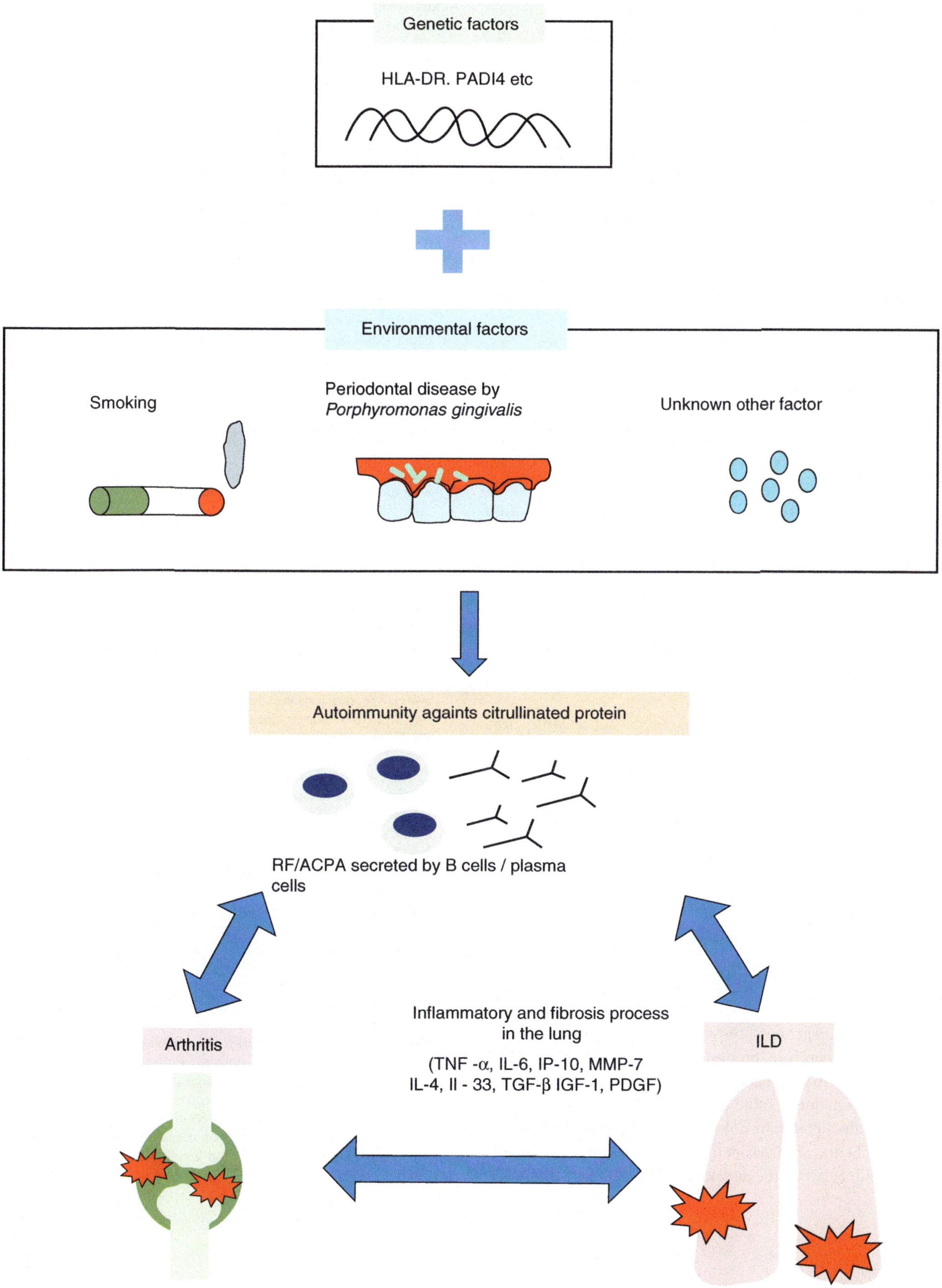

Fig. 6.4 Hypothesis of pathophysiology in RA-ILD

[57]. Factors such as age ≥ 60 years, smoking, and high titers of RF were associated with the presence of ILD in RA. In 6 of these 78 ILD patients, an acute exacerbation (AE) of ILD developed during treatment with TCZ. The median duration at the development of an AE was 48 weeks after the commencement of TCZ. There was no difference in clinical characteristics at baseline between ILD patients with an AE and those without an AE. The clinical disease activity index at 24 weeks after the initiation of TCZ was significantly higher in ILD patients with an AE than in those without an AE. A CDAI more than 10 was a risk factor for an AE. As mentioned previously, appropriate management of disease activity of RA might contribute to the prevention of an AE in patients with RA-ILD.

6.13.3 ABT and RA-ILD

In a retrospective study of RA-ILD patients being treated with ABT, no patient experienced worsening of ILD within 1 year after commencement of ABT [52]. Additionally, two patients with ILD showed complete resolution. Although this result should be interpreted carefully, treatment with ABT might provide a lower risk for progression of ILD in RA patients with pre-existing ILD than treatment with TNFi.

6.13.4 Rituximab and RA-ILD

Rituximab (RTX) has been reported to successfully treat RA-ILD [54]. A previous study showed that marked follicular B cell hyperplasia was detected in peribronchiolar lymphoid aggregates in RA-ILD [58]. The quantification of B cell cellularity was higher in RA-ILD than in IPF. These findings could suggest that RTX is a potential agent for improving RA-ILD.

Conclusion

There have been several unknown findings regarding RA-ILD. However, more recently, new findings have been observed in RA-ILD. ILD is one of the most important extra-articular symptoms and complications of RA because ILD is one of the main causes of mortality in RA patients. Therefore, prompt management of ILD in RA is necessary. Additionally, to provide a better prognosis for RA-ILD patients, more efforts need to be made to determine the pathophysiology and clinical features of RA-ILD, the biomarkers for RA-ILD, and the causal relationship between the development of ILD and DMARDs.

Acknowledgment I would like to thank Naohiro Sugitani for providing the chest imaging.

References

1. Nakajima A, Saito K, Kojima T, Amano K, Yoshio T, Fukuda W, Inoue E, Taniguchi A, Momohara S, Minota S, Takeuchi T, Ishiguro N, Tanaka Y, Yamanaka H. No increased mortality in patients with rheumatoid arthritis treated with biologics: results from the biologics register of six rheumatology institutes in Japan. Mod Rheumatol. 2013;23:945–52.
2. Bongartz T, Nannini C, Medina-Velasquez YF, Achenbach SJ, Crowson CS, Ryu JH, Vassallo R, Gabriel SE, Matteson EL. Incidence and mortality of interstitial lung disease in rheumatoid arthritis: a population-based study. Arthritis Rheum. 2010;62:1583–91.
3. Chen J, Shi Y, Wang X, Huang H, Ascherman D. Asymptomatic preclinical rheumatoid arthritis-associated interstitial lung disease. Clin Dev Immunol. 2013;2013:406927.
4. Mori S, Koga Y, Sugimoto M. Different risk factors between interstitial lung disease and airway disease in rheumatoid arthritis. Respir Med. 2012;106:1591–9.
5. Mori S, Cho I, Koga Y, Sugimoto M. Comparison of pulmonary abnormalities on high-resolution computed tomography in patients with early versus longstanding rheumatoid arthritis. J Rheumatol. 2008;35:1513–21.
6. Gochuico BR, Avila NA, Chow CK, Novero LJ, Wu HP, Ren P, MacDonald SD, Travis WD, Stylianou MP, Rosas IO. Progressive preclinical interstitial lung disease in rheumatoid arthritis. Arch Intern Med. 2008;168:159–66.
7. Wang JX, Du CG. A retrospective study of clinical characteristics of interstitial lung disease associated with rheumatoid arthritis in Chinese patients. Med Sci Monit. 2015;21:708–15.
8. Shidara K, Hoshi D, Inoue E, Yamada T, Nakajima A, Taniguchi A, Hara M, Momohara S, Kamatani N, Yamanaka H. Incidence of and risk factors for interstitial pneumonia in patients with rheumatoid arthritis in a large Japanese observational cohort, IORRA. Mod Rheumatol. 2010;20:280–6.
9. Pérez-Dórame R, Mejía M, Mateos-Toledo H, Rojas-Serrano J. Rheumatoid arthritis-associated interstitial lung disease: lung inflammation evaluated with high resolution computed tomography scan is correlated to rheumatoid arthritis disease activity. Reumatol Clin. 2015;11:12–6.
10. Koduri G, Norton S, Young A, Cox N, Davies P, Devlin J, Dixey J, Gough A, Prouse P, Winfield J, Williams P, ERAS (Early Rheumatoid Arthritis Study). Interstitial lung disease has a poor prognosis in rheumatoid arthritis: results from an inception cohort. Rheumatology (Oxford). 2010;49:1483–9.
11. Raghu G, Collard HR, Egan JJ, Martinez FJ, Behr J, Brown KK, Colby TV, Cordier JF, Flaherty KR, Lasky JA, Lynch DA, Ryu JH, Swigris JJ, Wells AU, Ancochea J, Bouros D, Carvalho C, Costabel U, Ebina M, Hansell DM, Johkoh T, Kim DS, King TE, Kondoh Y, Myers J, Müller NL, Nicholson AG, Richeldi L, Selman M, Dudden RF, Griss BS, Protzko SL, Schünemann HJ, ATS/ERS/JRS/ALAT Committee on Idiopathic Pulmonary Fibrosis. An official ATS/ERS/JRS/ALAT statement: idiopathic pulmonary fibrosis: evidence-based guidelines for diagnosis and management. Am J Respir Crit Care Med. 2011;183:788–824.
12. Suda T. Up-to-date information on rheumatoid arthritis-associated interstitial lung disease. Clin Med Insights Circ Respir Pulm Med. 2015;9:155–62.

13. Kelly CA, Saravanan V, Nisar M, Arthanari S, Woodhead FA, Price-Forbes AN, Dawson J, Sathi N, Ahmad Y, Koduri G, Young A, British Rheumatoid Interstitial Lung (BRILL) Network. Rheumatoid arthritis-related interstitial lung disease: associations, prognostic factors and physiological and radiological characteristics—a large multicentre UK study. Rheumatology (Oxford). 2014;53:1676–82.
14. Hozumi H, Nakamura Y, Johkoh T, Sumikawa H, Colby TV, Kono M, Hashimoto D, Enomoto N, Fujisawa T, Inui N, Suda T, Chida K. Acute exacerbation in rheumatoid arthritis-associated interstitial lung disease: a retrospective case control study. BMJ Open. 2013;3:e003132.
15. Assayag D, Lubin M, Lee JS, King TE, Collard HR, Ryerson CJ. Predictors of mortality in rheumatoid arthritis-related interstitial lung disease. Respirology. 2014;19:493–500.
16. Kim EJ, Elicker BM, Maldonado F, Webb WR, Ryu JH, Van Uden JH, Lee JS, King TE, Collard HR. Usual interstitial pneumonia in rheumatoid arthritis-associated interstitial lung disease. Eur Respir J. 2010;35:1322–8.
17. Dixon WG, Hyrich KL, Watson KD, Lunt M, Symmons DP, BSRBR Control Centre Consortium, British Society for Rheumatology Biologics Register. Influence of anti-TNF therapy on mortality in patients with rheumatoid arthritis-associated interstitial lung disease: results from the British Society for Rheumatology Biologics Register. Ann Rheum Dis. 2010;69:1086–91.
18. Solomon JJ, Ryu JH, Tazelaar HD, Myers JL, Tuder R, Cool CD, Curran-Everett D, Fischer A, Swigris JJ, Brown KK. Fibrosing interstitial pneumonia predicts survival in patients with rheumatoid arthritis-associated interstitial lung disease (RA-ILD). Respir Med. 2013;107:1247–52.
19. Takayanagi N. Biological agents and respiratory infections: causative mechanisms and practice management. Respir Investig. 2015;53:185–200.
20. Zamora-Legoff JA, Krause ML, Crowson CS, Ryu JH, Matteson EL. Risk of serious infection in patients with rheumatoid arthritis-associated interstitial lung disease. Clin Rheumatol. 2016;35:2585–9.
21. Roubille C, Haraoui B. Interstitial lung diseases induced or exacerbated by DMARDS and biologic agents in rheumatoid arthritis: a systematic literature review. Semin Arthritis Rheum. 2014;43:613–26.
22. Ohnishi H, Yokoyama A, Kondo K, Hamada H, Abe M, Nishimura K, Hiwada K, Kohno N. Comparative study of KL-6, surfactant protein-A, surfactant protein-D, and monocyte chemoattractant protein-1 as serum markers for interstitial lung diseases. Am J Respir Crit Care Med. 2002;165:378–81.
23. Nakajima H, Harigai M, Hara M, Hakoda M, Tokuda H, Sakai F, Kamatani N, Kashiwazaki S. KL-6 as a novel serum marker for interstitial pneumonia associated with collagen diseases. J Rheumatol. 2000;27:1164–70.
24. Lee YS, Kim HC, Lee BY, Lee CK, Kim MY, Jang SJ, Lee HS, Moon J, Colby TV, Kim DS. The value of biomarkers as predictors of outcome in patients with rheumatoid arthritis-associated usual interstitial pneumonia. Sarcoidosis Vasc Diffuse Lung Dis. 2016;33:216–23.
25. Richards TJ, Eggebeen A, Gibson K, Yousem S, Fuhrman C, Gochuico BR, Fertig N, Oddis CV, Kaminski N, Rosas IO, Ascherman DP. Characterization and peripheral blood biomarker assessment of anti-Jo-1 antibody-positive interstitial lung disease. Arthritis Rheum. 2009;60:2183–92.
26. Chen J, Doyle TJ, Liu Y, Aggarwal R, Wang X, Shi Y, Ge SX, Huang H, Lin Q, Liu W, Cai Y, Koontz D, Fuhrman CR, Golzarri MF, Hatabu H, Nishino M, Araki T, Dellaripa PF, Oddis CV, Rosas IO, Ascherman DP. Biomarkers of rheumatoid arthritis-associated interstitial lung disease. Arthritis Rheumatol. 2015;67:28–38.
27. Richards TJ, Kaminski N, Baribaud F, Flavin S, Brodmerkel C, Horowitz D, Li K, Choi J, Vuga LJ, Lindell KO, Klesen M, Zhang Y, Gibson KF. Peripheral blood proteins predict mortality in idiopathic pulmonary fibrosis. Am J Respir Crit Care Med. 2012;185:67–76.
28. Fujishima S, Shiomi T, Yamashita S, Yogo Y, Nakano Y, Inoue T, Nakamura M, Tasaka S, Hasegawa N, Aikawa N, Ishizaka A, Okada Y. Production and activation of matrix metalloproteinase 7 (matrilysin 1) in the lungs of patients with idiopathic pulmonary fibrosis. Arch Pathol Lab Med. 2010;134:1136–42.
29. Salmela MT, Pender SL, Karjalainen-Lindsberg ML, Puolakkainen P, Macdonald TT, Saarialho-Kere U. Collagenase-1 (MMP-1), matrilysin-1 (MMP-7), and stromelysin-2 (MMP-10) are expressed by migrating enterocytes during intestinal wound healing. Scand J Gastroenterol. 2004;39:1095–104.
30. Zuo F, Kaminski N, Eugui E, Allard J, Yakhini Z, Ben-Dor A, Lollini L, Morris D, Kim Y, DeLustro B, Sheppard D, Pardo A, Selman M, Heller RA. Gene expression analysis reveals matrilysin as a key regulator of pulmonary fibrosis in mice and humans. Proc Natl Acad Sci U S A. 2002;99:6292–7.
31. Shen H, Xia L, Lu J. Interleukin-4 in rheumatoid arthritis patients with interstitial lung disease: a pilot study. Indian J Med Res. 2013;138:919–21.
32. Jian XD, Guo GR, Ruan YJ, Zhao B, Wang YC, Ning Q, Zhang YC. [Clinical observation of rheumatoid arthritis associated interstitial lung disease patients and changes of serum cytokines thereof]. Zhonghua Yi Xue Za Zhi. 2008;88:1884–7.
33. Xiangyang Z, Lutian Y, Lin Z, Liping X, Hui S, Jing L. Increased levels of interleukin-33 associated with bone erosion and interstitial lung diseases in patients with rheumatoid arthritis. Cytokine. 2012;58:6–9.
34. Giles JT, Darrah E, Danoff S, Johnson C, Andrade F, Rosen A, Bathon JM. Association of cross-reactive antibodies targeting peptidyl-arginine deiminase 3 and 4 with rheumatoid arthritis-associated interstitial lung disease. PLoS One. 2014;9:e98794.
35. Harlow L, Rosas IO, Gochuico BR, Mikuls TR, Dellaripa PF, Oddis CV, Ascherman DP. Identification of citrullinated hsp90 isoforms as novel autoantigens in rheumatoid arthritis-associated interstitial lung disease. Arthritis Rheum. 2013;65:869–79.
36. Bernstein EJ, Barr RG, Austin JH, Kawut SM, Raghu G, Sell JL, Hoffman EA, Newell JD, Watts JR, Nath PH, Sonavane SK, Bathon JM, Majka DS, Lederer DJ. Rheumatoid arthritis-associated autoantibodies and subclinical interstitial lung disease: the Multi-Ethnic Study of Atherosclerosis. Thorax. 2016;71:1082–90.
37. Paulin F, Doyle TJ, Fletcher EA, Ascherman DP, Rosas IO. Rheumatoid arthritis-associated interstitial lung disease and idiopathic pulmonary fibrosis: shared mechanistic and phenotypic traits suggest overlapping disease mechanisms. Rev Investig Clin. 2015;67:280–6.
38. Reynisdottir G, Karimi R, Joshua V, Olsen H, Hensvold AH, Harju A, Engström M, Grunewald J, Nyren S, Eklund A, Klareskog L, Sköld CM, Catrina AI. Structural changes and antibody enrichment in the lungs are early features of anti-citrullinated protein antibody-positive rheumatoid arthritis. Arthritis Rheumatol. 2014;66:31–9.
39. Giles JT, Danoff SK, Sokolove J, Wagner CA, Winchester R, Pappas DA, Siegelman S, Connors G, Robinson WH, Bathon JM. Association of fine specificity and repertoire expansion of anti-citrullinated peptide antibodies with rheumatoid arthritis associated interstitial lung disease. Ann Rheum Dis. 2014;73:1487–94.
40. Sokolove J, Bromberg R, Deane KD, Lahey LJ, Derber LA, Chandra PE, Edison JD, Gilliland WR, Tibshirani RJ, Norris JM, Holers VM, Robinson WH. Autoantibody epitope spreading in the pre-clinical phase predicts progression to rheumatoid arthritis. PLoS One. 2012;7:e35296.

41. Furukawa H, Oka S, Shimada K, Sugii S, Ohashi J, Matsui T, Ikenaka T, Nakayama H, Hashimoto A, Takaoka H, Arinuma Y, Okazaki Y, Futami H, Komiya A, Fukui N, Nakamura T, Migita K, Suda A, Nagaoka S, Tsuchiya N, Tohma S. Association of human leukocyte antigen with interstitial lung disease in rheumatoid arthritis: a protective role for shared epitope. PLoS One. 2012;7:e33133.
42. Laki J, Lundström E, Snir O, Rönnelid J, Ganji I, Catrina AI, Bengtsson C, Saevarsdottir S, Wick MC, Alfredsson L, Klareskog L, Padyukov L. Very high levels of anti-citrullinated protein antibodies are associated with HLA-DRB1*15 non-shared epitope allele in patients with rheumatoid arthritis. Arthritis Rheum. 2012;64:2078–84.
43. Ikari K, Kuwahara M, Nakamura T, Momohara S, Hara M, Yamanaka H, Tomatsu T, Kamatani N. Association between PADI4 and rheumatoid arthritis: a replication study. Arthritis Rheum. 2005;52:3054–7.
44. Scher JU, Abramson SB. Periodontal disease, Porphyromonas gingivalis, and rheumatoid arthritis: what triggers autoimmunity and clinical disease? Arthritis Res Ther. 2013;15:122.
45. Scher JU, Ubeda C, Equinda M, Khanin R, Buischi Y, Viale A, Lipuma L, Attur M, Pillinger MH, Weissmann G, Littman DR, Pamer EG, Bretz WA, Abramson SB. Periodontal disease and the oral microbiota in new-onset rheumatoid arthritis. Arthritis Rheum. 2012;64:3083–94.
46. Mikuls TR, Payne JB, Yu F, Thiele GM, Reynolds RJ, Cannon GW, Markt J, McGowan D, Kerr GS, Redman RS, Reimold A, Griffiths G, Beatty M, Gonzalez SM, Bergman DA, Hamilton BC, Erickson AR, Sokolove J, Robinson WH, Walker C, Chandad F, O'Dell JR. Periodontitis and Porphyromonas gingivalis in patients with rheumatoid arthritis. Arthritis Rheumatol. 2014;66:1090–100.
47. Hitchon CA, Chandad F, Ferucci ED, Willemze A, Ioan-Facsinay A, van der Woude D, Markland J, Robinson D, Elias B, Newkirk M, Toes RM, Huizinga TW, El-Gabalawy HS. Antibodies to porphyromonas gingivalis are associated with anticitrullinated protein antibodies in patients with rheumatoid arthritis and their relatives. J Rheumatol. 2010;37:1105–12.
48. Makrygiannakis D, Hermansson M, Ulfgren AK, Nicholas AP, Zendman AJ, Eklund A, Grunewald J, Skold CM, Klareskog L, Catrina AI. Smoking increases peptidylarginine deiminase 2 enzyme expression in human lungs and increases citrullination in BAL cells. Ann Rheum Dis. 2008;67:1488–92.
49. Gabbay E, Tarala R, Will R, Carroll G, Adler B, Cameron D, Lake FR. Interstitial lung disease in recent onset rheumatoid arthritis. Am J Respir Crit Care Med. 1997;156:528–35.
50. Moazedi-Fuerst FC, Kielhauser S, Brickmann K, Tripolt N, Meilinger M, Lufti A, Graninger W. Sonographic assessment of interstitial lung disease in patients with rheumatoid arthritis, systemic sclerosis and systemic lupus erythematosus. Clin Exp Rheumatol. 2015;33:S87–91.
51. Cogliati C, Antivalle M, Torzillo D, Birocchi S, Norsa A, Bianco R, Costantino G, Ditto MC, Battellino M, Sarzi Puttini PC, Montano N. Standard and pocket-size lung ultrasound devices can detect interstitial lung disease in rheumatoid arthritis patients. Rheumatology (Oxford). 2014;53:1497–503.
52. Nakashita T, Ando K, Takahashi K, Motojima S. Possible effect of abatacept on the progression of interstitial lung disease in rheumatoid arthritis patients. Respir Investig. 2016;54:376–9.
53. Wang Y, Xu SQ, Xu JH, Ding C. Treatment with etanercept in a patient with rheumatoid arthritis-associated interstitial lung disease. Clin Med Insights Case Rep. 2011;4:49–52.
54. Hartung W, Maier J, Pfeifer M, Fleck M. Effective treatment of rheumatoid arthritis-associated interstitial lung disease by B-cell targeted therapy with rituximab. Case Reports Immunol. 2012;2012:272303.
55. Horai Y, Miyamura T, Shimada K, Takahama S, Minami R, Yamamoto M, Suematsu E. Eternacept for the treatment of patients with rheumatoid arthritis and concurrent interstitial lung disease. J Clin Pharm Ther. 2012;37:117–21.
56. Nakashita T, Ando K, Kaneko N, Takahashi K, Motojima S. Potential risk of TNF inhibitors on the progression of interstitial lung disease in patients with rheumatoid arthritis. BMJ Open. 2014;4:e005615.
57. Akiyama M, Kaneko Y, Yamaoka K, Kondo H, Takeuchi T. Association of disease activity with acute exacerbation of interstitial lung disease during tocilizumab treatment in patients with rheumatoid arthritis: a retrospective, case-control study. Rheumatol Int. 2016;36:881–9.
58. Atkins SR, Turesson C, Myers JL, Tazelaar HD, Ryu JH, Matteson EL, Bongartz T. Morphologic and quantitative assessment of CD20+ B cell infiltrates in rheumatoid arthritis-associated nonspecific interstitial pneumonia and usual interstitial pneumonia. Arthritis Rheum. 2006;54:635–41.

Pathology of Interstitial Lung Disease in Patients with Rheumatoid Arthritis

7

Tamiko Takemura

Abstract

Interstitial lung d isease (ILD) and airway diseases are thought to be important prognostic factors of rheumatoid arthritis (RA). Although the classification used for idiopathic interstitial pneumonias has been applied to describe the histological patterns of RA-ILD, mixtures of these histological patterns, hyperplasia of bronchus-associated lymphoid tissue, and variable bronchiolar diseases complicate a pathological diagnosis. We investigated pathological features of RA-ILD and detected characteristic cystic lesions in the pulmonary lobules of long-standing RA patients with ILD. Cystic lesions in the lung with long-standing RA that were tentatively identified as cystic bronchiolectasis were closely associated with intralobular bronchiolar damage and the subsequent alveolar reconstruction resulting from inflammatory change. Indeterminate peribronchiolar metaplasia and splitting of alveolar walls similar to the conditions observed in patients with emphysema and resulting in cystic changes in lobules were also seen in the lungs of patients with long-standing RA. The exact mechanism of peribronchiolar metaplasia with intralobular cystic alteration in the never smokers with RA still remains to be resolved. Here, we emphasize that intralobular bronchiolar lesion and cystic consequences are important for the prognosis and treatment of RA-ILD.

Keywords

Rheumatoid arthritis • Interstitial lung disease • Idiopathic interstitial pneumonia • Bronchus-associated lymphoid tissue • Intralobular bronchiolitis • Cystic bronchiolectasis

7.1 Introduction

Rheumatoid arthritis (RA) is a systemic destructive inflammatory disease. RA patients frequently suffer from extra-articular disease, especially pulmonary manifestations [1, 2]. RA affects all the anatomic compartments of the lung, i.e., pleural, broncho-bronchiolar, parenchymal involvement, as well as interstitial lung diseases [3]. Among them, interstitial pneumonia and airway diseases are thought to be the important prognostic factors for patients with RA [4–10].

T. Takemura, M.D., Ph.D.
Department of Pathology, Japanese Red Cross Medical Center, Tokyo, Japan
e-mail: byori@med.jrc.or.jp

The classification used for idiopathic interstitial pneumonias (IIPs) has been applied to describe the histological patterns of RA-associated interstitial lung disease (RA-ILD), i.e., usual interstitial pneumonia (UIP), nonspecific interstitial pneumonia (NSIP), organizing pneumonia (OP), desquamative interstitial pneumonia (DIP), and so on [11, 12]. However, mixture of these histological patterns, hyperplasia of bronchus-associated lymphoid tissue, and variable bronchiolar diseases complicate the pathological diagnosis. Furthermore, the adequacy of using RA-ILD histological patterns based on the classification for IIPs and the exact pathogenesis of interstitial pneumonia of RA have not yet been sufficiently evaluated.

A few reports have discussed the difference between the pathogenesis of interstitial pneumonia in patients with

T. Gono et al. (eds.), *Lung Disease Associated with Rheumatoid Arthritis*, https://doi.org/10.1007/978-981-10-6750-1_7

connective tissue disease (CTD-ILD) and IIPs [13, 14]. The earliest event in CTD-ILD is considered to be inflammation including alveolar epithelial injury induced by environmental pathogens or inflammation [13]. Paulin suggested that RA-ILD with a non-UIP pattern may be related to the immune response against citrullinated peptide in the lung, while RA-ILD with a UIP pattern may represent a disease process in which an IPF-like pathology triggers an immune response against citrullinated proteins [14]. Recently, the crucial role of anti-citrullinated protein/peptide antibodies (ACPA) in the lung has been reported, and these antibodies might participate in the pathogenesis of airway and parenchymal lung diseases in RA [15–18].

In this chapter, classical interstitial alterations occurring in the lung, i.e., pleural change, rheumatoid nodules, and hyperplasia of bronchus-associated lymphoid tissue, are described. Then, recent pathological advances in our knowledge of interstitial pneumonia associated with RA are discussed, i.e., new observations of the early phase of interstitial lung disease and intralobular bronchiolar damage, as well as consecutive cystic changes, are presented.

7.2 Pleural Involvement

Pleural involvement is common intrathoracic manifestation of RA, occurring in about 5% of patients [19], and pleural effusion is commonest manifestation. Pleuritis is commonly seen in autopsies of patients with RA. Histologically, nonspecific inflammatory changes are seen in the visceral pleura, i.e., fibrinous exudates, fibrosis, and chronic inflammatory cell infiltration with lymphocyte and plasma cells (Fig. 7.1a). The rupture of rheumatoid nodules in the visceral pleura and the subpleural region can result in pneumothorax (Fig. 7.1b, c).

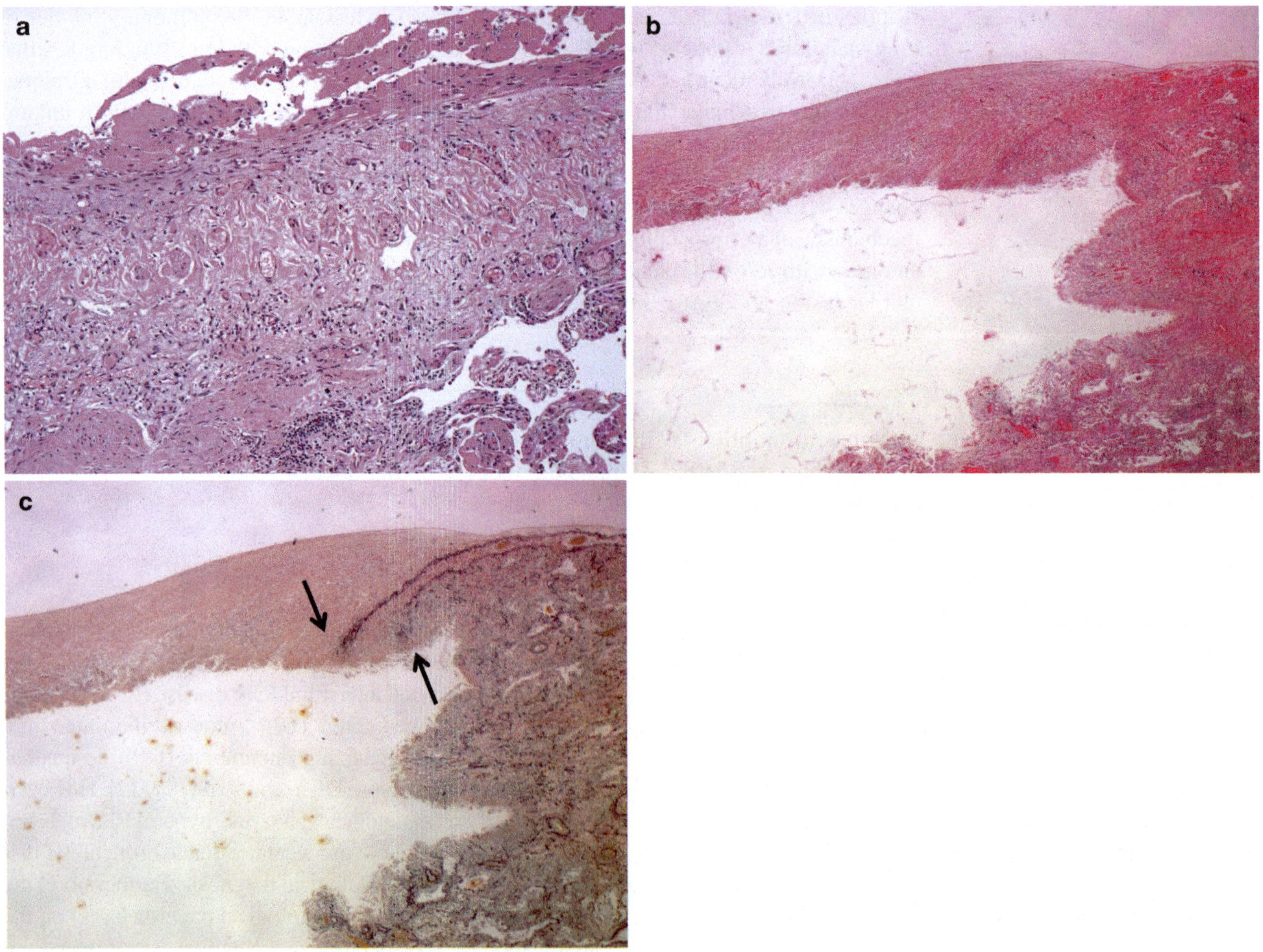

Fig. 7.1 Pleural diseases. (**a**) Fibrinous exudate is visible on the visceral pleural surface with marked fibrosis and infiltration of lymphocytes and plasma cells (HE, ×10). (**b**) Cavitary rheumatoid nodule is located just at the subpleural region with dense pleural fibrosis (HE, ×2.5). (**c**) Disruption of the external and internal elastic lamina (arrows) is seen in the subpleural rheumatoid nodule (EVG, ×2.5)

7.3 Rheumatoid Nodules

Rheumatoid nodules in the lung are seen about 20% of patients [20]. These nodules are similar to those of observed outside the lung. They may occur as singles or multiples, usually measuring 1–2 cm, and they are preferentially located in the subpleural region, consisting of central necrosis and fibrinoid necrosis with a rim of palisading histiocytes and giant cells (Fig. 7.2). Cavitary formation in the subpleural RA nodule can lead to rupture into the thoracic cavity (Fig. 7.1b, c).

7.4 Hyperplasia of Bronchus-Associated Lymphoid Tissue

Bronchus-associated lymphoid tissue (BALT) was originally described as a submucosal lymphoid organ, located along the bifurcations of the bronchi and lying between an artery and a bronchus [21, 22]. Although BALT is not conspicuous in healthy normal lung tissue, pulmonary infection or inflammation leads to the development of BALT in the lung [23]. Sato et al. described BALT as an immunological defense mechanism resulting in the production of IgA in patients with RA [24, 25]. Inducible BALT (iBALT) appears in the lung after infection or inflammation and has B-cell follicles and T-cell areas [26, 27]. iBALT is preferentially observed in patients with connective tissue disease, especially patients with RA or primary Sjögren syndrome. Rangel-Moreno demonstrated B-cell and dendritic cell proliferation and the production of various cytokines, chemokines, and ACPA in iBALT [28]. He suggested that the presence of iBALT might be correlated with tissue damage in the lungs of patients with RA.

Hyperplastic BALT, with an enlarged germinal center, are distributed along the pulmonary lymphatic vessels in the lungs, i.e., broncho-vascular bundle, interlobular septa, and pleura, of patients with RA (Fig. 7.3a). In areas of iBALT located in the bronchiolar walls, the loss of the elastic lamina

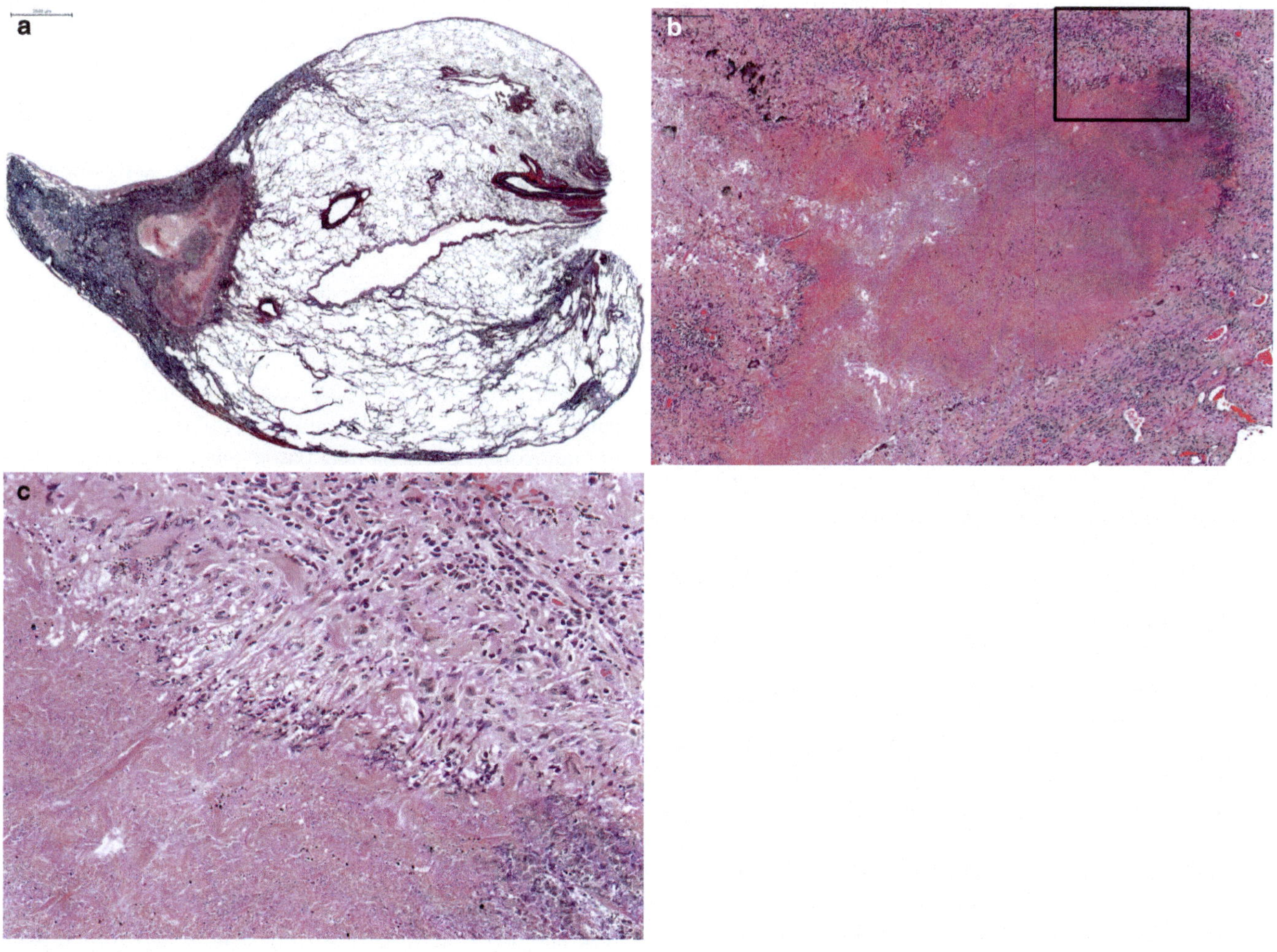

Fig. 7.2 Rheumatoid nodule. (**a**) A rheumatoid nodule is located in the atelectatic region of right S6 (EVG, ×1). (**b**) Coagulation necrosis with eosinophilic granular materials in a rheumatoid nodule is surrounded by chronic inflammatory granulation tissue (HE, ×4). (**c**) Palisading histiocytes and occasional giant cells are visible near the rim of the area of necrosis (square of **b**) (HE, ×20). (Courtesy of Dr. U. Sakurai)

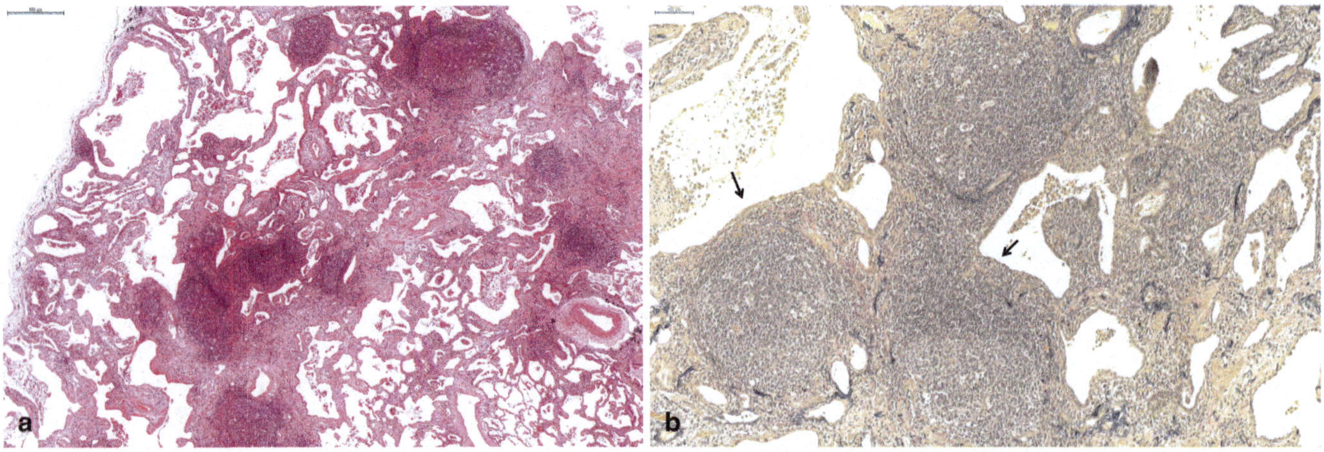

Fig. 7.3 Hyperplasia of BALT. (**a**) Hyperplasia of BALT is observed in the lung with interstitial pneumonia of RA (HE, ×4.5). (**b**) Loss of elastic fibers (arrows) are detected in the bronchiolar wall involved by BALT (EVG, ×10)

and fibrosis are also observed (Fig. 7.3b). iBALT is also observed in alveoli with indiscernible alveolar structure. Histological alterations of surgical lung biopsy specimens of RA lungs suggest the participation of iBALT in the destruction of the lung architecture. Tissue damage with iBALT and inflammatory cell infiltration in the lungs of RA patients will be further discussed in Sect. 7.6.

7.5 Interstitial Pneumonia in Patients with RA

7.5.1 Current Understanding

The radiological and pathological patterns of interstitial pneumonia in patients with RA have been reported by applying the classification used for IIPs [11, 12, 29–36]. Recent studies have reported a higher incidence of UIP than NSIP or OP [2, 33–38]. The prognosis of RA patients with UIP has been reported to be poorer than that of patients with other histological patterns [35–37, 40]. However, Zamora-Legoff reported that survival of the patients with RA-ILD did not differ between UIP, NSIP, and OP using with GAP (gender, age, lung physiology) model [39].

Pathologically, lymphoid follicles with germinal centers, pleuritis, bronchiolitis, and plasma cell infiltration are more prominent in RA-UIP than in IPF/UIP, while fibroblastic foci are less common in RA-ILD [40–43].

We recently examined the characteristic cystic bronchiolar lesions found in patients with RA-ILD. Although these pathological alterations until now were classified as honeycomb cyst in a so-called UIP pattern in patients with RA, they were not the same as honeycomb lesion seen in IPF/UIP. These findings are crucial to understanding remodeling and prognosis of RA patients with interstitial lung disease. These bronchiolar alterations are discussed further in Sect. 7.6.

7.5.2 Nonspecific Interstitial Pneumonia in Patients with RA

7.5.2.1 What Constitutes the Early Stage of Interstitial Pneumonia in Patients with RA?

Figure 7.4 shows slight ground-glass opacification on a high-resolution CT (HRCT) image of a young patient with a high titer of ACPA (258 U/mL) and high rheumatoid factor. A surgical lung biopsy revealed slight thickening of the alveolar septa and good preservation of the alveolar structures (Fig. 7.5).

Another site of poorly aerated lung tissue of the same specimen showed the infiltration of plasma cells into the alveolar walls with collagen deposition with preserved alveolar structure (Fig. 7.6). These histological features are compatible with those of NSIP pattern (cellular and fibrotic) and immunocompetent cells may participate in the early lesions of interstitial pneumonia in patients with RA. In this case, the bronchioles are slightly involved. Gochuico et al. also reported the characteristics of preclinical interstitial lung disease in patients with RA [44]. Overall, 33% of patients with RA without dyspnea or a cough had preclinical ILD as identified using HRCT and exhibited a NSIP histology. The presence of ACPA is associated with parenchymal lung abnormalities [45] and histological findings of interstitial plasm cell infiltration reflect circulating ACPA-specific plasma cells [46].

7.5.2.2 Progressive Stage of NSIP in Patients with RA

Fibrosing NSIP (f-NSIP) in patients with RA appears as diffuse panlobular fibrosis of the alveolar walls with temporal homogeneity and is frequently accompanied by BALT hyperplasia. Interlobular and broncho-vascular bundle fibrosis and bronchiolitis are often observed in surgical lung

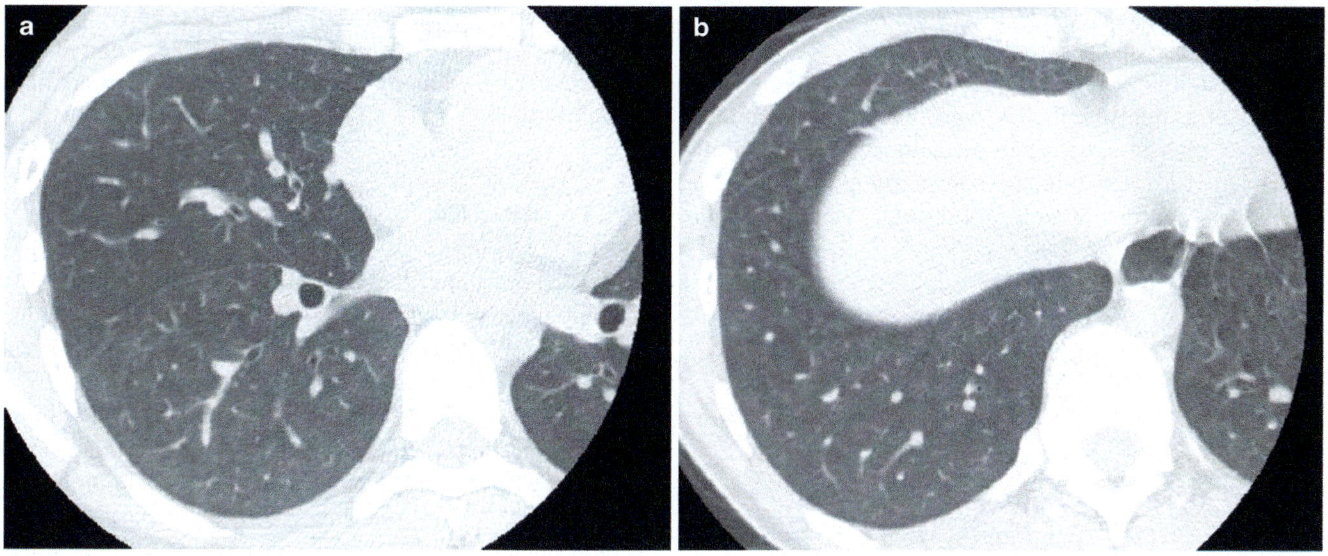

Fig. 7.4 HRCT of an early stage of NSIP pattern. HRCT of a young woman with rheumatoid arthritis shows mild ground-glass opacity of the right upper lobe (**a**) and lower lobe (**b**). Courtesy of Dr. H. Sugimoto

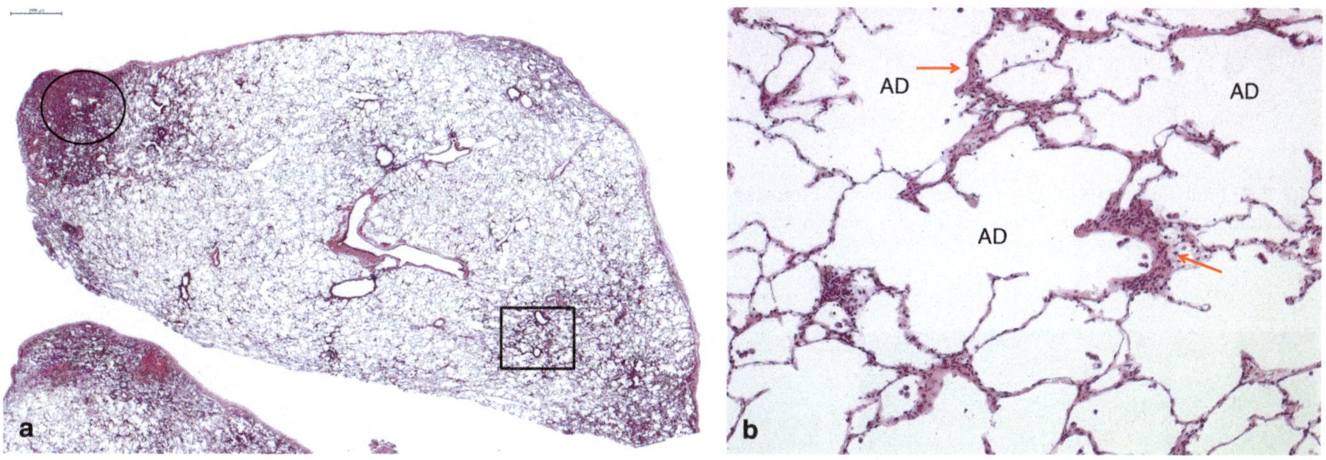

Fig. 7.5 Early stage of NSIP. (**a**) A panoramic view of the lower lobe of a case shown in Fig. 7.4. Alveolar structures are well preserved (HE, ×1). (**b**) A square of the figure (**a**) shows slight thickening of the alveolar walls (arrows) with mild mononuclear cell infiltration (HE, ×10). *AD* alveolar duct

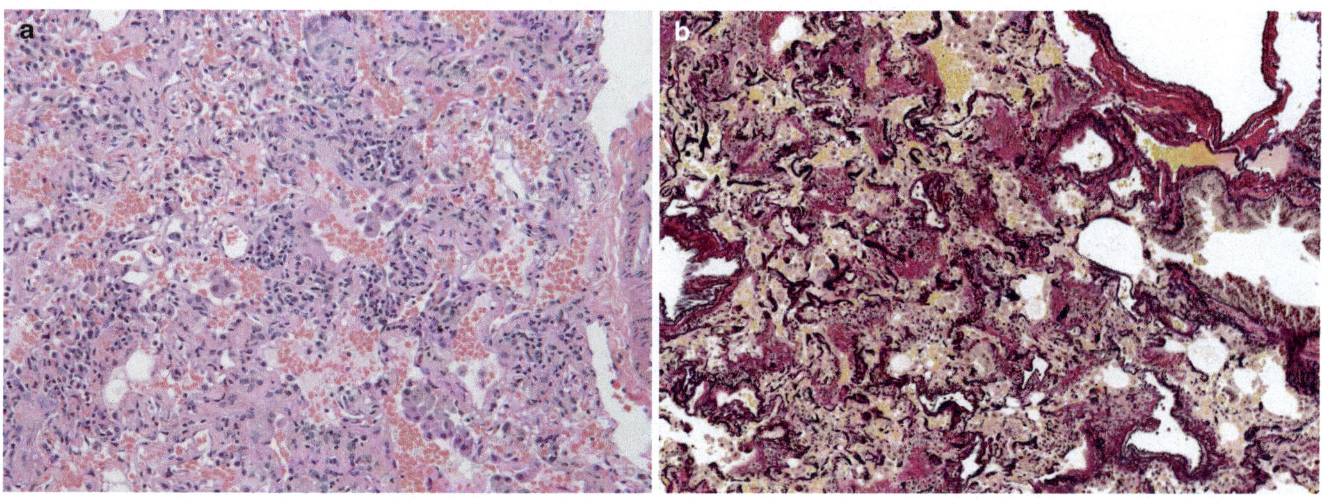

Fig. 7.6 Poorly aerated lesion (a circled area) shown in Fig. 7.5a. (**a**) Poorly aerated area shows infiltration of plasma cells in the alveolar walls (HE, ×20). (**b**) Mural-incorporated fibrosis is visible in the alveolar walls (EVG, ×10)

biopsy specimens (Fig. 7.7). Bronchiolitis, especially cellular and destructive types, is often coexistent.

The pathological subsequent changes arising from f-NSIP in patients with RA were examined in autopsy cases. In one case in which an autopsy was performed 8 years after a surgical biopsy shown in Fig. 7.7, the lower lobes were contracted with prominent broncho-bronchiolectasis and subpleural alveoli had collapsed (Fig. 7.8a). The secondary lobules revealed the airspace enlargement with dilatation of membranous and terminal bronchioles (Fig. 7.8b).

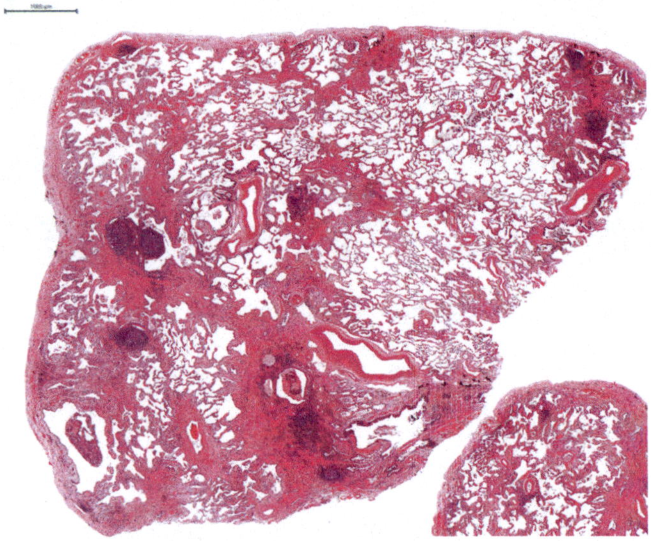

Fig. 7.7 Fibrosing NSIP in RA of a man in his 50s. Fibrosing NSIP with cellular bronchiolitis and lymphoid follicles. Note interlobular and broncho-vascular fibrosis (HE, ×1)

7.5.3 UIP in RA

UIP is the most prevalent pattern of RA-ILD, preferentially involving men with older age [34–38]. It is important to discriminate UIP from non-UIP patterns, because of clinical implications with regard to treatment and prognosis.

UIP/IPF is characterized by perilobular fibrosis with an abrupt transition to normal lung tissue resulting in a patchwork-like appearance, honeycombing, and fibroblastic foci [11]. RA/UIP is characterized by hyperplasia of lymphoid follicles with germinal centers, and interstitial infiltration of the lymphocytes and plasma cells are frequently observed in addition to the common feature of UIP [40, 42, 43], while fibroblastic foci are less common than IPF/UIP [41, 42]. Histopathological comparison between RA/UIP and IPF/UIP is presented in Table 7.1.

7.5.3.1 Early Stage of UIP in RA

A preclinical early phase of UIP has been occasionally observed in patients with RA. Figure 7.9 shows the early stage of a UIP pattern in an RA patient. The patient had a history of smoking and high ACPA titer (753 U/mL), and a

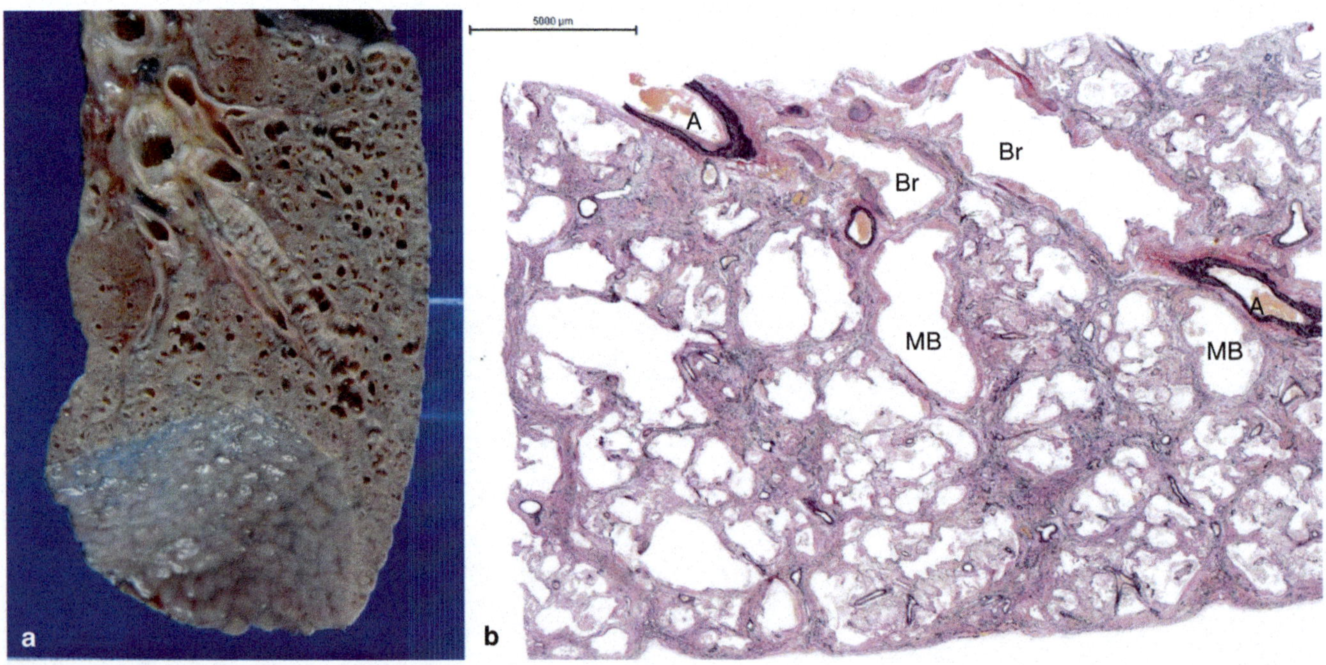

Fig. 7.8 Autopsy lung, 6 years after a surgical lung biopsy shown in Fig. 7.7. (**a**) Gross feature of the left lower lobe shows bronchiolectasis. (**b**) Broncho-bronchiolectasis and airspace enlargement are visible (EVG, ×3.5). *Br* bronchus, *MB* membranous bronchiole, *A* pulmonary artery

reticular pattern in the lower lobe was observed using HRCT. However, the patient did not have any apparent respiratory symptoms.

Although a panoramic view of the histology was consistent with UIP, a centrilobular bronchiolar change was observed in one lobule (Fig. 7.10a).

The centrilobular lesion exhibited chronic inflammation involving the terminal and respiratory bronchioles with destruction of alveolar structure (Fig. 7.10b). Adjacent lobule separated by the interlobular septum appeared normal. Mucus filling and neutrophil infiltration were observed in the centrilobular area. Cystic lesions resembling honeycombing were located in an adjacent lobule. The centrilobular bronchiolar destruction suggests to represent the initial cystic changes of the lobules in RA/UIP.

Intralobular bronchiolar inflammation and destruction are important contributors to disease progression in RA. This intralobular bronchiolar damage cannot be observed in IPF/UIP. After inflammation, such lesions can progress to intralobular cystic lesions in patients with RA.

As for the histogenesis of honeycomb cyst in the lungs of patients with IPF/UIP, the first events are perilobular fibrosis and collapse and alveolar structural destruction without inflammation, followed by dilatation of the alveolar ducts and respiratory bronchioles [47]. Thus, the honeycomb lesions observed in IPF/UIP are completely different from those arising from bronchiolar inflammation and destruction in the lobule in patients with RA. To my knowledge, the histogenesis of the honeycomb-like cysts occurring in RA-ILD has not been reported. In the less affected upper lobe of the present case of Fig. 7.10, infiltration of plasma cells in the interlobular septum and focal alveolar wall fibrosis are observed (Fig. 7.11).

Table 7.1 Comparison of pathological features between RA/UIP and IPF/UIP

	RA/UIP	IPF/UIP
Interstitial inflammation	Marked	Mild
Plasma cell infiltration	Marked	Mild
Fibroblastic foci	Occasional	Frequent
Lymphoid follicles with germinal center	Prominent	Occasional ~ absent
Bronchiolitis, cellular, and destructive	Frequent	Occasional ~ absent
Organizing pneumonia	Often	Occasional ~ absent
Bronchiolectasis	Marked	Occasional ~ marked
Honeycomb	Occasional	Frequent
Cyst connecting to the bronchioles	Frequent	Occasional
Pleuritis	Frequent	Occasional

7.5.3.2 Progressive Stage of UIP in RA

The most common HRCT image of UIP in patients with RA is shown in Fig. 7.12. This case was an elder woman who was diagnosed as having RA 3 years previously and who had a high ACPA titer (690 U/mL). The upper lobe exhibited dense subpleural fibrosis with inflammatory cell infiltration and an abrupt transition to normal alveoli (Fig. 7.13a).

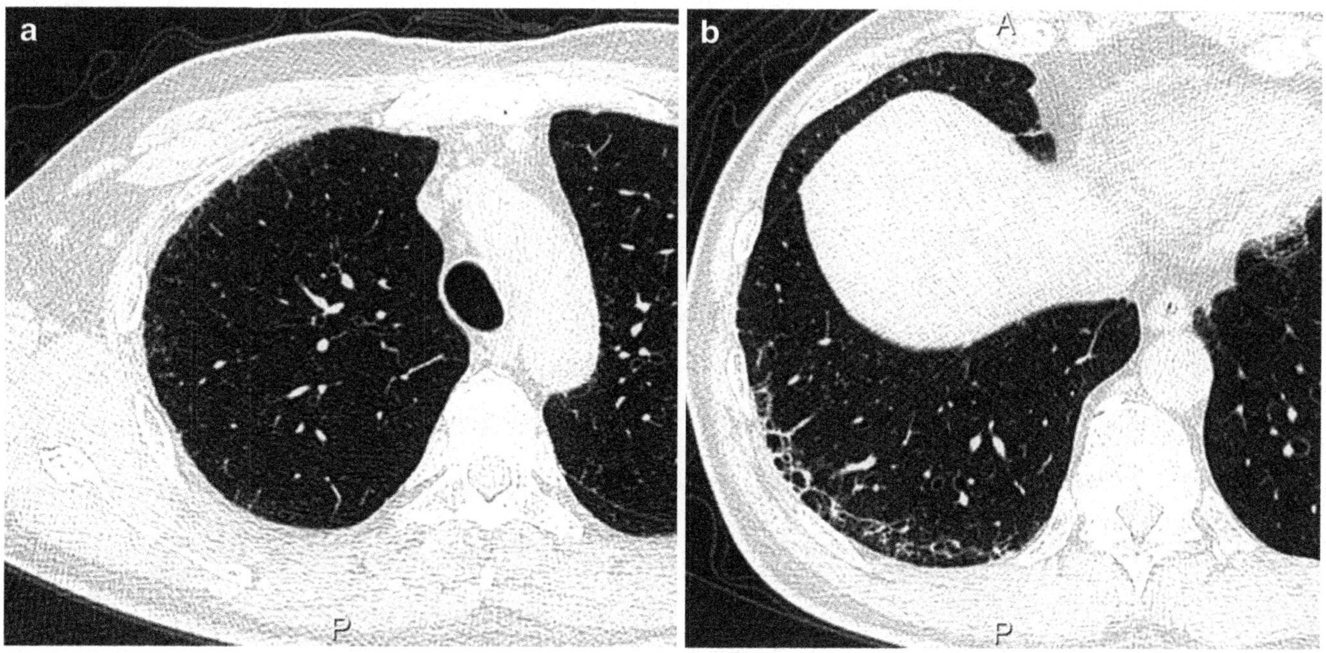

Fig. 7.9 Early stage of UIP in a male smoker with RA. (**a**) HRCT shows a ground-glass opacity in the right upper lobe. (**b**) A linear reticular pattern in the inner zone is observed in the right lower lobe

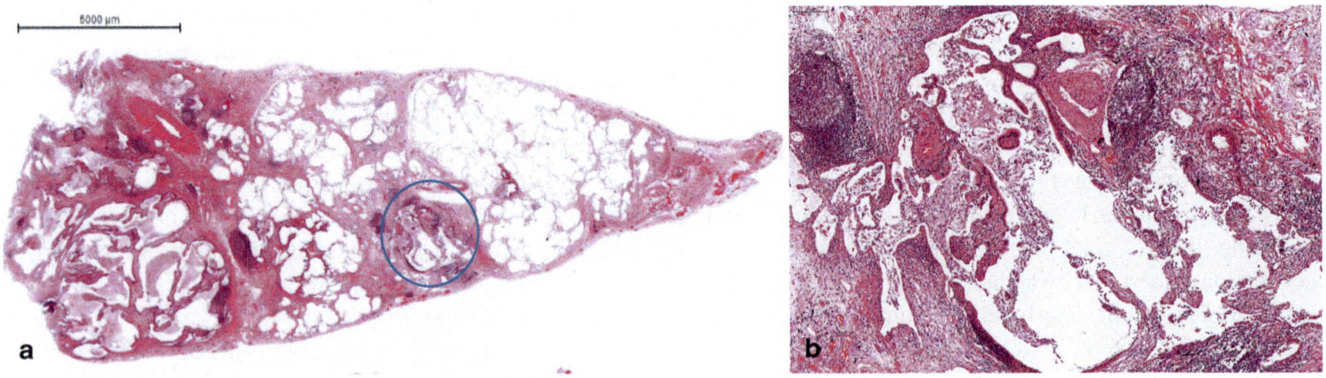

Fig. 7.10 UIP pattern with early bronchiolar lesion of right lower lobe. (**a**) A panoramic view of the right lower lobe (HE, ×1). Perilobular fibrosis is observed with an abrupt transition to the normal alveoli. A micro-honeycomb lesion is visible on the left side. Note a bronchiolar lesion in a lobule (circle). (**b**) Bronchiolitis involving a terminal and respiratory bronchioles with destruction of the bronchiolar walls and alveoli. Mucus repletion and infiltration of neutrophils are seen in the dilated airspace (HE, ×8.5). Courtesy of Dr. S. Izumi

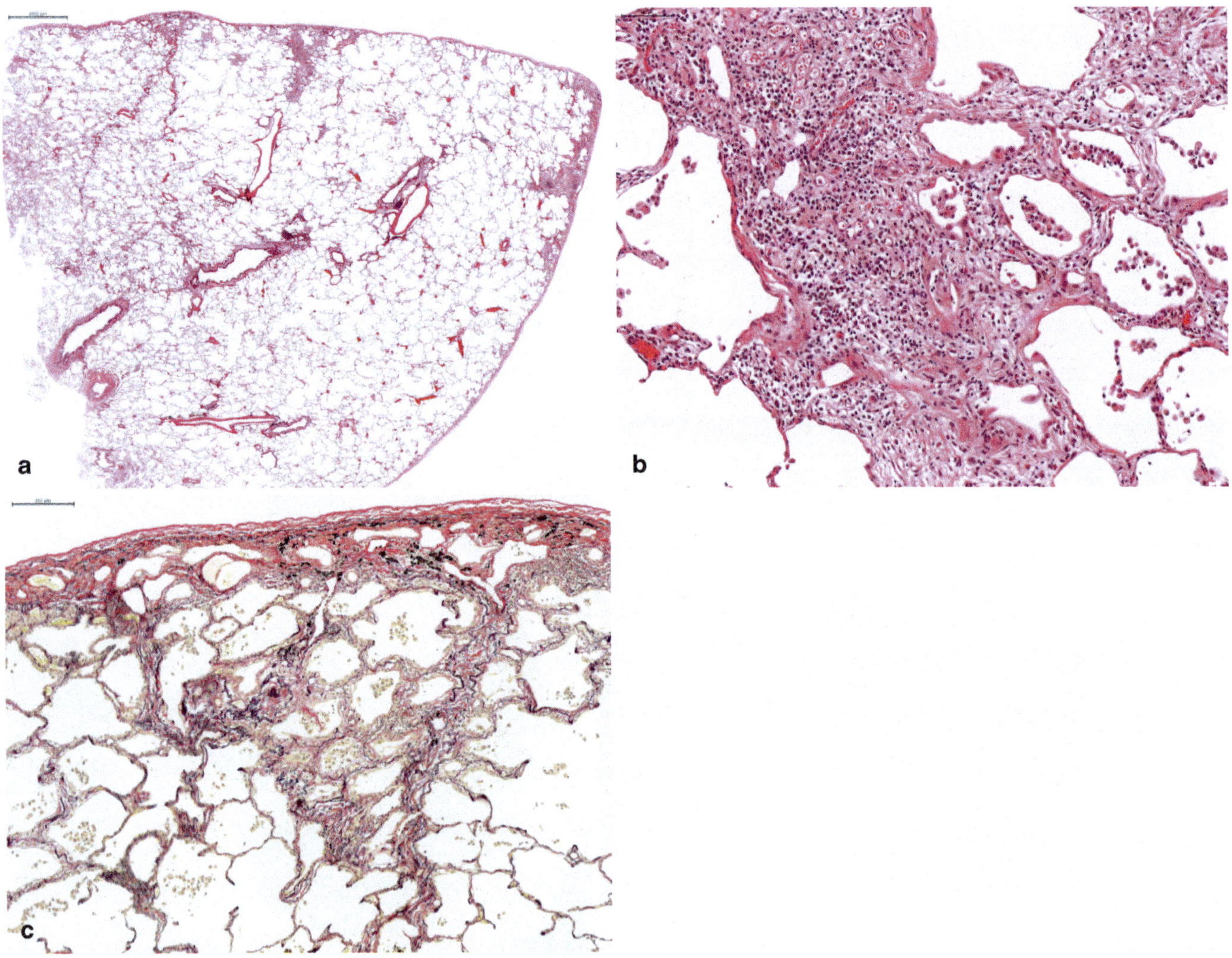

Fig. 7.11 Upper lobe of the same patient shown in Figs. 7.9 and 7.10. (**a**) A panoramic view of the upper lobe (HE, ×1). (**b**) Plasma cells infiltrate to the interlobular septum (HE, ×20). (**c**) Focal alveolar wall fibrosis is visible (EVG, ×10)

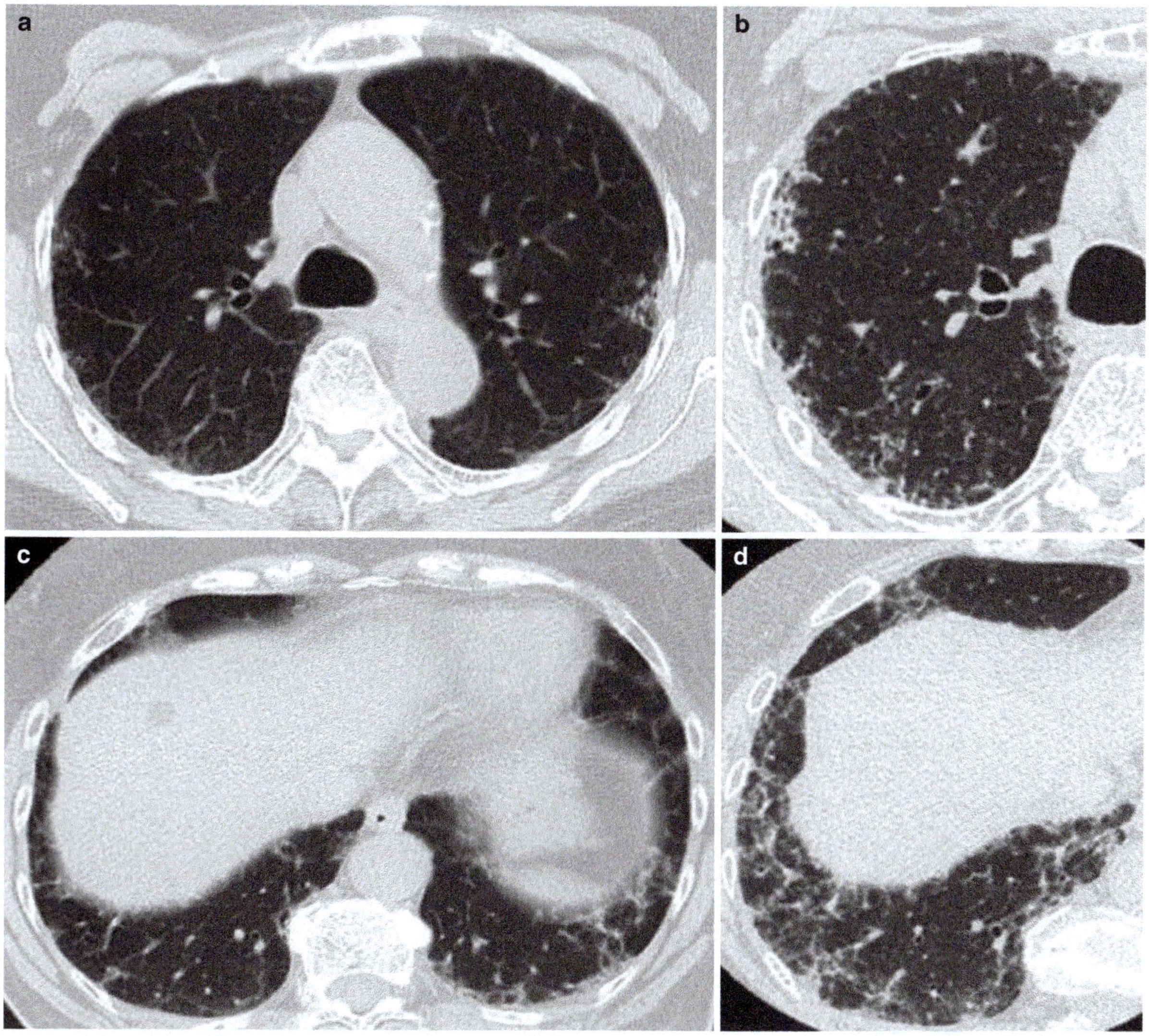

Fig. 7.12 HRCT of RA-UIP of a woman in her 60s with a 4-year history of RA and a high ACPA titer (690 U/mL). (**a**, **b**) Reticular opacities predominantly are seen in the subpleural region and perilobular opacities of the upper lobe. (**c**, **d**) Reticular and ground-glass opacities along bronchovascular bundle and honeycombing are seen in the lower lobe

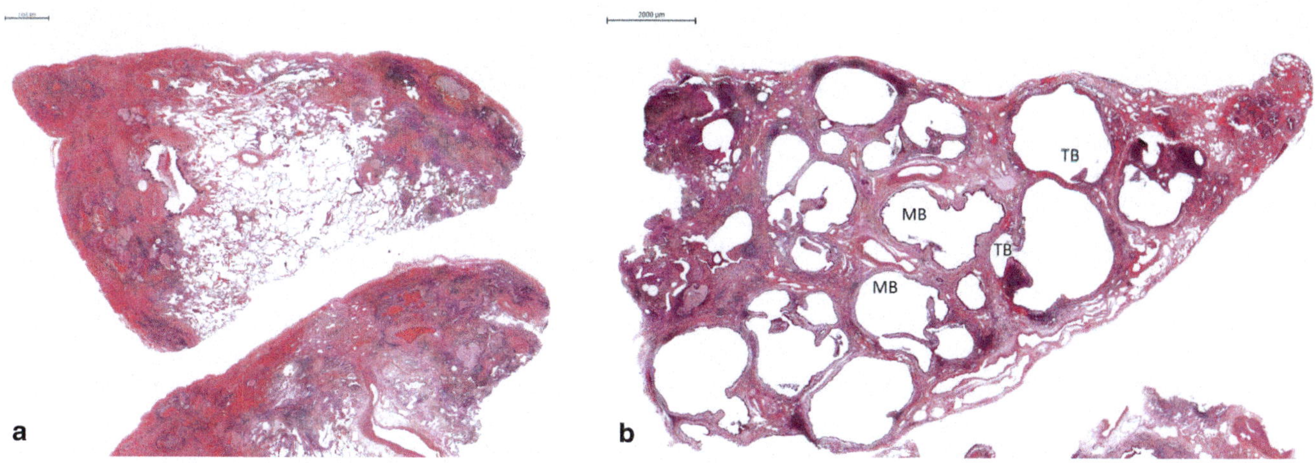

Fig. 7.13 Histology of RA-UIP of the same case shown in Fig. 7.12. (**a**) Upper lobe shows dense subpleural fibrosis with inflammatory cell infiltration and abrupt transition to the normal alveoli (HE, ×1.5). (**b**) The lower lobe of the same case shows multiple up to 3-mm-size cysts like honeycombing with lymphoid aggregates (HE, ×1). *MB* membranous bronchiole, *TB* terminal bronchiole

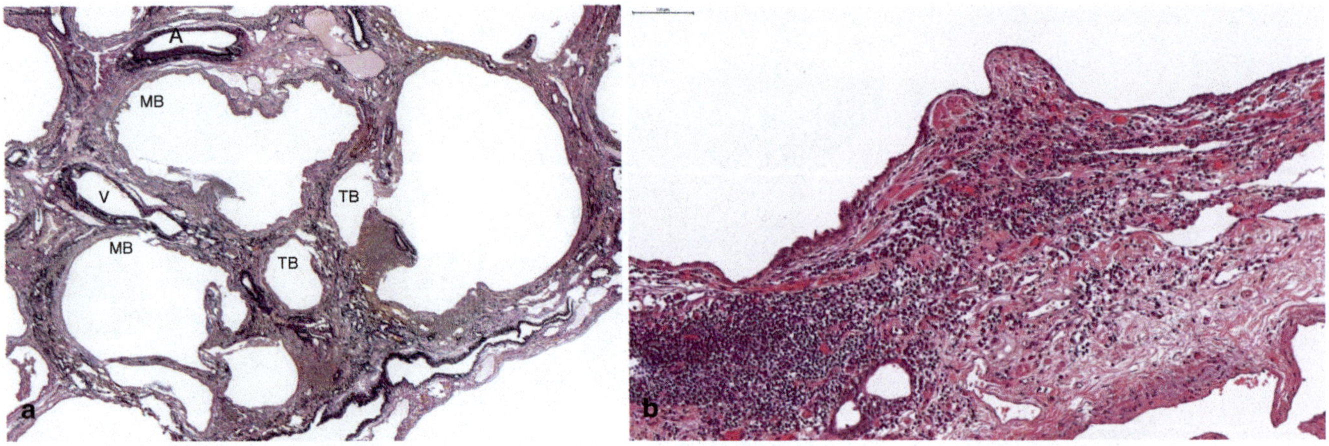

Fig. 7.14 Characteristics of the cystic lesion. (**a**) Cysts are identified as bronchioles by wall component and bronchiolar epithelial lining. Continuous dilatation of respiratory bronchiole and alveoli (EVG, ×3.3). *MB* membranous bronchiole, *TB* terminal bronchiole, *A* pulmonary artery, *V* pulmonary vein. (**b**) Subpleural area of the cyst wall shows marked infiltration of lymphocytes and plasma cells (HE, ×20). Courtesy of Dr. T. Ogura

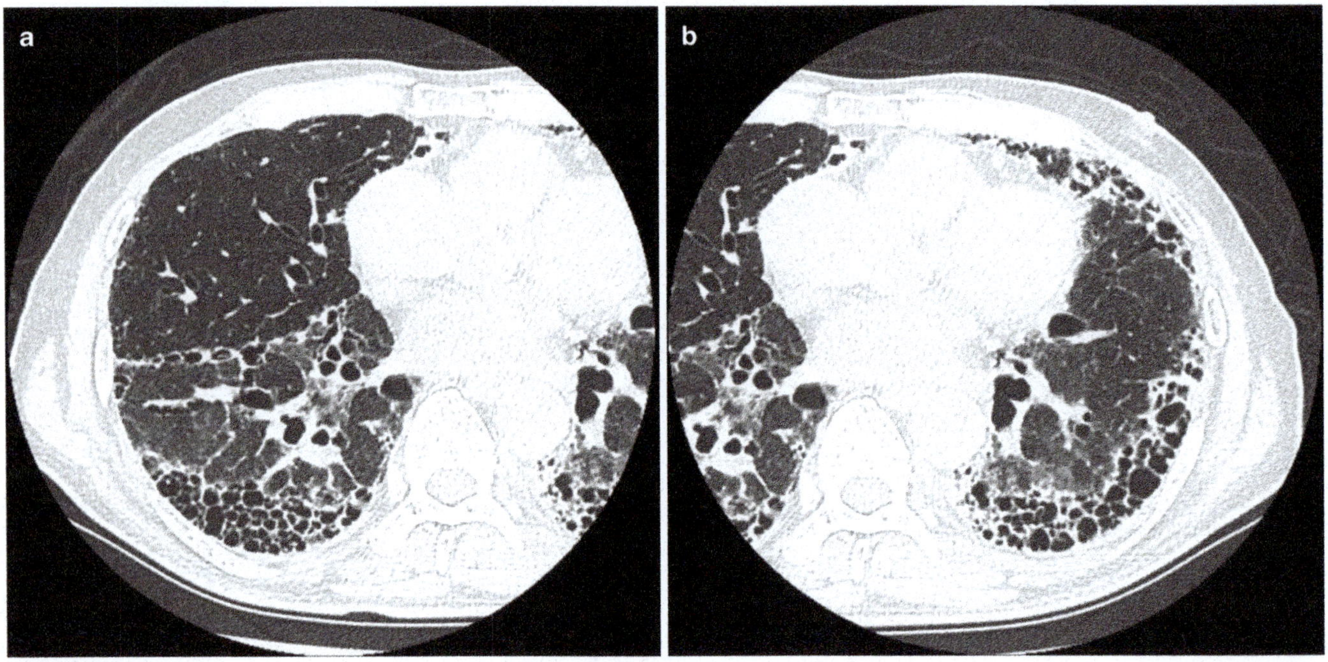

Fig. 7.15 HRCT of multiple cystic changes like honeycomb cysts in a man in his 70s with a 13-year history of RA. (**a**) Right lung. (**b**) Left lung. Courtesy of Dr. S. Izumi

The lower lobe showed multiple cystic lesions, resembling honeycombing (Fig. 7.13b). The cystic lesions measured up to 3 mm in size, and most were in communication with the membranous bronchioles. Smooth muscle cells and lamina elastic belonging to the bronchiolar wall were observed (Fig. 7.14a). However, all areas of the cyst walls were not consistent with those of bronchiolar walls, but destroyed alveoli were detected in some area of the cystic wall. The subpleural area exhibited collapse and chronic inflammatory cell infiltration (Fig. 7.14b). These cystic lesions were thought to represent the process of intralobular bronchiolar inflammation with destruction of the walls and loss of alveolar structures. After inflammation, the cystic lesions became lined by bronchiolar epithelia with fibrous walls. Figure 7.15 shows multiple cysts in the subpleural area of bilateral lower lobe on HRCT, resulting from persistent airway inflammation in a man in his 70s with a 13-year history of RA. An autopsied lung with RA-UIP showed distinctly

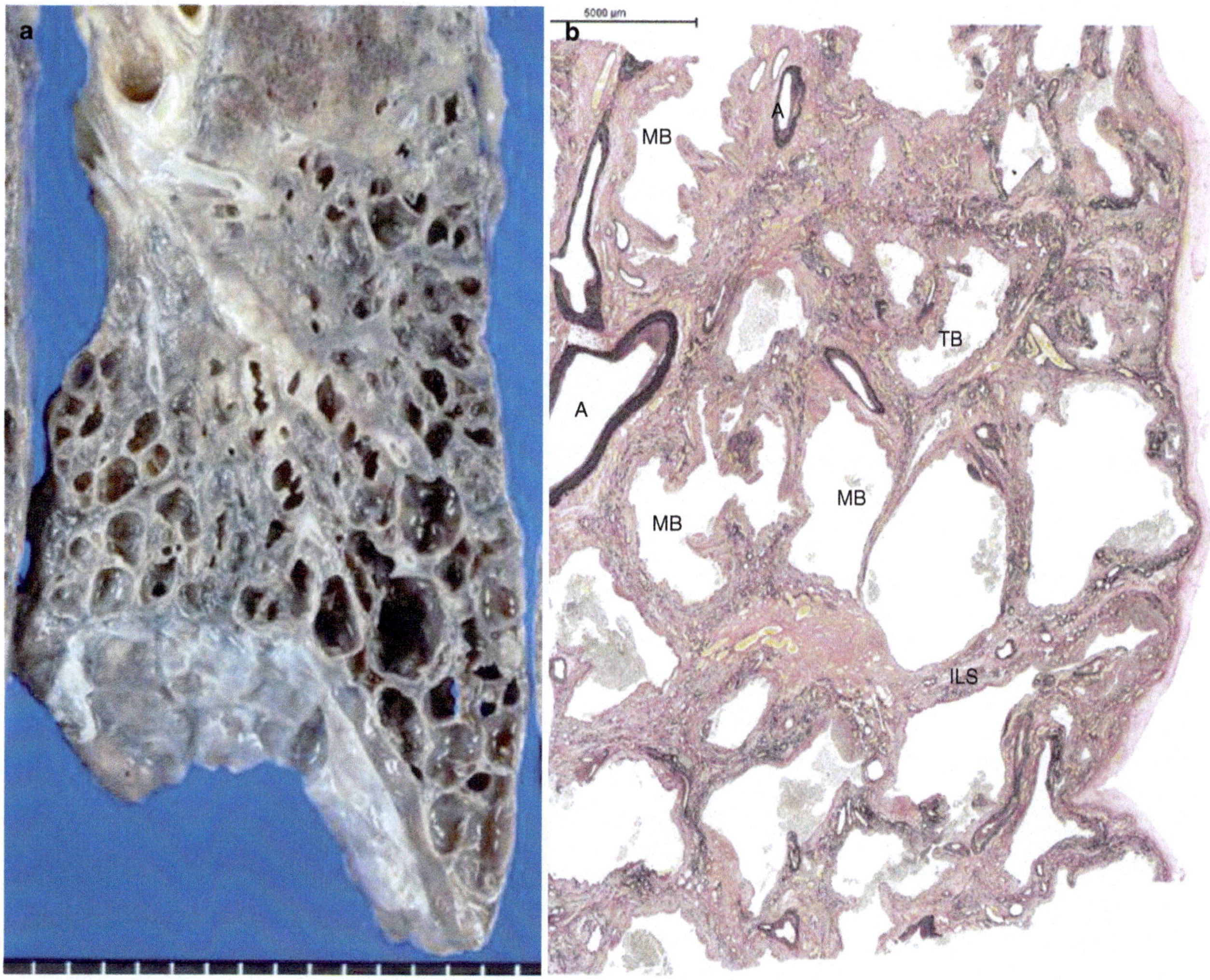

Fig. 7.16 Autopsied lung of the same patient shown in Fig. 7.15. (**a**) Marked broncho-bronchiolectasis of the left lower lobe. 5 mm; interspace. (**b**) Irregular dilatation of membranous bronchioles and continuous dilatation of the terminal and respiratory bronchioles and collapsed alveoli (EVG, ×3.3). *MB* membranous bronchiole, *TB* terminal bronchiole, *ILS* interlobular septum, *A* pulmonary artery.

visible cystic bronchioles reaching to the visceral pleura (Figs. 7.15 and 7.16). Cystic broncho-bronchiolectasis had involved almost all of the lower lobe with the destruction of the bronchiolar walls and alveolar structure.

Thus, the most cystic lesions in the lung with RA-UIP are composed of dilated bronchioles, not identical to honeycomb cysts observed in IPF/UIP.

7.6 Peripheral Airway Diseases Associated with Interstitial Pneumonia in Patients with RA

As the detailed pathological descriptions of broncho-bronchiolar diseases are described in Sect. 2.3, intralobular small airway diseases (namely, terminal and respiratory bronchiolar diseases) associated with interstitial pneumonia in patients with RA will be discussed in this section. Bronchiolitis, i.e., follicular bronchiolitis and constrictive bronchiolitis, is frequently observed in patients with RA [48–51].

Intralobular bronchiolitis, especially cellular and destructive bronchiolitis often involving the adjacent alveolar structure, can result in reconstruction of the alveolar structure with subsequent cystic formation.

7.6.1 Cystic Changes Coexisting in Chronic Fibrosing Interstitial Pneumonia

RA patients with interstitial pneumonia frequently have bronchiolitis [42, 43]. Figure 7.17 shows f-NSIP pattern with cellular and destructive bronchiolitis involving a respiratory bronchiole. Although the patient had been treated with steroid and methotrexate, cystic lesions gradually developed (Fig. 7.18). Six years later, an autopsy revealed multiple thick-walled cysts in the upper lobes (Fig. 7.19). A histologi-

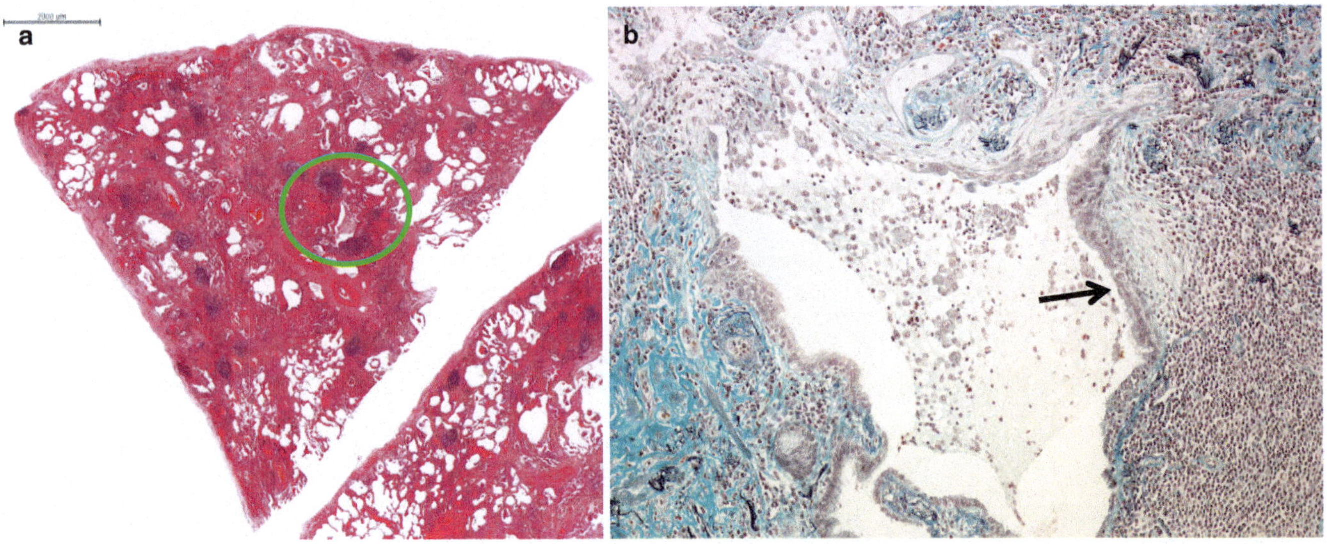

Fig. 7.17 f-NSIP with cellular and destructive bronchiolitis of a man in his 50s. (**a**) A panoramic view of f-NSIP of a man who was a current smoker (HE, ×1.5). (**b**) The circled area of figure (**a**) shows cellular and destructive bronchiolitis. Fibroblastic focus (arrow) is located at the respiratory bronchiole (Elastica-Masson, ×10)

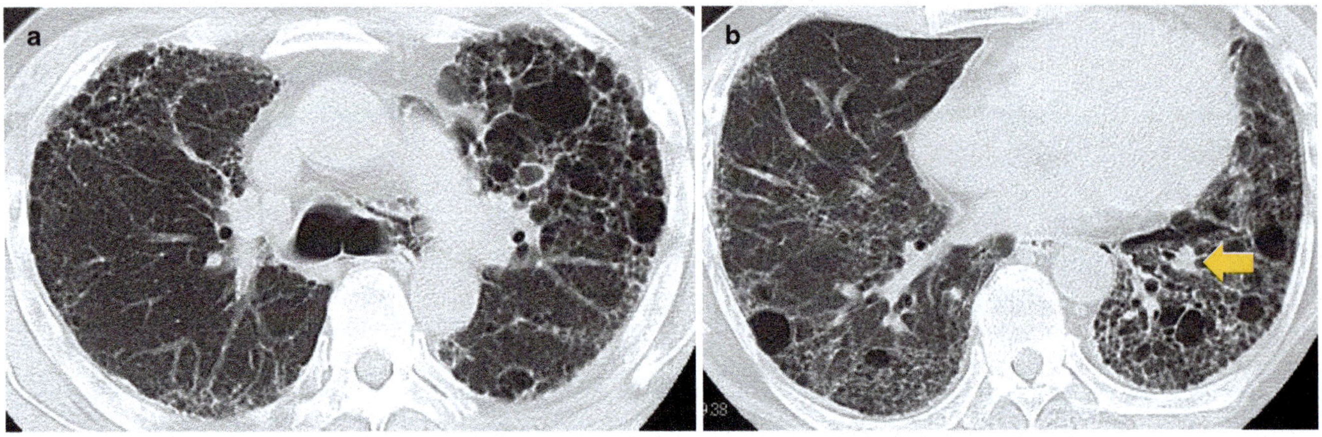

Fig. 7.18 Progressive cystic lesions on HRCT during 6 years. Thin-walled cystic lesions are located prominently in the inner zone and subpleural areas with diffuse reticular opacities. (**a**) Upper lobe; (**b**) lower lobe. Note nodular consolidation in the left S6 which was identified as *Mycobacterium avium* infection (arrow)

cal examination revealed the cysts to be connected to the terminal bronchioles with dense collagen deposition in the walls. The surrounding alveoli had collapsed.

In long-standing RA patients, cystic lesions involving a whole pulmonary lobule, similar to honeycombing in IPF/UIP, are frequently observed.

Figure 7.20 shows interstitial pneumonia and multiple ring shadows involving peripheral airways in the lungs in a man in his 50s. An early lesion of the lingula occurred in the centrilobular area with inflammatory involvement of respiratory bronchiole and destruction of the alveoli (Fig. 7.21). These findings represent the initial change occurring in a respiratory bronchiole in the centrilobular (centriacinar) region. The other area of the lingula exhibited interstitial pneumonia of NSIP and cystic peripheral lobule with marked inflammatory cell infiltration (Fig. 7.22).

In the lower lobe in the present case, the membranous bronchiole was completed destroyed and replaced by thick fibrous tissue with loss of elastic fibers of the bronchiolar walls and loss of alveolar structure (Fig. 7.23a, b). The area of the lobule with prominent inflammation showed marked destruction of the alveolar structures (Fig. 7.24), unlike honeycombing in UIP/IPF.

Cystic lesions in RA-ILD originating from bronchiolitis become enlarged with the progressive destruction of the bronchiolar walls and alveolar structures.

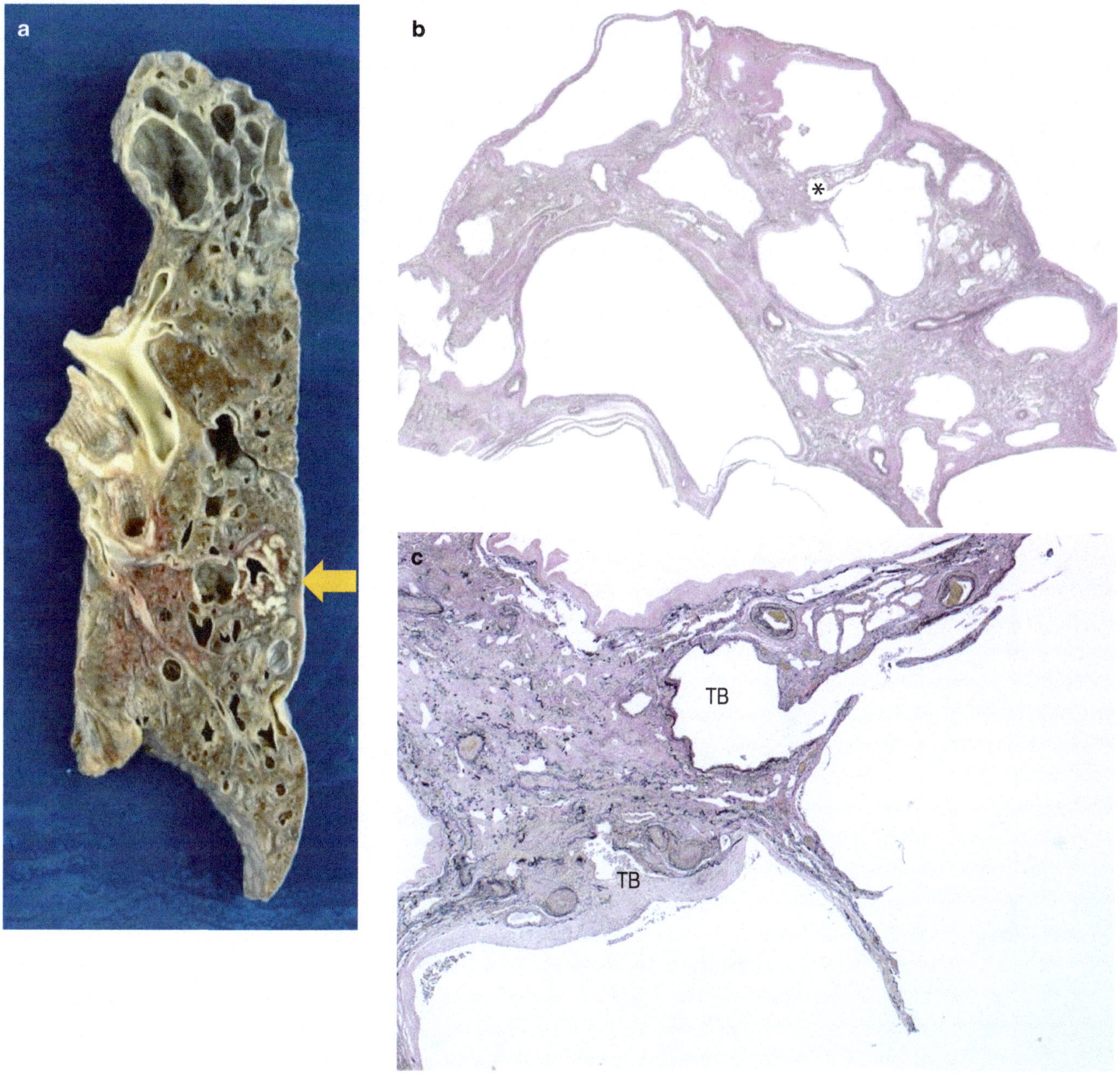

Fig. 7.19 Autopsied lung from the same case. (**a**) Up to 5 cm cystic lesions located in the upper lobe. Note caseous necrosis in the cystic lesion of left S6 (arrow). (**b**) A panoramic view of the left upper lobe shows multiple cysts and atelectasis of alveoli in between cysts (EVG, ×1). *Terminal bronchiole (**c**) Cysts communicate with the terminal bronchus (*). (EVG, ×5). *TB* terminal bronchiole

Cystic involvement of the bronchioles was more prominent in the lower lobes, most of which are induced by intralobular bronchiolar destruction with inflammation.

Generally, the pathogenesis of bronchiectasis is considered to be infection, mucosal inflammation, and the production of elastases and matrix metalloproteinases with the resulting destruction of bronchial structures [52–56]. Mori reported that bronchial dilatation is a common radiological change observed in early and long-standing RA patients [53]. Thus, intralobular inflammatory bronchiolar disease with subsequent bronchiolectasis with destruction of intralobular bronchiolar and alveolar structures should be emphasized in the lung with RA-ILD.

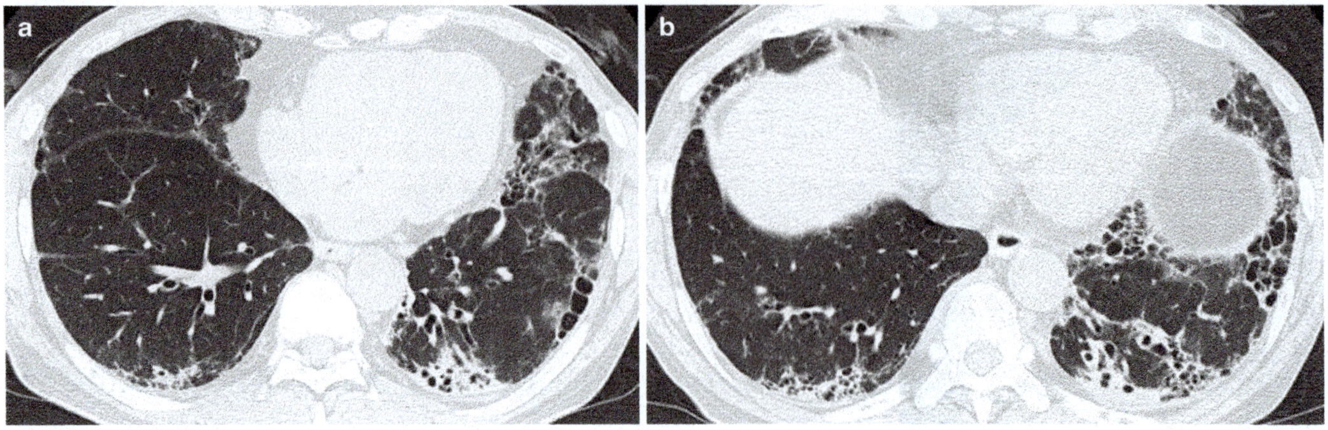

Fig. 7.20 HRCT of a man in his 50s with poorly controlled RA. (**a**) Lingula shows bronchiectasis with surrounding ground-glass opacity. (**b**) Basal area shows marked bronchiectasis with subpleural cystic lesions similar to honeycombing. Courtesy of Dr. H. Tokuda

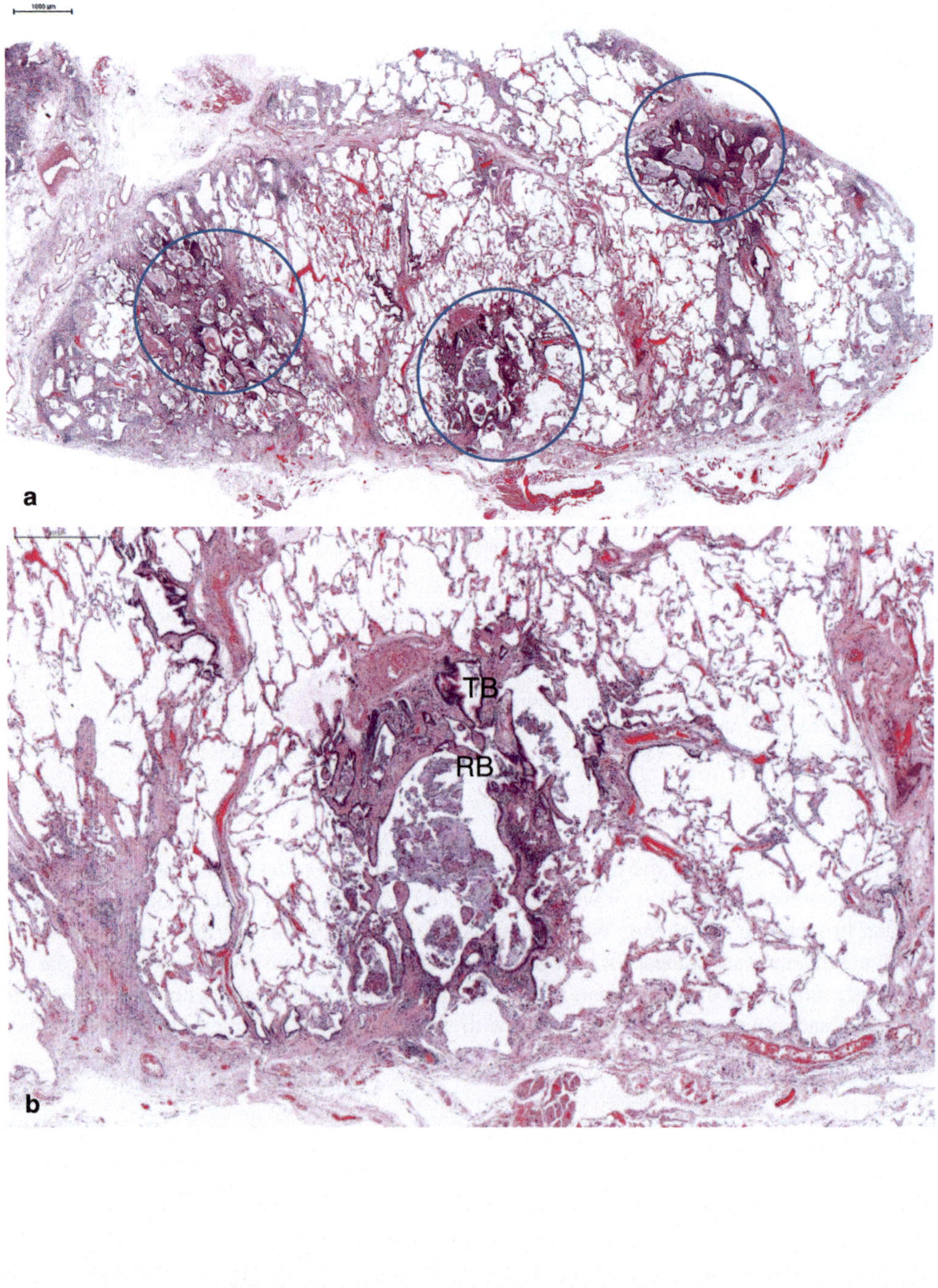

Fig. 7.21 Bronchiolar disease of the lingula of this case. (**a**) A panoramic view of the lingula. Centrilobular inflammatory changes (circles) involving a terminal and respiratory bronchiole can be observed (HE, ×1.5). (**b**) Intralobular bronchiolar involvement reveals the inflammatory cells and mucus retention with neutrophil infiltration. Destruction of the respiratory bronchiole and alveolar structure can be observed in the centrilobular area (HE, ×5). *TB* terminal bronchiole, *RB* respiratory bronchiole

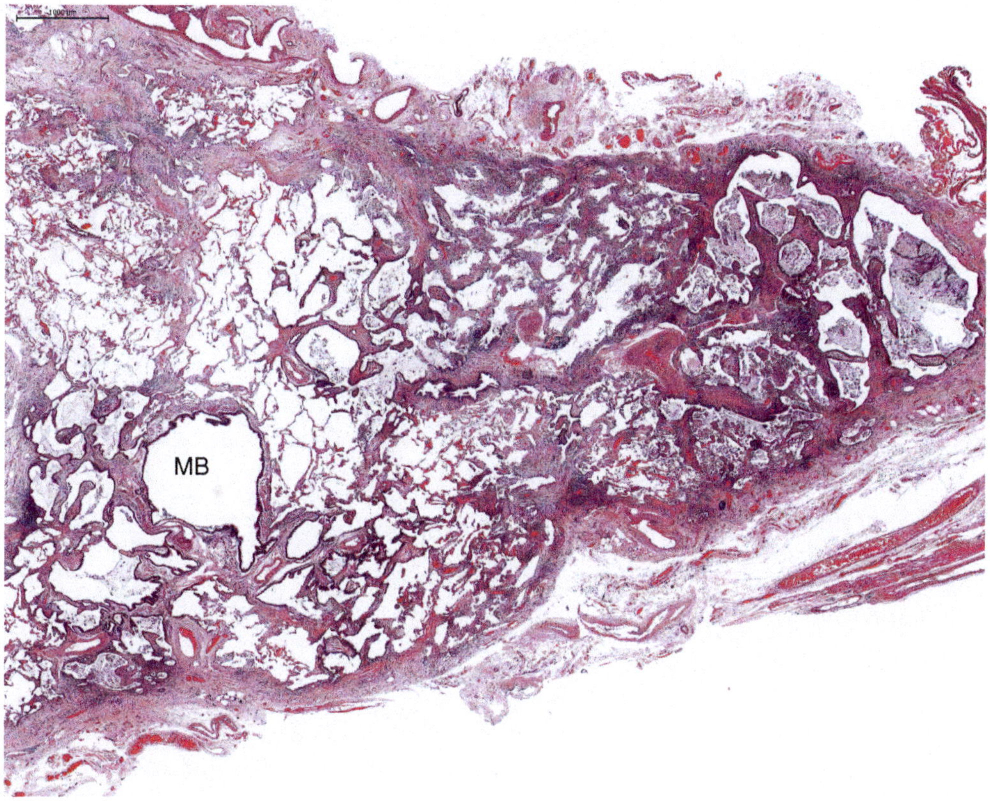

Fig. 7.22 Coexistent interstitial pneumonia (NSIP/p) and peripheral cystic change of the lingula (HE,×2). Note mucus repletion with neutrophils in the irregularly dilated lobular structure. *MB* membranous bronchiole

7.6.2 Indeterminate Peribronchiolar Metaplasia and Cystic Intralobular Bronchiolectasis

Peribronchiolar metaplasia (PBM) is a nonspecific histological feature, called lambertosis (communication between terminal or respiratory bronchioles and adjacent alveoli), and it is often observed in cases with a history of smoking or some inhalational events [57]. Fukuoka described 15 cases of interstitial pneumonia with PBM, including two cases with RA, but the details were not presented [57]. Figure 7.25 shows multiple cystic lesions in the basal area on an HRCT image of a never-smoker woman in her 70s with a history of RA for about 30 years. A pathological examination revealed cystic bronchiolectasis involving almost the entire secondary lobule (Fig. 7.26a) and PBM involving a respiratory bronchiole (thick arrow). In this case, the cysts often involved one lobule with a remnant of lung tissue (including a pulmonary artery and interstitium) within the cystic lesion, similar to an emphysematous bulla (Fig. 7.26b). The cyst wall reveals dense fibrosis without bronchial smooth muscle layer and destruction of the alveolar structure.

In the PBM, increase in bronchiole-alveolar communication and marked splitting of the alveolar walls are observed, resulting in the airspace enlargement (Fig. 7.27). Both the intralobular cystic lesion and PBM showed minimal inflammatory cell infiltration. In these instances, the intralobular cystic lesions with thick fibrous walls were directly connected to the intralobular bronchioles, so-called "mm pattern" of Reid [58] (Fig. 7.28). These cystic lesions show bronchiolar epithelial lining, with occasional smooth muscle layer, loss of the bronchiolar elastic lamina, and dense fibrosis. Figure 7.29 shows a schematic representation of the intralobular cystic bronchiolectasis. PBM and cystic dilatation at the respiratory bronchioles are sometimes coexistent (Fig. 7.30).

Whether PBM may promote the cystic bronchiolectasis in the lobule remains to be resolved.

7.6.3 Intralobular Bronchiolar and Alveolar Inflammation Inducing Alveolar Structural Remodeling

As for the alveolar structural remodeling in RA lung, the terminal and respiratory bronchioles are often involved by dense inflammatory cells. BALT in the lung parenchyma also participates in the remodeling of lung structure. Figure 7.31 shows a case of 60s woman with BALT hyperplasia in the alveoli and plasma cell infiltration to the alveolar walls with loss of elastic fibers, which developed into a large cystic lesion over the course of 7 years.

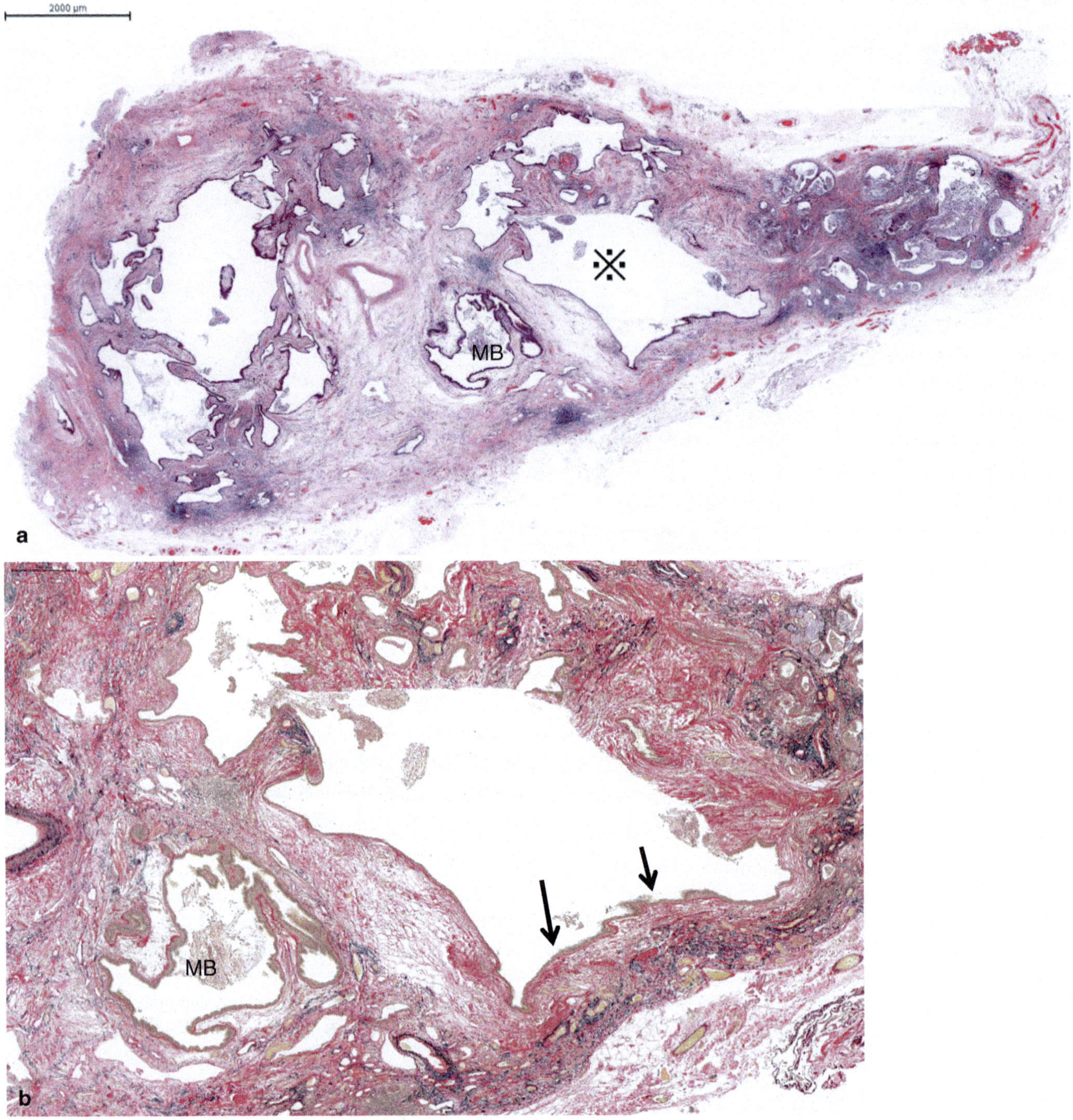

Fig. 7.23 Basal segment of the lower lobe of the same case shown in Figs. 7.21 and 7.22. (**a**) Irregular cystic lesion involving the lobules without normal alveoli (HE, ×1). (**b**) Cyst (indicating *Reference mark* of **a**) originating from a destructive membranous bronchiole with thick collagenous fiber deposition in the wall (arrows). A normal bronchiolar component has been lost and inflammatory cells are scant (EVG, ×4). *MB* membranous bronchiole

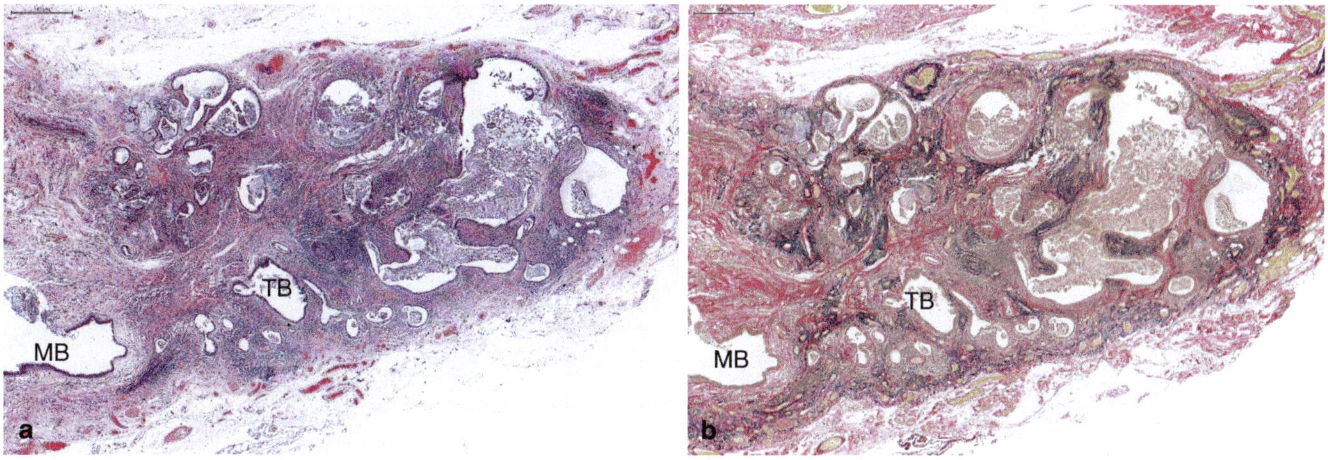

Fig. 7.24 Tip of the basal segment of the lower lobe. Note destruction of alveolar structure with mucopurulent exudates. (**a**: HE, ×5, **b**: EVG, ×5). *MB* membranous bronchiole, *TB* terminal bronchiole

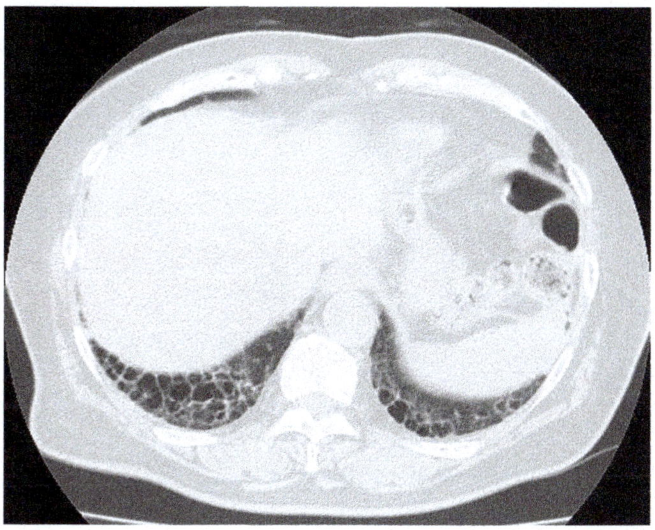

Fig. 7.25 An elderly never smoker woman in her 70s with a 30-year history of RA. HRCT shows multiple large cystic lesions mimicking honeycombing in the basal segments

The above findings suggest that appropriate therapy for the bronchiolar and alveolar inflammation is important to prevent the destruction of the alveolar structure.

7.7 Interstitial Pneumonia Preceding RA

Interstitial pneumonia, especially idiopathic NSIP, can be the first or only manifestation of connective tissue disease (CTD) prior to diagnosis [59–61]. Figure 7.32 shows an NSIP pattern in a woman in her 60s; 8 years after surgical lung biopsy, she was diagnosed as having RA based on a high ACPA titer. UIP also precedes CTD including RA and is often initially diagnosed as IPF [62]. Such patients tend to be younger and are often women, and they are thought to have a better prognosis than patients with IPF. Fischer reported 74 patients with lung diseases and positive ACPA in the absence of existing RA or other CTD [63]. Most of the patients were women, and three patients with a high ACPA titer developed articular RA. The histopathological results showed airway inflammation and UIP with lymphoplasmacytic interstitial infiltration.

7.8 Other Histological Patterns of RA-ILD

As there are multifaceted aspects of RA-ILD, other forms than UIP and NSIP pattern will be discussed in this section.

7.8.1 Organizing Pneumonia in RA

Organizing pneumonia (OP) frequently affects RA patients and sometimes precedes the articular symptoms of RA [64, 65]. In the consecutive study in Japan, the prevalence of OP is 4% of RA patients, which occurs independently from articular disease [66]. OP may arise from various clinical settings such as drug use, infection, aspiration, and so on [11]. The histological features of OP in patients with RA are not different from those with cryptogenic OP or other connective tissue diseases [67]. The patchy distribution of a polypoid intra-alveolar organization with well-preserved alveolar structures and slight mononuclear cell infiltration

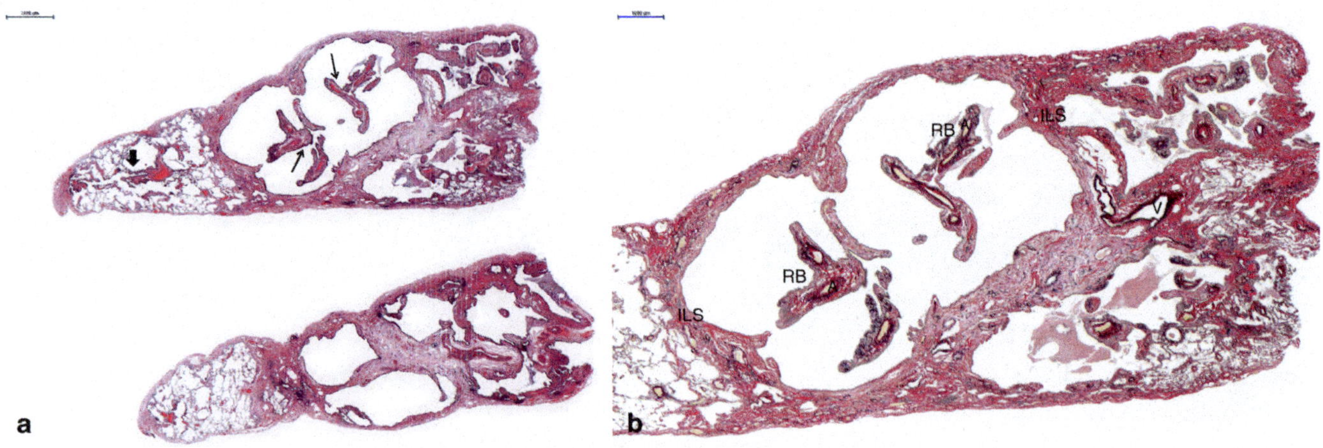

Fig. 7.26 Prominent cystic lesions in the basal area. (**a**) Large cysts involving the entire lobules with floating remnant of lung tissue (arrows) like emphysema are visible. A thick arrow shows peribronchiolar metaplasia (HE, ×1). (**b**) Cystic lesions involve the lobules with remnant of artery and lung interstitium within it. *ILS* interlobular septum, *A* pulmonary artery, *V* pulmonary vein, *RB* respiratory broncnhiole

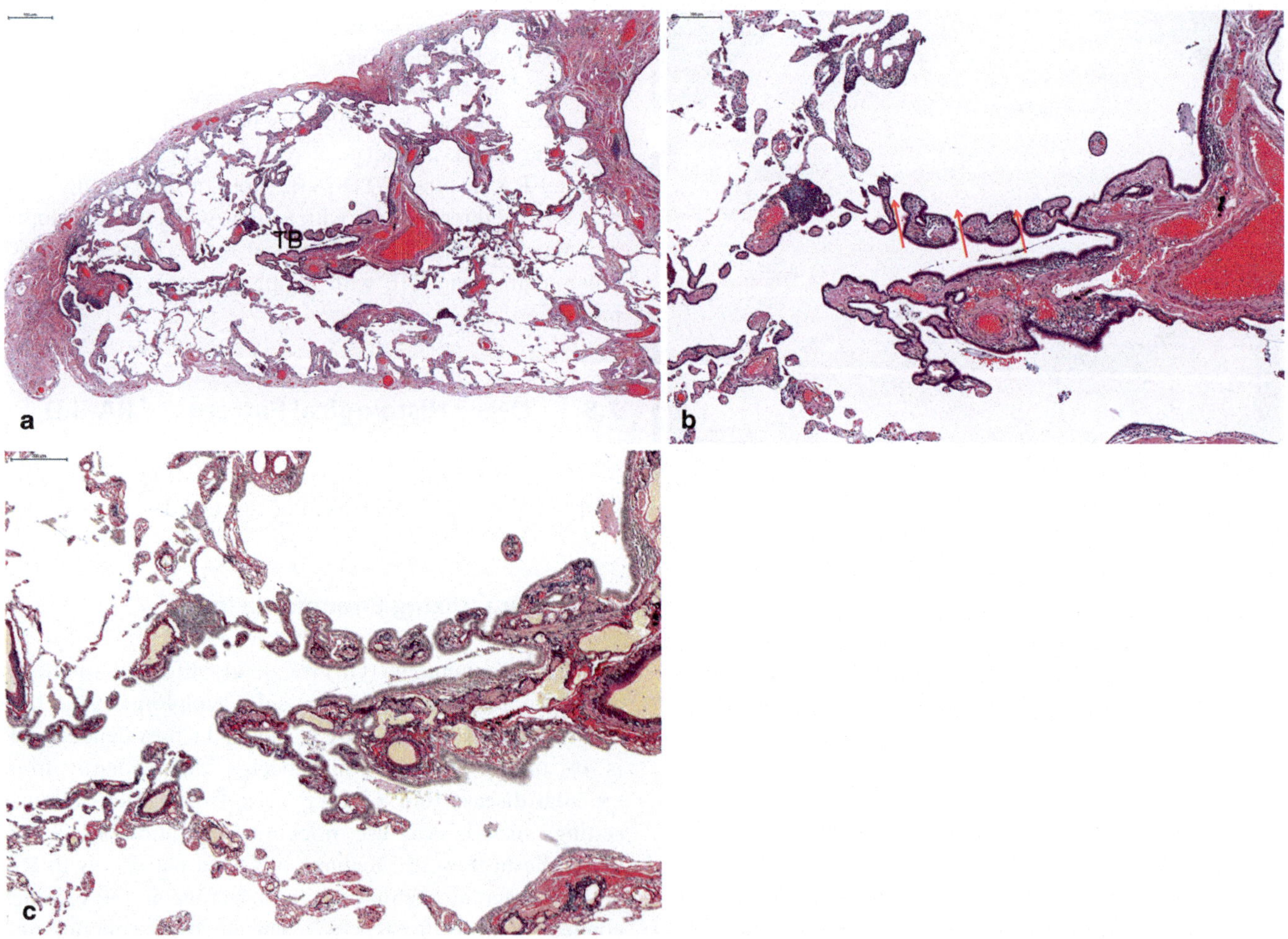

Fig. 7.27 Peribronchiolar metaplasia of the same section. (**a**) Peribronchiolar metaplasia just beneath the respiratory bronchioles. (HE, ×10). TB terminal bronchiole. (**b**, **c**) Increase in the number of bronchiole-alveolar communications (arrows) and splitting of the alveolar walls (HE, ×10). (**c**) (EVG, ×10)

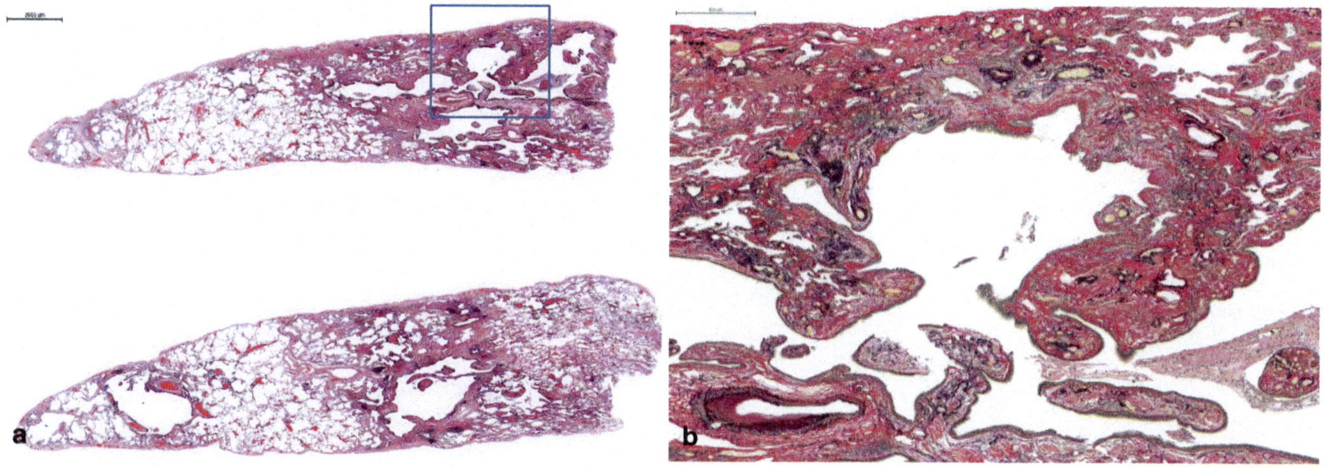

Fig. 7.28 Cystic bronchiolectasis in the lobule. (**a**) Intralobular "mm pattern" bronchioles showing air ballon-like dilatation with wall fibrosis and slight mononuclear cell infiltration (HE, ×1). (**b**) Loss of bronchiolar walls with dense collagen deposition and loss of alveolar structure (square of **a**) (EVG, ×5)

Fig. 7.29 Schematic representation of cystic bronchiolectasis "mm" pattern bronchioles become destroyed and cystic change, involving a lobule. *MB* membranous bronchiole, *A* pulmonary artery, *V* pulmonary vein, *TB* terminal bronchiole. *Brown* smooth muscle belonging to the bronchiole, *Green* lining bronchiolar epithelium

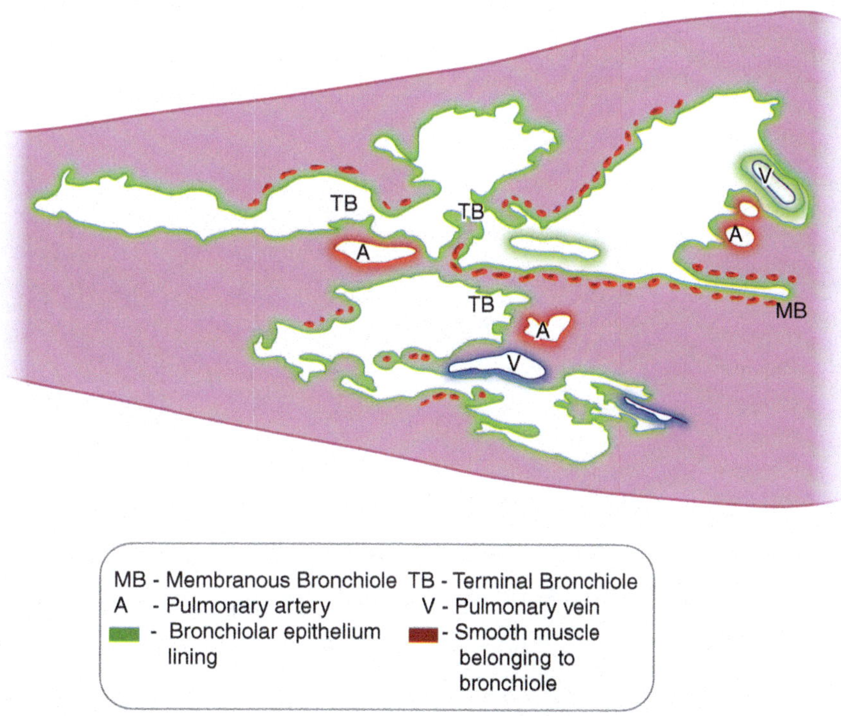

in the alveolar walls, often involving centriacinar area (Fig. 7.33) OP in RA patients, is accompanied by cellular NSIP, with peribronchovascular consolidation, which sometimes results in a twisted appearance on HRCT images [68] (Fig. 7.34).

7.8.2 Desquamative Interstitial Pneumonia in RA

Desquamative interstitial pneumonia (DIP) is a rare disease that is typically associated with smoking [11]. Ishii reported a case of DIP associated with RA [69]. DIP may be related to autoimmune disease. DIP reaction can be observed in some cases of RA.

7.8.3 Fibroelastosis in RA

RA has been depicted as one of the secondary causes of pleuroparenchymal fibroelastosis (PPFE) [70]. However, the detailed histopathological studies have not been reported, except clinical observation of upper lobe fibrosis and cavitation [71]. Figure 7.35 shows subpleural atelectasis with marked elastosis involving the upper lobe of the right lung, histologically consistent with PPFE, accompanying aspergillus infection in the left apex.

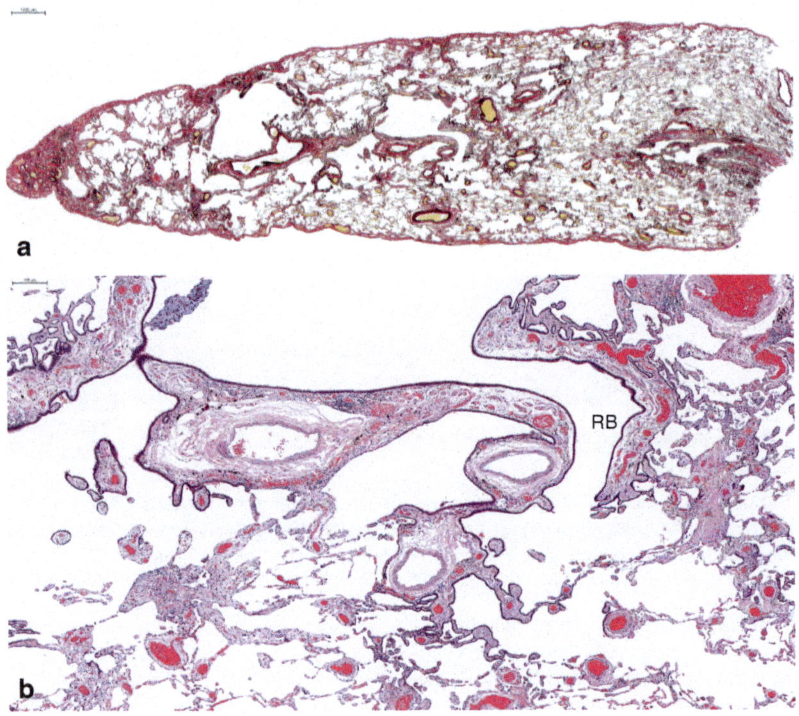

Fig. 7.30 Coexistence of peribronchiolar metaplasia and dilatation of respiratory bronchiole. (**a**) Dilatation of a respiratory bronchiole, resembling centriacinar emphysema (EVG, ×1). (**b**) Peribronchiolar metaplasia is seen around a dilated respiratory bronchiole (HE, ×7). *RB* respiratory bronchiole

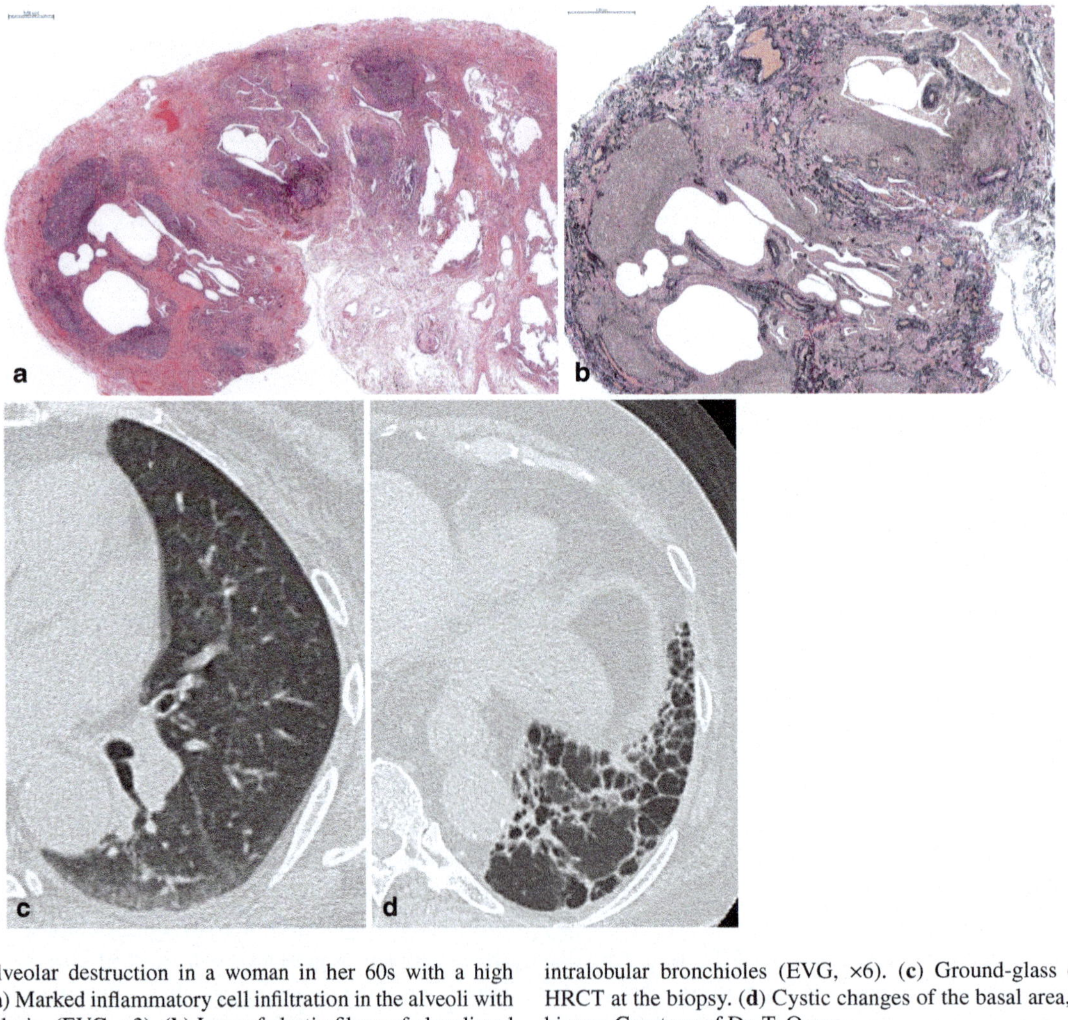

Fig. 7.31 Alveolar destruction in a woman in her 60s with a high ACPA titer. (**a**) Marked inflammatory cell infiltration in the alveoli with BALT hyperplasia. (EVG, ×3). (**b**) Loss of elastic fibers of alveoli and intralobular bronchioles (EVG, ×6). (**c**) Ground-glass opacity on a HRCT at the biopsy. (**d**) Cystic changes of the basal area, 7 years after biopsy. Courtesy of Dr. T. Ogura

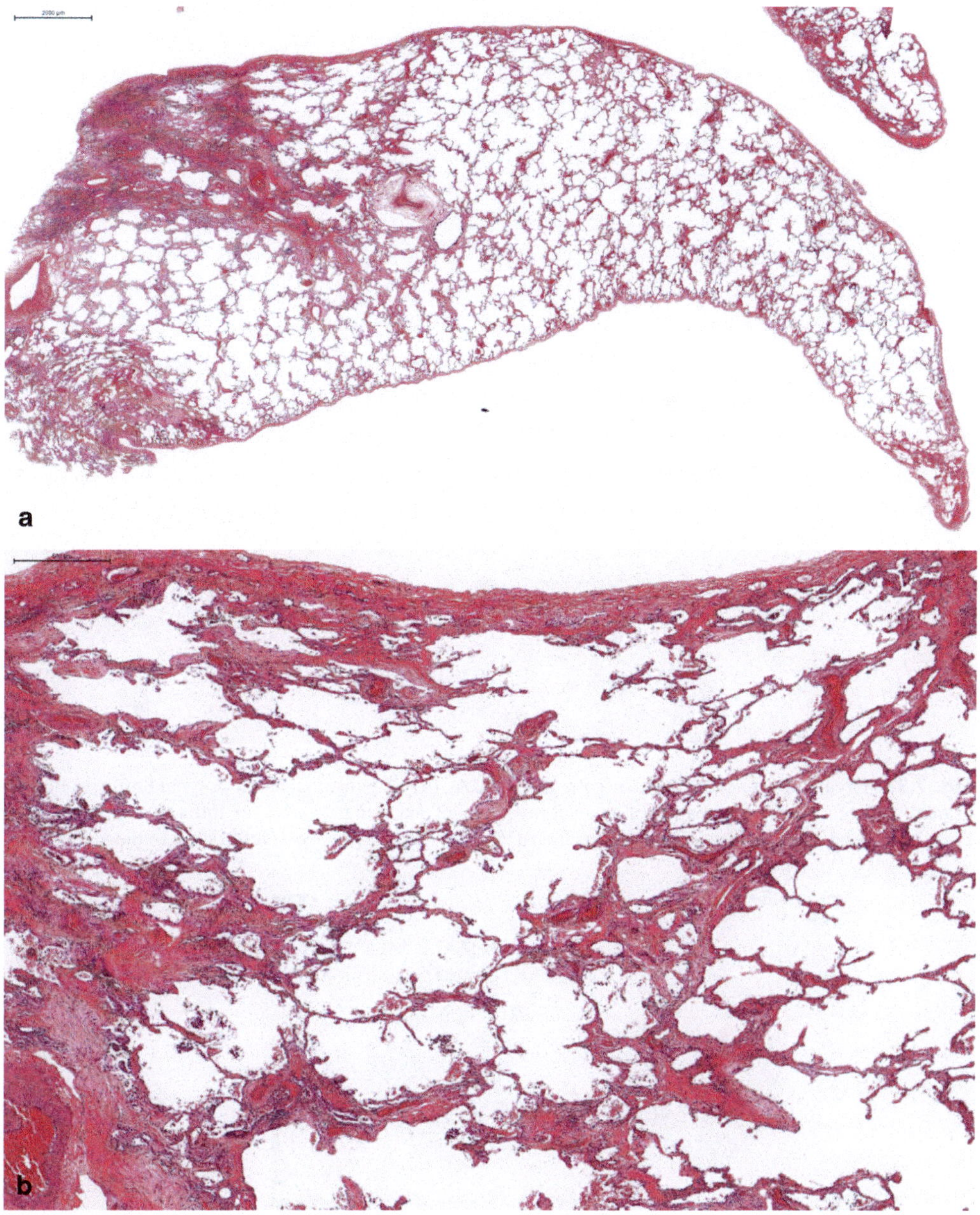

Fig. 7.32 NSIP preceding RA. (**a**) A woman in her 60s exhibited an NSIP pattern. Eight years later, she was diagnosed as having RA based on high ACPA and MMP3 titers (HE, ×1). (**b**) Cellular NSIP with slight mural incorporation fibrosis (HE, ×5)

7.8.4 Diffuse Alveolar Damage in RA

Diffuse alveolar damage (DAD) occurs in interstitial lung disease in patients with RA, especially those with a preexisting UIP pattern, and is associated with a poor prognosis [72, 73].

Overall, the incidence of DAD is reportedly 20~22% of patients with RA-ILD [74, 75]. Preexisting ILD, methotrexate usage, and an elderly age are associated with the development of acute exacerbation [72]. The histology of acute exacerbation of RA is similar to that of IIPs (Fig. 7.36), namely, acute and organizing diffuse alveolar damage [11]. In the 2013 revised classification [12], acute exacerbation occurs in chronic fibrosing IP (UIP/IPF and f-NSIP), connective tissue disease, and chronic hypersentivity pneumonia, and it is important to exclude infection, left heart failure, and other identifiable causes of acute lung injury. Acute exacerbation occurs mostly in patients with RA-UIP and is associated with a poor outcome, while acute exacerbation in patients with RA-NSIP is associated with a better prognosis [72]. Patients treated with leflunomide in Japan reportedly suffered from diffuse alveolar damage [76].

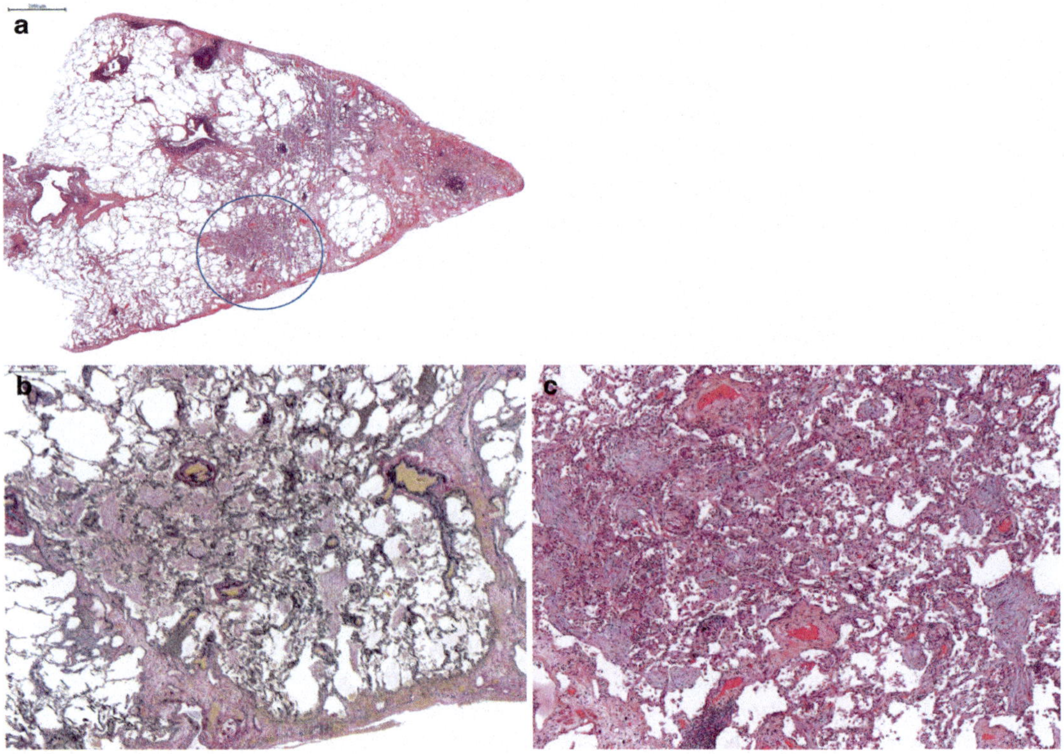

Fig. 7.33 Organizing pneumonia in a patient with RA. (**a**) A panoramic view of a patchy distribution of alveolar involvement. Follicular bronchiolitis and bronchiectasis are also visible (HE, ×1). (**b**) Intra-alveolar polypoid organization with preserved alveolar structure (EVG, ×4). (**c**) Intra-alveolar polypoid organization with mild mononuclear cell infiltration to the alveolar walls (HE, ×10)

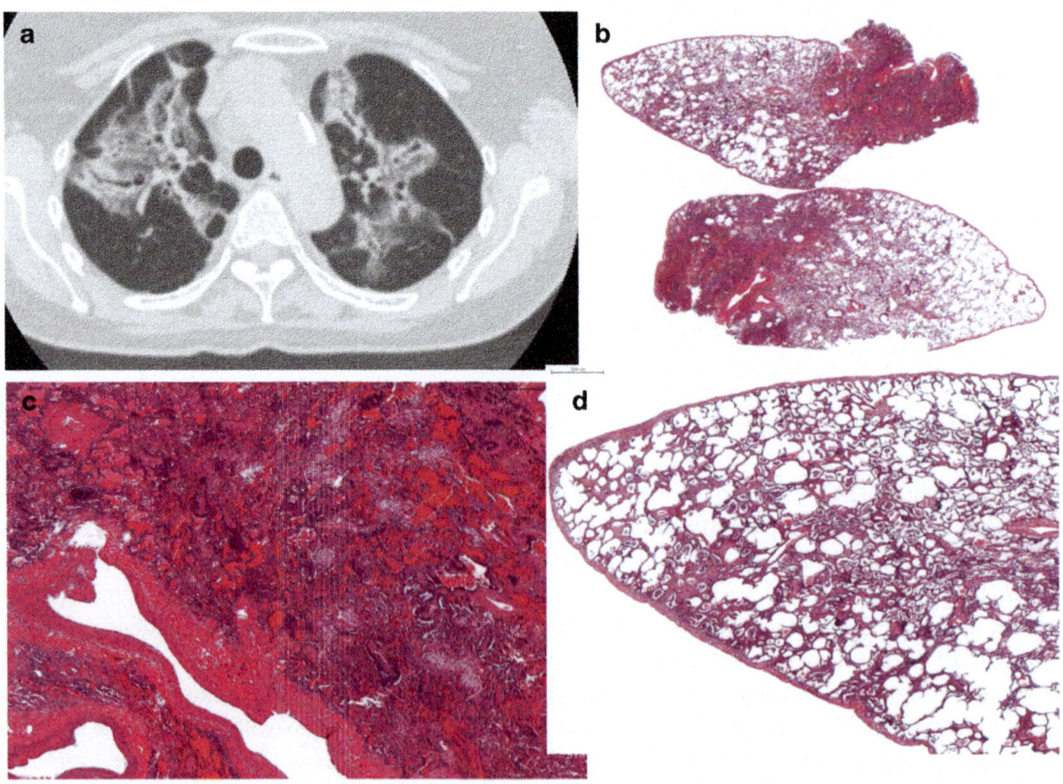

Fig. 7.34 A woman in her 60s with RA showing a twisted consolidation. (**a**) Bilateral airspace consolidation along the airways is visible on a HRCT image. (**b**) A panoramic view shows peribronchiolar OP pattern and cellular NSIP (HE, ×1). (**c**) Intra-alveolar polypoid fibrosis (HE, ×10). (**d**) Cellular NSIP in the periphery of the lobule (HE, ×2)

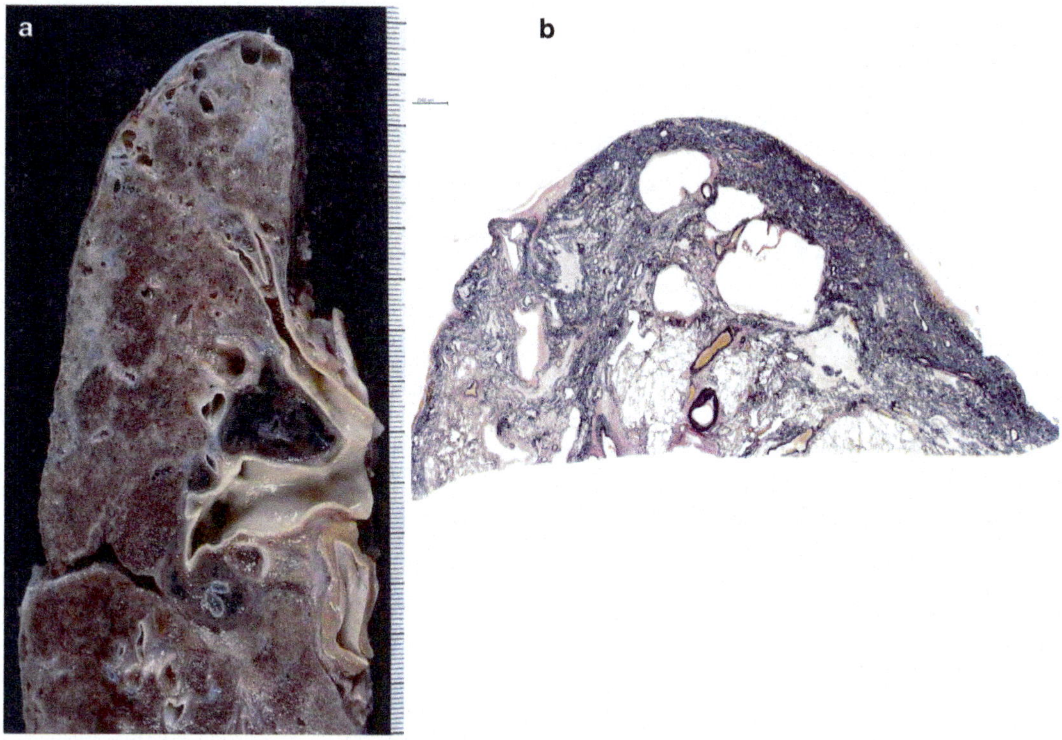

Fig. 7.35 Upper lobe contraction of the lung in a man in his 70s. (**a**) Gross feature of the right upper lobe shows apical and subpleural band-like atelectatic fibrosis. (**b**) Subpleural fibroelastosis of the left apex is visible (EVG, ×1)

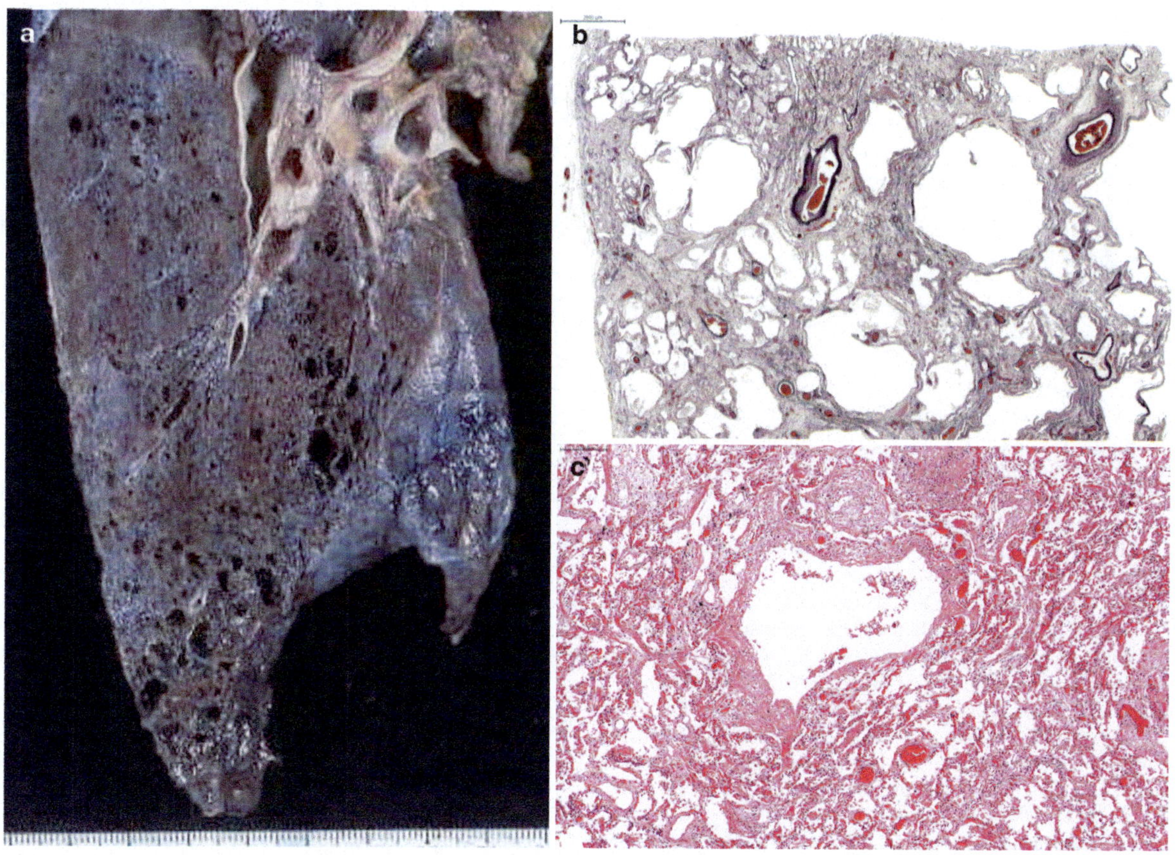

Fig. 7.36 Diffuse alveolar damage associated with RA. (**a**) Gross feature of an autopsied lung shows homogeneous viscid parenchyma and cystic changes in the basal region. (**b**) Honeycomb-like cystic lesion of the basal segment (HE, ×1). (**c**) Hyaline membranes along the alveolar ducts (HE, ×5)

Conclusion

Histopathological patterns of RA-ILD have been described using the classification for IIPs. We described the early phase of RA-ILD in a patient with high ACPA titer but no distinct respiratory symptoms and found that it corresponded to cellular NSIP and early bronchiolar damage in UIP. Patients with RA-ILD also exhibit bronchiolitis and BALT hyperplasia, in addition to interstitial pneumonia. Intralobular chronic inflammatory bronchiolar damages promoting the destruction of not only the intralobular bronchioles, but also the alveoli can result in unexpected cystic lesions in a considerable number of cases with long-standing RA.

Thus, awareness of intralobular chronic bronchiolar damage, destructive bronchiolar inflammation, and consequent cystic change in the lobule should be promoted to ensure an adequate therapeutic strategy.

Acknowledgment The author greatly appreciates Dr. Takashi Ogura, Kanagawa Cardiovascular and Respiratory Center; Dr. Hideyasu Sugimoto, Tokushuukai Kamakura General Hospital; Dr. Sinyu Izumi, Respiratory Medicine, National Center for Global Health and Medicine; and Dr. Hitoshi Tokuda, JCHO Tokyo Yamate Medical Center, for their valuable specimens and comments.

References

1. Turesson C, O'Fallon WM, Crowson CS, Gabriel SE, Matteson EL. Extraarticular disease manifestations in rheumatoid arthritis. Incidence trends and risk factors over 46 years. Ann Rheum Dis. 2003;62:722–7.
2. Brown KK. Rheumatoid lung disease. Proc Am Thorac Soc. 2007;4:443–8.
3. Schneider F, Gruden J, Tazelaar HD, Leslie KO. Pleuropulmonary pathology in patients with rheumatic disease. Arch Pathol Lab Med. 2012;136:1242–52.
4. Koudri G, Norton S, Young A, Cox N, Davies P, Devlin J, Dixey J, Gough A, et al. Interstitial lung disease has a poor prognosis in rheumatoid arthritis: results from an inception cohort. Rheumatology (Oxford). 2010;49:1483–9.
5. Bongartz T, Nannini C, Medina-Velasquez YF, et al. Incidence and mortality of interstitial lung disease in rheumatoid arthritis: a population-based study. Arthritis Rheum. 2010;62:1583–91.
6. Olson AL, Swigris JJ, Sprunger DB, Fischer A, Fernadez-Perez ER, Solomon J, Murphy J, Cohen M, Raghu G, Brown K. Rheumatoid arthritis-interstitial lung disease-associated mortality. Am J Respir Crit Care Med. 2011;183:32–378.
7. Nannini C, Medina-Velasquez YF, Achenbach SJ, Crowson CS, Ryu JH, Vassallo R, Gabrile SE, Matteson EL, Bongartz R. Incidence and mortality of obstructive lung disease in rheumatoid arthritis: a population-based study. Arthritis Care Res. 2013;65:1243–50.
8. Solomon JJ, Ryu JH, Tazelaar HD, Myers JL, Tuder R, Cool CD, Curran-Everette D, Fischer A, Swigris JJ, Brown KK. Fibrosing interstitial pneumonia predicts survival in patients with rheumatoid arthritis-associated interstitial lung disease (RA-ILD). Res Med. 2013;107:1247–52.
9. Kelly CA, Saravanan V, Nisar M, Arthanari S, Woodhead FA, Price-Forbes AN, Dawson J, Sathi N, Ahmad Y, Koduri G, Young A, on behalf of the British Rheumatoid Interstitial Lung (BRILL) Network. Rheumatoid arthritis-related interstitial lung disease: associations, prognostic factors and physiological and radiological characteristics—a large multicentre UK study. Rheumatology. 2014;53:1676–82.
10. Puechal X, Genin E, Bienvenue T, Jeunne CL, Dusser DJ. Poor survival in rheumatoid arthritis associated with bronchiectasis: a family-based cohort study. PLoS One. 2014;9:1–8, e110066.
11. American Thoracic Society; European Respiratory Society. American Thoracic Society/European Respiratory Society International Multidisciplinary Consensus Classification of the idiopathic interstitial pneumonias. Am J Respir Crit Care Med. 2002;165:277–304.
12. Travis WD, Costabel U, Hansell DM, King TE, Lynch DA, Nicholson AG, et al. An official American Thoracic Society/ European Respiratory Society statement: update of the international multidisciplinary classification of the idiopathic interstitial pneumonias. Am J Respir Crit Care Med. 2013;188:733–48.
13. Wells AU, Denton CP. Interstitial lung disease in connective tissue disease-mechanisms and management. Nature Rev Rheumatology. 2014;10:728–39.
14. Paulin F, Doyle TJ, Fletcher EA, Ascherman DP, Rosas IO. Rheumatoid arthritis-associated interstitial lung disease and idiopathic pulmonary fibrosis: shared mechanistic and phenotypic traits suggest overlapping disease mechanisms. Rev Investig Clin. 2015;67:280–6.
15. Bongartz T, Cantaert T, Atkins SR, Harle P, Myers JL, Turesson C, Ryu JH, Baeten D, Matteson EL. Citrullination in extra-articular manifestations of rheumatoid arthritis. Rheumatology (Oxford). 2007;46:70–5.
16. Giles JT, Danoff SK, Sokolove J, Wagner CA, Winchester R, Pappas DA, Siegelman S, Connors G, Robinson WH, Bathon JM. Association of fine specificity and repertoire expansion of anticitrullinated peptide antibodies with rheumatoid arthritis associated interstitial lung disease. Ann Rheum Dis. 2014;73: 1487–94.
17. Reynisdotti G, Karimi R, Joshua V, Olsen H, Hensvold AH, Harju A, Engtrom M, Grunewald J, et al. Structural changes and antibody enrichment in the lungs are early features of anti-citrullinated protein antibody-positive rheumatoid arthritis. Arthrithis Rheum. 2014;66:31–9.
18. Perry E, Kelly C, Eggleton P, Soyza AD, Hutchinson D. The lung in ACPA-positive rheumatoid arthritis: an initiating site of injury? Rheumatology (Oxford). 2014;53:1940–50.
19. Joseph J, Sahn SA. Connective tissue disease and the pleura. Chest. 1993;104:262–70.
20. Walters MN, Ojeda VJ. Pleuropulmonary necrobiotic rheumatoid nodule. A review and clinicopathological study of six patients. Med J Aust. 1986;144:648–51.
21. Bienenstock J, Johnston N, Perey DY. Bronchial lymphoid tissue. I. Morphologic characteristics. Lab Investig. 1973;29:686–92.
22. Sminia T, van der Brugge-Gamelkoorn GL, Jeurissen SH. Structure and function of bronchus-associated lymphoid tissue (BALT). Crit Rev Immunol. 1989;9:119–50.
23. Tschernig T, Pabst R. Bronchus-associated lymphoid tissue (BALT) is not present in the normal adult lung but in different diseases. Pathobiology. 2000;68:1–8.
24. Sato A, Chida K, Hayakawa H. Cellular distribution of bronchus-associated lymphoid tissue in rheumatoid arthritis. Am J Respir Crit Care Med. 1996;154:1903–7.
25. Sato A. Basic and clinical aspects of bronchus-associated lymphoid tissue. Nihon Kokyuki Gakkai Zasshi. 2000;38:3–11. (in Japanese with English abstract).
26. Moyron-Quiroz JE, Rangel-Moreno J, Kusser K, Harton L, Sprague F, Goodrich S, Woodland DL, Lung FE, Randall TD. Role of inducible bronchus associated lymphoid tissue (iBALT) in respiratory immunity. Nat Med. 2004;10:927–34.

27. Foo SY, Phipps S. Regulation of inducible BALT formation and contribution to immunity and pathology. Mucosal Immunol. 2010;3:537–44.
28. Rangel-Moreno J, Hartson L, Navarro C, Gaxiola M, Selman M, Randall TD. Inducible bronchus-associated lymphoid tissue (iBALT) in patients with pulmonary complications of rheumatoid arthritis. J Clin Invest. 2006;116:3183–94.
29. Nakamura Y, Chida K, Suda Y. Nonspecific interstitial pneumonia in collagen vascular disease: comparison of the clinical characteristics and prognostic significance with usual interstitial pneumonia. Sarcoidosis Vasc Diffuse Lung Dis. 2003;20:235–41.
30. Tansey D, Wells AU, Colby TV. Variations in histological patterns of interstitial pneumonia between connective tissue disorders and their relationship to prognosis. Histopathology. 2004;44: 585–96.
31. Tanaka N, Kim JS, Newell JD, et al. Rheumatoid arthritis-related lung diseases: CT findings. Radiology. 2004;232:81–91.
32. Yoshinouchi T, Ohtsuki Y, Fujita J. Nonspecific interstitial pneumonia pattern as pulmonary involvement of rheumatoid arthritis. Rheumatol Int. 2005;26:121–5.
33. Lee HK, Kim DS, Yoo B. Histopathologic pattern and clinical features of rheumatoid arthritis-associated interstitial lung disease. Chest. 2005;127:2019–27.
34. Tsuchiya Y, Takayanagi N, Sugiura H, Miyahara Y, Tokunaga D, Kawabata Y, Sugita Y. Lung diseases directly associated with rheumatoid arthritis and their relationship to outcome. Eur Respir J. 2011;37:1411–7.
35. Nakamura Y, Suda T, Kaida Y. Rheumatoid lung disease: prognostic analysis of 54 biopsy-proven cases. Respir Med. 2012;106: 1164–9.
36. Assyag D, Elicker BM, Urbania TH, Colby TV, Ryu JH, King TE Jr, Collard HR, Kim DS, Lee JS. Rheumatoid arthritis-associated interstitial lung disease; radiologic identification of usual interstitial pneumonia pattern. Radiology. 2014;270:583–8.
37. Solomon JJ, Chung JH, Cosgrove GP, Demoruelle MK, Fernandez-Perez ER, Fishcer A, Frankel SK, et al. Predictors of mortality in rheumatoid arthritis-associated interstitial lung disease. Eur Respir J. 2016;47:588–96.
38. Suda T. Up-to-date information on rheumatoid arthritis-associated interstitial lung disease. Clin Med Insights Circular Pulm Med. 2016;9:155–62.
39. Zamore-Legoff JA, Krause ML, Crowson CS, Ryu JH, Matteson EL. Patterns of interstitial lung disease and mortality in rheumatoid arthritis. Rheumatology (Oxford). 2017;56(3):344–50.
40. Park JH, Kim DS, Park IN. Prognosis of fibrotic interstitial pneumonia: idiopathic versus collagen vascular disease-related subtypes. Am J Respir Crit Care Med. 2007;175:705–11.
41. Enomoto N, Suda T, Kato M. Quantitative analysis of fibroblastic foci in usual interstitial pneumonia. Chest. 2006;130:22–9.
42. Song JW, Do K-H, Kim M-Y, Jang SJ, Colby TV, Kim DS. Pathologic and radiologic differences between idiopathic and collagen vascular disease-related usual interstitial pneumonia. Chest. 2009;136:23–30.
43. Smith M, Dalurzo M, Panse P, Parish J, Leslie K. Usual interstitial pneumonia-pattern fibrosis in surgical lung biopsies. Clinical, radiological and histopathological clues to aetiology. J Clin Pathol. 2013;66:896–903.
44. Gochuico BR, Avila NA, Chow CK, Novero LJ, Wu H-P, Ren P, MacDonald SD, Travis WD, Stylianou MP, Rosas IO. Progressive preclinical interstitial lung disease in rheumatoid arthritis. Arch Intern Med. 2008;168:159–66.
45. Reynisdottir G, Karimi R, Joshua V, Olsen H, Hensvold AH, Harju A, Engstrom M, Grunewald J, Nyren S, Eklund A, et al. Structural changes and antibody enrichment in the lungs are early features of anti-citrullinated protein antibody-positive rheumatoid arthritis. Arthritis Rheum. 2014;66:31–9.
46. Kerkman PF, Rombouts Y, van der Voort EIH, Trouw LA, Huizinga TWJ, Toes REM, Scherer HU. Circulating plasmablasts/plasma cells as a source of anticitrullinated protein antibodies in patients with rheumatoid arthritis. Ann Rheum Dis. 2013;72: 1259–63.
47. Takemura T. Pathology of chronic interstitial pneumonia and honeycombing. In: Sakai F, Jokoh T, Noma S, editors. Imaging diagnosis of idiopathic pulmonary fibrosis. Tokyo: Medial Science International; 2015. p. 25–56. (in Japanese).
48. Yousem SA, Colby RV, Carrington CB. Follicular bronchitis/bronchiolitis. Hum Pathol. 1985;16:700–6.
49. Hebisawa A, Asakawa K, Sugino K, Tamura A, Homma S. Pathology of bronchiolitis obliterans. Kokyu. 2008;27:265–74. (in Japanese).
50. Allen TC. Pathology of small airways disease. Arch Pathol Lab Med. 2010;134:702–18.
51. Debouassoux G, Cottin V, Liote H, Marchand E, Frachon I, Schuller A, Bejui-Thivolet F, Cordier JF, Group d'Etudes et de Recherche sur les Maladie d' Orphelines" Pulmonaires. Characterisation of severe obliterative bronchiolitis in rheumatoid arthritis. Eur Respir J. 2009;33:1053–61.
52. Fuschillo S, De Felice A, Balzano G. Mucosal inflammation in idiopathic bronchiectasis: cellular and molecular mechanisms. Eur Respir J. 2008;31:396–406.
53. Mori S, Chuo I, Koga Y, Sugimoto M. Comparison of pulmonary abnormalities on high-resolution computed tomography in patients with early versus longstanding rheumatoid arthritis. J Rheumatol. 2008;35:1513–21.
54. Demoruelle MK, Weisman MH, Simonian PL, Lynch DA, Sachs PB, Pedraza IF, Harrington AR, Kolfenbach JR, et al. Airway abnormalities and rheumatoid arthritis-related autoantibodies in subjects without arthritis: early injury or initiating site of autoimmunity? Arthritis Rheum. 2012;64:1756–61.
55. Tokuda H. Airway disease in rheumatoid arthritis. Nihon Kyoubu Rinsho. 2016;75:396–406, 528–537. (in Japanese).
56. Boyton RJ, Altman DM. Bronchiectasis: current concepts in pathogenesis, immunology, and microbiology. Annu Rev Pathol Mech Dis. 2016;11:523–54.
57. Fukuoka J, Franks TJ, Colby TV, Flaherty KR, Galvin JR, Hayden D, Gochuico BR, Kazerooni EA, Martinez F, Travis WD. Peribronchiolar metaplasia: a common histologic lesion in diffuse lung disease and a rare cause of interstitial kung disease. Am J Surg Pathol. 2005;29:948–54.
58. Reid L, Simon G. The peripheral patterns in the normal bronchogram and its relation to peripheral pulmonary anatomy. Thorax. 1958;13:103–9.
59. Sato T, Fujita J, Yamadori I, Ohtsuki Y, Yoshinouchi T, et al. Nonspecific interstitial pneumonia: as the first clinical presentation of various collagen vascular disorders. Rheumatol Int. 2006;26: 551–5.
60. Park IN, Jegal Y, Kim DS, Do KH, Yoo B, et al. Clinical course and lung function change of idiopathic nonspecific interstitial pneumonia. Eur Respir J. 2009;33:68–76.
61. Romagnoli M, Nannini C, Piciucchi S, Girelli F, Gurioli C, et al. Idiopathic nonspecific interstitial pneumonia: an interstitial lung disease associated with autoimmune disorders? Eur Respir J. 2011;38:384–91.
62. Kono M, Nakamura Y, Enomoto N, Hashimoto D, Fujisawa T, Inui N, Maekawa M, Suda T, Colby TV, Chida K. Usual interstitial pneumonia preceding collagen vascular disease: a retrospective case control study of patients initially diagnosed with idiopathic pulmonary fibrosis. PLoS One. 2014;9(4):e94775, 1–10.
63. Fischer A, Solomon JJ, du Bois RM, Deane KD, Olson AL, Fernadez-Perez ER, Huie TJ, Stevens AD, et al. Lung disease with anti-CCP antibodies but not rheumatoid arthritis or connective tissue disease. Respir Med. 2012;106:1040–70.

64. Mori S, Koga Y, Sugimoto M. Organizing pneumonia in rheumatoid arthritis patients: a case-based review. Respir Pulm Med. 2015;9(S1):69–80.
65. Komiya K, Teramoto S, Kurosaki Y, Kashizaki F, Kawashima M, Masuda K, Akagawa S, Hebisawa A, Ishii H, Kadota J. Organizing pneumonia with a positive result for anti-CCP antibodies as the first clinical presentation of rheumatoid arthritis. Intern Med. 2010;49:1605–7.
66. Okada H, Kurasawa K, Yamazaki R, Tanaka A, Arai S, Owada T, Maezawa R, Ishii Y. Clinical features of organizing pneumonia associated with rheumatoid arthritis. Mod Rheumatol. 2016;4:1–6.
67. Yoo JW, Song JW, Jang SJ, Lee CK, Kim M-Y, Lee HK, Jegal Y, Kim DS. Comparison between cryptogenic organizing pneumonia and connective tissue disease-related organizing pneumonia. Rheumatology (Oxford). 2011;50:932–8.
68. Watanabe E, Kawamura T, Mochizuki Y, Nakahara Y, Sasaki S, Okamoto A, Higashino T. Consolidation with a twisted appearance along the airways: a report of five cases of interstitial pneumonia. Respir Invest. 2014;52:213–8.
69. Ishii H, Iwata A, Sakamoto N, Mizunoe S, Mukae H, Kadota J. Desquamative interstitial pneumonia (DIP) in a patient with rheumatoid arthritis: is DIP associated with autoimmune disorders? Intern Med. 2009;48:827–30.
70. Watanabe K. Pleuroparenchymal fibroelastosis: its clinical characteristics. Curr Res Med Rev. 2013;9:229–37.
71. Petrie GR, Bloomfield P, Grant IWB, Crompton GK. Upper lobe fibrosis and cavitation in rheumatoid disease. Br J Dis Chest. 1980;74:263–7.
72. Parambil JG, Myers JL, Ryu JH. Diffuse alveolar damage. Uncommon manifestation of pulmonary involvement in patients with connective tissue diseases. Chest. 2006;130:553–8.
73. Park I-N, Kim DS, Shim TS, Lim c-M, Lee SD, Koh Y, Kim WS, Kim WD, Jan SJ, Colby TV. Acute exacerbation of interstitial pneumonia other than idiopathic pulmonary fibrosis. Chest. 2007;132:214–20.
74. Suda T, Kaida Y, Nakamura Y, Enomoto N, Fujisawa T, Imokawa S, Hashimizu H, Naito T, Hashimoto D, et al. Acute exacerbation of interstitial pneumonia associated with collagen vascular diseases. Respir Med. 2009;103:846–53.
75. Hozumi H, Nakamura Y, Jokoh T, Sumikawa H, Colby TV, Kono M, Hashimoto D, Enomoto N, Fujisawa T, Inui N, Suda T, Chida K. Acute exacerbation in rheumatoid arthritis-associated interstitial lung disease: a retrospective case control study. BMJ Open. 2013;3:e003132.
76. Sawada T, Inokuma S, Sato T, Otsuka Y, Saeki Y, Takeuchi T, Matsuda T, Takemura T, Sagawa A, Study Committee for Leflunomide-induced Lung injury, Japan College of Rheumatology. Leflunomide-induced interstitial lung disease: prevalence and risk factors in Japanese patients with rheumatoid arthritis. Rheumatology (Oxford). 2009;48:1069–72.

8 Radiological Characteristics of Interstitial Lung Diseases in Patients with Connective Tissue Disease: Focus on Rheumatoid Arthritis

Kiminori Fujimoto

Abstract

Impairments/comorbidities of the respiratory system are important extra-articular features in patients with rheumatoid arthritis (RA) and represent a major cause of mortality. Interstitial lung disease (ILD) in RA (RA-ILD) and other types of connective tissue diseases (CTDs) is categorized using the international consensus classification of an idiopathic interstitial pneumonia. Unlike other types of CTDs, RA-ILD most often shows a usual interstitial pneumonia-like pattern on high-resolution computed tomography (HRCT), and less often, it displays patterns of nonspecific interstitial pneumonia, organizing pneumonia (OP), diffuse alveolar damage, and variants of OP. In addition, airway impairment (including bronchiectasis, follicular bronchiolitis, and bronchiolitis obliterans) and pleural disease are well-known comorbidities in patients with RA. In clinical practice, these lung lesions are problematic, because they are often difficult to distinguish from pulmonary infections and drug-induced lung injury. This chapter describes CTD-ILDs and mainly focuses on RA-ILD. HRCT images and histopathological patterns are reviewed and illustrated. Acute exacerbations of CTD-ILD/RA-ILD and ILDs that precede CTDs are also discussed.

Keywords

Rheumatoid arthritis • Connective tissue disease • Interstitial lung disease • Idiopathic interstitial pneumonia • Computed tomography

8.1 Introduction

Idiopathic interstitial pneumonia (IIP) is an exclusion diagnosis classification that temporarily includes interstitial lung diseases (ILDs) of unknown cause. IIP is classified as a disease unit based on multidisciplinary discussion (MDD), and even now its clinical validity has been continuing to be verified. An ILD that is associated with an underlying disease, such as a connective tissue disease (CTD), is categorized as a "secondary ILD," and it is called "ILD associated with CTD (CTD-ILD)." Therefore, in classifying IIPs, it is necessary to exclude all "secondary" ILDs, and needless to say, the exclusion diagnosis is also very important. Furthermore, in excluding secondary ILDs and to classifying IIPs, a comprehensive diagnosis is necessary to evaluate changes over time (disease behavior), and a multidisciplinary consensus should be conducted to consider clinical, radiological, and pathological diagnoses [1–4].

CTDs are inflammatory diseases caused by autoimmune mechanisms, which mainly involve the connective tissues, like collagen fibers and blood vessels that surround organs and tissues. Although symptoms in joints and muscles are conspicuous, CTDs comprise a so-called group of diseases or a set of several diseases that could cause multiple visceral lesions simultaneously. In recent years, a number of characteristic autoantibodies have been identified, and the detection of these antibodies contributes to the diagnosis of each type of CTD (Table 8.1) [3–9].

K. Fujimoto, M.D., Ph.D.
Department of Radiology, Kurume University School of Medicine, Kurume, Japan
e-mail: kimichan@med.kurume-u.ac.jp

T. Gono et al. (eds.), *Lung Disease Associated with Rheumatoid Arthritis*, https://doi.org/10.1007/978-981-10-6750-1_8

Table 8.1 Frequency and characteristics of pulmonary manifestations of connective tissue diseases

	RA	SSc	PM-DM	SjS	SLE	MCTD
No. of patients (×10^3)[a]	700–1000	20	17–20	100	60–100	11
Age range of onset (year)	20–50	30–50	10–/30–60	40–60	20–40	30–50
Woman-to-man ratio	3	12	3	9–14	10	13–16
Related autoimmune antibodies	Anti-CCP Ab	Anti-centromere Ab (limited disease) Anti-SLC-70 Ab (diffuse type) Anti-RNP polymerase Ab (diffuse type) Anti-RNP Ab (anti-U1-RNP Ab)	ASS: anti-ARS Ab (anti-Jo-1, other seven types) Anti-SRP Ab Anti-MDA5 Ab (anti-CADM-140Ab)	Anti-SS-A (Ro) Ab anti-SS-B (La) Ab	Anti-dsDNA Ab Anti-Smith Ab Anti-phospholipid Ab ANA (nonspecific) Anti-SS-A Ab	Anti-RNP Ab (anti-U1-RNP Ab) Anti-dsDNA Ab Anti-Smith Ab
UIP	+++	+	+	+	+	+
NSIP	++	+++	+++	++	++	++
OP	++	+	+++	++	+	+
DAD	+	±	++	±	+	±
DLH (or LIP)	±			++	+	
DPH					+++	
PH	+	++	±	+	++	+
Bronchiectasis	++			++		
BO	++			+	+	
FB	+			+		+
Pleural diseases	++	+		+	+++	+

Adopted and modified from [3–5, 7]

Symbols in columns indicate the frequency with which a feature or pattern of features occurs, with "+" indicating the lowest and "+++" the highest frequency; with a blank of column indicating absence of feature or pattern; and with "±" meaning rare but possible cause

Abbreviations: *Ab* antibody, *ANA* antinuclear antibody, *ARS* aminoacyl-transfer tRNA synthetase, *ASS* antisynthetase syndrome, *BO* bronchiolitis obliterans, *CADM* clinical amyopathic dermatomyositis, *CCP* cyclic citrullinated peptide, *DAD* diffuse alveolar damage, *DLH* diffuse lymphoid hyperplasia, *DPH* diffuse pulmonary hemorrhage, *DsDNA* double-standed deoxyribonucleic acid, *FB* follicular bronchiolitis, *LIP* lymphoid interstitial pneumonia, *MCTD* mixed connective tissue disease, *MDA-5* melanoma differentiation-associated gene 5, *NSIP* nonspecific interstitial pneumonia, *OP* organizing pneumonia, *PH* pulmonary hypertension, *PM-DM* polymyositis/dermatomyositis, *RA* rheumatoid arthritis, *RNP* ribonuclear protein, *SjS* Söjgren syndrome, *SLC* scleroderma, *SLE* systemic lupus erythematosus, *SRP* signal recognition particle, *SSc* systemic sclerosis, *UIP* usual interstitial pneumonia

[a]The estimation of the number of patients was quoted from the website of the Japan Intractable Diseases Information Center by the Japan Ministry of Health, Labor and Welfare (http://www.nanbyou.or.jp/; accessed on February 26, 2017)

Lung lesions in CTD cause various pathological conditions, including ILD and vascular lesions (e.g., vasculitis and pulmonary hypertension), nodular lesions (e.g., rheumatic nodules), airway lesions (e.g., follicular or constrictive bronchiolitis), pleural lesions, and lymphatic diseases; and often, multiple lesions appear. In addition, CTD-related lung conditions may display a number of features on diagnostic imaging, including signs of opportunistic infections, drug-induced lung lesions, or malignant neoplasms. Thus, all these lung lesions have been collectively called the "CTD lung" [3, 4].

High-resolution or thin-section computed tomography (HRCT or TSCT, respectively) is useful for evaluating the extent of interstitial fibrotic changes, disease severity, and the fibrotic/inflammatory lesion ratio. Moreover, semiquantitative and qualitative data obtained from HRCT have shown significant correlations with pulmonary function tests. HRCT plays an important role in understanding the characteristics of ILD, which present with various clinical features. HRCT is also an effective method for evaluating responses to ILD treatments. Therefore, HRCT examinations should be actively performed in patients with CTD-ILD [5, 6].

In this chapter, among the lung lesions likely to develop in each type of CTD, RA-ILD is the primary focus; HRCT images and the histopathological patterns are reviewed and illustrated. In addition, this chapter considers conditions of rapidly progressive interstitial pneumonia (acute exacerbation of CTD-ILD) and interstitial pneumonia that precedes CTD (interstitial pneumonia with autoimmune features).

8.2 Interstitial Lung Diseases in Connective Tissue Disease

8.2.1 Frequency of CTD-ILD

The most common CTDs that cause ILDs include systemic sclerosis (SSc), RA, polymyositis/dermatomyositis (PM/DM), Sjögren syndrome (SjS), systemic lupus erythematosus

(SLE), and mixed connective tissue disease (MCTD) (Table 8.1). The frequency of identifying pulmonary lesions based on clinical findings varies widely among studies. Generally, pulmonary lesions are found most commonly in patients with SSc (60–70%). The next highest frequencies have been reported in PM/DM (40–50%), RA, and MCTD (both 30–40%); lower frequencies were reported in SjS and SLE (20–30%) [5–9]. Acute respiratory failure is commonly attributed to acute deterioration of interstitial pneumonia. The incidence of rapidly progressive deterioration of ILD is particularly high in patients with PM/DM (approximately 30%) [10], followed by patients with RA (10–20%) [11, 12] and SSc (approximately 10%) [13].

8.2.2 Undifferentiated Forms of CTD-ILD

Patients with PM/DM, RA, and SSc, in particular, frequently experience preceding ILDs, which present clinically before the condition meets the American College of Rheumatology (ACR) diagnostic criteria for a definitive diagnosis of a specific CTD subtype [14]. It has been proposed by different research groups that this condition should be termed "unclassifiable CTD (UCTD)" [15], "lung-dominant CTD (LD-CTD)" [16], or "autoimmune features with interstitial lung disease (AIF-ILD)" [17]. Recently, the European Respiratory Society (ERS)/American Thoracic Society (ATS) task force proposed that this condition should be termed "interstitial pneumonia with autoimmune features" [18] (IPAF, described below, part 8.4). However, even if it is termed IPAF, there is currently no choice but to classify it into IIPs.

8.2.3 Classification of CTD-ILDs

Most parenchymal manifestations of CTD-ILD are similar to those found in IIPs. Indeed, currently, the pattern classification of CTD-ILD in evaluating radiological (HRCT) and histological data is the same as those used for subtyping IIPs. In addition, a recent study described a new manifestation of CTD-ILD, which displayed a rare pattern of pleuroparenchymal fibroelastosis (PPFE); this pattern has not yet been completely characterized clinically [2, 5, 7].

8.2.4 Histopathological Patterns of CTD-ILD

CTD-ILD shows various histopathological patterns like IIPs including usual interstitial pneumonia (UIP), nonspecific interstitial pneumonia (NSIP), organizing pneumonia (OP), diffuse alveolar damage (DAD), lymphoid interstitial pneumonia (LIP), and diffuse lymphoid hyperplasia (DLH). Discordant UIP (e.g., UIP and NSIP coexisting in the surgical lung biopsy specimens) and multiple mixed patterns are also occasionally observed. Furthermore, conditions difficult to classify into any histological pattern are often observed, and these are categorized as "unclassifiable" ILDs (e.g., NSIP with OP variant [or fibrosing OP] and airway-centered fibrosis [or bronchiolocentric interstitial fibrosis]). Of these, NSIP was shown to be the most common histological pattern in CTD-ILD [3–8] (Table 8.1).

Other histological findings characteristic of CTD-ILD include interstitial lymphoid aggregates with germinal centers, diffuse lymphoplasmacytic infiltration, dense perivascular collagen, and extensive pleuritis [16–18]. CTD-ILD is strongly suggested when these findings are found in combination with a basic histological finding, such as NSIP.

8.2.5 Three Pathological Patterns of Pulmonary Fibrosis

There are three distinctive pathological patterns of pulmonary fibrosis, including UIP, fibrotic NSIP, and airway-centered fibrosis (ACF) [19]. Their distinctive histology is primarily based on the distribution of the fibrosis (diffuse versus patchy) as well as the anatomic location of the fibrosis (subpleural/paraseptal vs. interstitial vs. airway centered, respectively) (Fig. 8.1) [19].

UIP pattern is a form of diffuse parenchymal lung disease, characterized by patchy subpleural/paraseptal and basal predominance remodeling of lung tissue with honeycombing. The characteristic histological findings of UIP have been referred to as being "temporal heterogeneity" or having "patchwork quilt" appearance. In other words, the biopsy specimens appear to transition from dense scar tissue (the "past" or an established fibrosis) to normal lung tissue (the "future" or lung tissue not yet involved) [20].

In contrast, the inflammatory process in NSIP is diffuse and uniform, mainly involving the alveolar wall and variably affecting the bronchovascular sheaths and pleura. When fibrosis occurs in NSIP, it is usually mild and preserves lung structure, but it may proceed to extensive disease. Variable extents of peribronchiolar metaplasia may be present, but microscopic honeycombing is characteristically absent [20].

The ACF pattern is recently defined as surgical lung biopsy showing interstitial fibrosis centered on, and extending around, the bronchioles, with or without bronchiolar inflammation, and the presence of peribronchiolar metaplasia [19–21]. The initial reports referred to a lesion termed bronchiolocentric interstitial fibrosis or centrilobular fibrosis [22, 23]. The clinical condition resulting in the ACF pattern is chronic hypersensitivity pneumonitis. The other major conditions to consider include chronic aspiration and CTD

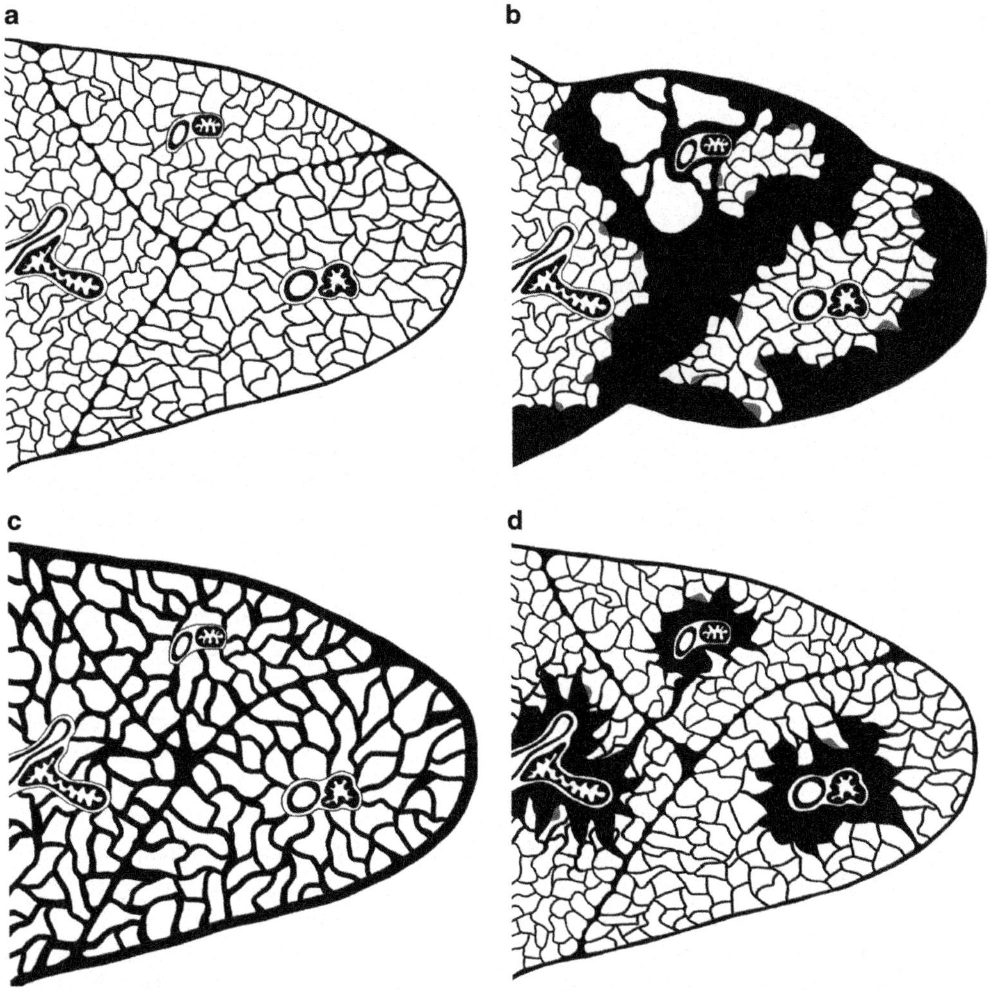

Fig. 8.1 Schematic representation of the three basic patterns of pulmonary fibrosis and their comparison to healthy lung (Illustrations of histopathologic specimen obtained from surgical lung biopsy). Adopted and modified from Smith ML [19]. (**a**) Healthy lung with thin alveolar walls and pleura, bronchovascular bundles located at the center of the lobules, and barely perceptible interlobular septae. (**b**) Usual interstitial pneumonia pattern of fibrosis with marked irregular fibrosis in a peripheral and subpleural distribution. The fibrosis transitions to completely normal alveolar walls abruptly, with numerous fibroblast foci at the interface zone. In some lobules, microscopic honeycombing change has occurred (upper lobule). (**c**) Fibrotic nonspecific interstitial pneumonia pattern of fibrosis showing diffuse involvement of the alveolar walls with thickening, fusion, and simplification. The pleura is similarly affected. In areas, there is more significant fusion and thickening lending a suggestion of heterogeneity, despite it being a diffuse process. (**d**) Airway-centered pattern of fibrosis with centrilobular stellate-appearing fibrosis, occasional bridges from one airway to another, and scattered fibroblast foci. Note the marked heterogeneity from field to field

(in particular, RA and SjS) [19–21]. Smoking and other inhalational exposures are also contributors to chronic airway-centered pathology [19].

8.2.6 CT UIP Pattern Based on the Current IPF Guideline

According to the IPF guidelines established by the ATS/ERS/Japanese Respiratory Society (JRS)/Latin American Thoracic Association (ALAT), published in 2011 [24], UIP pattern on HRCT images (actually, this means IPF-UIP) is characterized by the presence of reticular opacities, often associated with traction bronchiolectasis/bronchiectasis (hereafter, bronchiectasis). Honeycombing is common in UIP, and it is critical for making a definite diagnosis (Fig. 8.2) [24]. On HRCT images, honeycombing is manifested as clustered cystic airspaces, typically of compatible diameters on the order of 3–10 mm, but occasionally, they may be as large as 2.5 cm. Honeycombing is typically observed in subpleural areas, and it is characterized by well-defined walls (Fig. 8.3) [25]. However, a recent study suggested that there were variabilities of interobservers' agreements in diagnosing honeycombing on HRCT, and there were several mimickers, such as emphysema, airspace enlargement with fibrosis (Fig. 8.4), and cross-sectional images of traction bronchiectasis (Fig. 8.5) [26, 27].

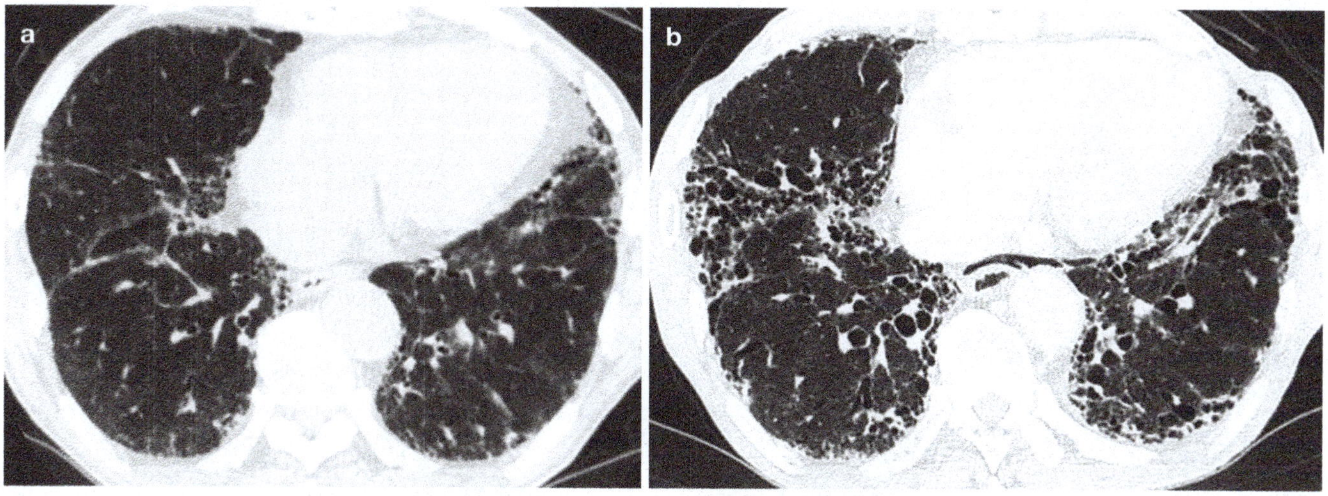

Fig. 8.2 60-year-old man with IPF/UIP. A patient had symptoms of persistent dry cough and breathlessness on exertion for 2 years. (**a**) Thin-section CT (lower lung zone) shows patchy areas of intralobular reticular opacities and vertical doted lines predominantly in bilateral subpleural regions. No honeycombing is present, and CT pattern based on the IPF guideline is the "possible UIP." (**b**) Thin-section CT (2 years later) shows extending of reticular opacities and irregular linear opacities with subpleural aircysts, and architectural distortion, which are thought to be deterioration of fibroproliferative changes. Areas of established fibrotic changes (reticular opacities with traction bronchiectasis and honeycombing) and nearly normal lung are coexistent and adjacent to each other. This pattern is called "temporal heterogeneity" or "abrupt change." On this time, CT pattern should be changed to the "UIP pattern"

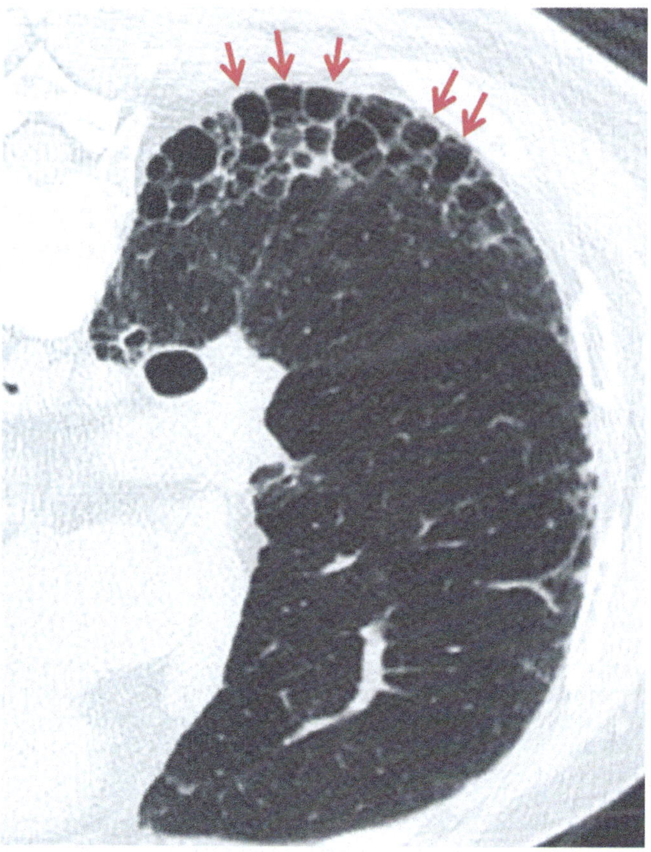

Fig. 8.3 Typical CT findings of "honeycombing" in a patient with IPF. HRCT image of right lung (lower zone) at prone position shows typical findings of "honeycombing," which consist of clustered cystic airspaces (diameters on the order of 3–10 mm, indicates by arrows) characterized by well-defined walls, observed in subpleural areas

With HRCT pattern based on the IPF guideline [24], UIP pattern is defined as having all following four items: (1) subpleural and basal predominance, (2) reticular abnormality, (3) honeycombing with/without traction bronchiectasis, and (4) absence of any seven features that are inconsistent with UIP pattern. The seven inconsistent features with UIP pattern are (1) upper or mid-lung predominance, (2) peribronchovascular predominance, (3) extensive ground-glass abnormality (extent > reticular abnormality), (4) profuse micronodules (bilateral, predominantly in the upper lobes), (5) discrete cysts (multiple, bilateral, away from areas of honeycombing), (6) diffuse mosaic attenuation (bilateral, in three or more lobes), or (7) consolidation in bronchopulmonary segment(s) or lobe(s). When "honeycombing" is absent, it is categorized as "possible UIP" pattern (Table 8.2). Due to the importance of "honeycombing," interpretations of the presence or absence of honeycombing often require multiplanar reconstruction (MPR) images and, ultimately, a multidisciplinary discussion (MDD) [26, 27].

With recent discussion of update version by the ATS/ERS/JRS/ALTA IPF guideline committee [28], CT patterns for UIP diagnosis will be changed into four categories as follows: (1) typical UIP CT pattern, (2) probable UIP CT pattern, (3) CT pattern indeterminate for UIP pattern, and (4) CT features most consistent with non-IPF diagnosis. New typical UIP CT pattern is defined as having all following five items: (1) CT distribution is basal (occasionally diffuse) and subpleural predominant and (2) distribution is often heterogenous; CT features show (3) presence of honeycombing, (4) reticular pattern with peripheral traction bronchiectasis or

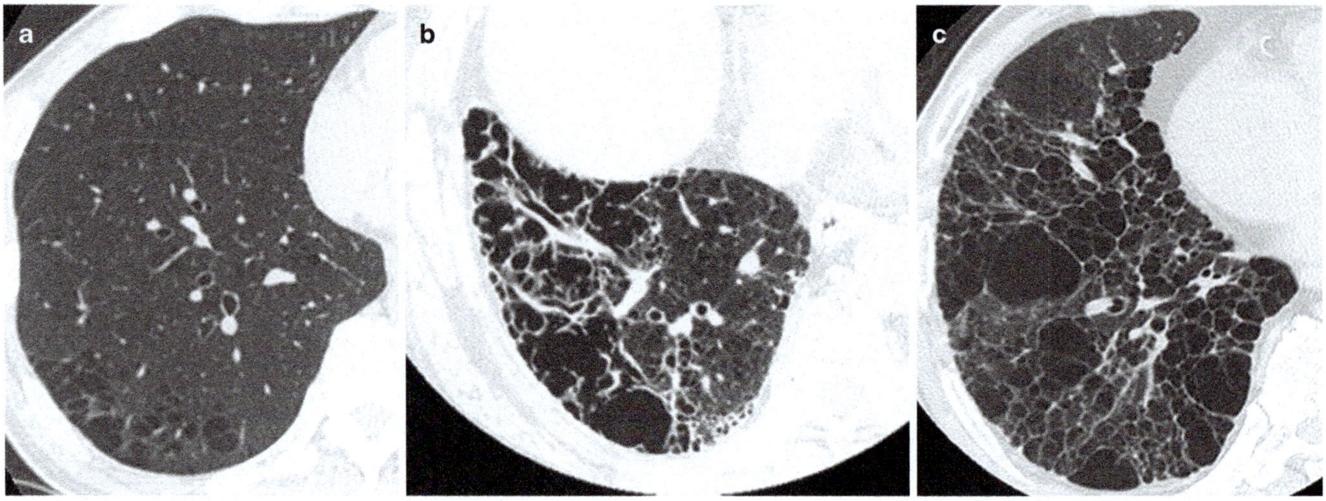

Fig. 8.4 Mimickers of honeycombing on HRCT (right basilar lung zone). (**a**) HRCT shows emphysematous air cysts (low-attenuation areas without well-defined wall), but some of them have thin walls, which may be related to slight fibrotic changes. (**b**) HRCT shows small to large aircysts with continuity, and cysts have thin or thick walls, which resemble airspace enlargement with fibrosis. (**c**) HRCT shows small to large multiple aircysts suspicious of emphysematous air cysts, but all of them have thin wall, and reticular opacities are also presented. Some of them in subpleural regions may be honeycobming

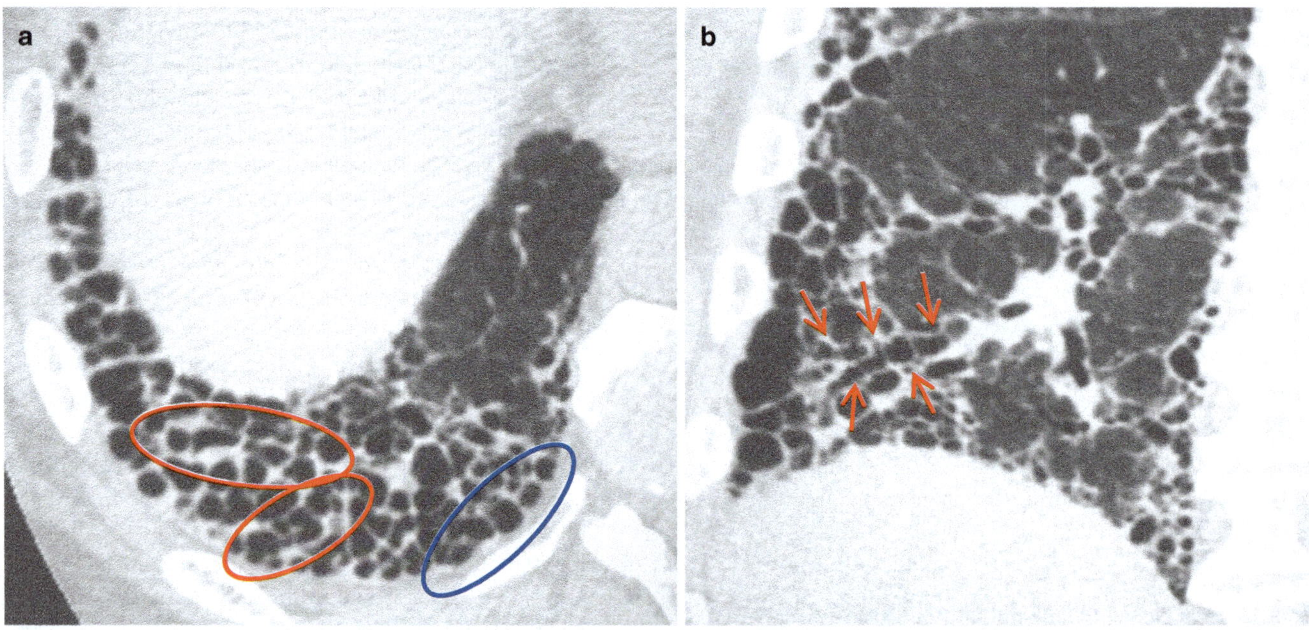

Fig. 8.5 Traction bronchiectasis versus honeycombing in a 65-year-old man with IPF/UIP. (**a**) HRCT transaxial image (right basal segment) shows aggregated multiple aircysts in subpleural region. Note continuous airspaces with continuity in the x-axis like dilated bronchioles (highlighted in red circles). Multiple aircysts (honeycombing, highlighted in blue circle) in subpleural area show well-definite wall sharing each other. (**b**) HRCT MPR coronal image shows traction bronchiectasis (red arrows, corresponding to red circle in **a**). (**c, d**) Microscopic images (HE, low power). (**c**) Honeycombing and traction bronchiolectasis are shown. (**d**) Typical findings of microscopic honeycombing. Size of honeycomb cystic space is 2 mm in diameter

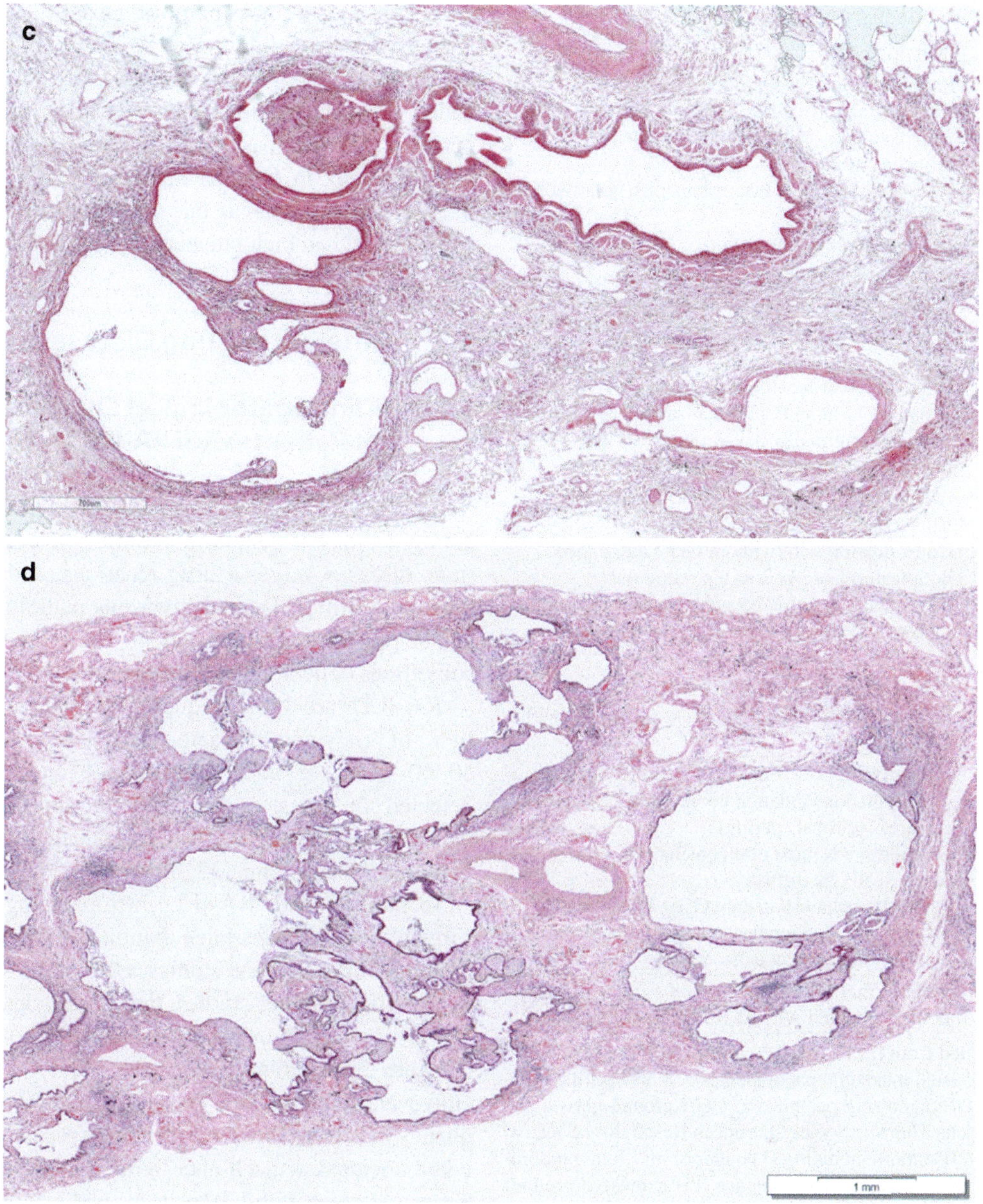

Fig. 8.5 (continued)

bronchiolectasis, and (5) absence of features to suggest an alternative diagnosis. Probable UIP CT pattern is defined as having all four items without honeycombing. An alternative diagnosis includes for example systemic autoimmune disease, chronic hypersensitivity pneumonitis, occupational and environmental lung disease, drug-induced pulmonary toxicity, or asbestosis. Since it was reported that subjects with probable UIP CT pattern on CT were more likely to have histologic probable/definite UIP than those with indeterminate UIP on CT [29], it is considered that the term "possible" on CT would be better to change to "probable." With this change the discrepancy of term between CT and pathological findings will be resolved.

8.2.7 CT Patterns of CTD-ILD

According to the ATS/ERS/JRS/ALAT IPF guidelines [24], HRCT patterns of CTD-ILD may often lead to classify into "inconsistent with UIP" pattern. Namely, HRCT patterns of CTD-ILD often display one or more of the seven findings listed as "inconsistent with UIP," and these findings are important as the common characteristics of CTD-ILD (Table 8.2).

HRCT findings characteristic of NSIP, which is pathologically the most frequent pattern in CTD-ILD, are ground-glass opacities (GGOs); reticular opacities, which typically represent fibrosis; and traction bronchiectasis. These features are predominantly observed in the lower lung zones and/or

Table 8.2 Definition of HRCT pattern

HRCT pattern	Definition
UIP	Subpleural and basal predominance Reticular abnormalities Honeycombing with/without traction bronchiectasis Absence of features listed as inconsistent with UIP pattern[a]
Possible UIP	Subpleural and basal predominance Reticular abnormalities Absence of features listed as inconsistent with UIP pattern[a]
NSIP	Diffuse or peribronchovascular distribution Bilateral lower lobe predominance Broad GGO more than reticulation with/withouot minimal honeycombing without prominent consolidation
NSIP with OP	Diffuse or peribronchovascular distribution Bilateral lower lobe predominance Consolidation with/without GGO associated with features of fibrosis (e.g., reticular abnormality, traction bronchiectasis, or lower lobe volume loss)
OP	Subpleural, peribronchial Distribution or band-like pattern Patchy consolidation commonly associated with GGO
DAD	Exudative phase = bilateral patchy GGO or often with consolidation geographic appearance (by areas of focal sparing) Distribution is most often basilar but occasionally be diffuse Organizing phase = mainly GGO, distortion of bronchovascular bundles, traction bronchiectasis, cysts, or other lucent areas of lung
Unclassifiable	Patterns that could be classified as those listed in 2015 updated ATS/ERS IIPs classification

Adopted and modified from [2, 12, 24]
Abbreviations: *UIP* usual interstitial pneumonia, *NSIP* nonspecific interstitial pneumonia, *OP* organizing pneumonia, *GGO* ground-glass opacity, *ATS/ERS* American Thoracic Society/European Respiratory Society
[a]Inconsistent with UIP pattern including (1) upper or mid-lung predominance, (2) peribronchovascular predominance, (3) extensive ground-glass abnormality (extent > reticular abnormality), (4) profuse micronodules (bilateral, predominantly upper lobes), (5) discrete cysts (multiple, bilateral, away from areas of honeycombing), (6) diffuse mosaic attenuation (bilateral, in three or more lobes), or (7) consolidation in bronchopulmonary segment(s)/lobe(s)

along peribronchovascular bundles; additionally, these findings are bilateral and symmetric in most patients (Fig. 8.6).

HRCT findings characteristic of CTD-UIP (histopathologically the most frequent pattern in RA-ILD) are reticular opacities and honeycombing with/without traction bronchiectasis, predominantly present in subpleural and lower lung zones, similar to IPF/UIP. However, patients with CTD-UIP showed less extensive emphysema, more prevalence of non-typical UIP pattern without honeycombing, and a tendency for less honeycombing compared to patients with IPF/UIP [30].

Although histopathological findings appear similar to UIP patterns, concluding them as UIP is sometimes difficult on HRCT due to the possibility of mixed histological findings. Namely, corresponding to the coexistence of various histological findings, high-attenuation lesions such as GGO and consolidation are seen on HRCT relatively in peribronchiolar area or outside of the lung basal zones, and disease progression seems homogenously in the bilateral lung (Fig. 8.7). Furthermore, mosaic attenuation areas (air trapping), due to airway lesions superimposed on high-attenuation areas, are also seen [3, 4].

8.3 Interstitial Lung Disease in RA

8.3.1 Clinicopathological Characteristics of Patients with RA-ILD

Various lung lesions are associated with RA, including ILD, airway lesions, rheumatoid nodules, pleural diseases, infectious diseases, adverse drug reactions, and malignant neoplasms. Additionally, these various pathological conditions can be present in a single patient. Therefore, this condition is sometimes collectively called the "rheumatoid lung" [4].

RA-ILDs are found frequently among patients with a high titer of rheumatoid factor and commonly in men of 50–60 years of age. Evidence of interstitial fibrosis is detected on chest radiographs in approximately 5% of patients with RA [31, 32], but it is detected on HRCT images in 30–40% of patients [33, 34].

In patients with RA-ILD, histopathological analyses of surgical lung biopsies have exhibited different trends in different cohorts. In some studies, UIPs were found more often than NSIPs; in other studies, the frequencies of finding UIPs and NSIPs were nearly equal. The next most common findings are bronchiolar impairments and OP patterns [3–8]. However, unlike other CTDs, RA-ILD has shown a high frequency of UIP patterns. According to recent reports, RA-ILD was associated with a higher frequency of UIP than NSIP patterns, and cases with UIP patterns had a poor prognosis [35].

Although patients with RA-ILD commonly follow a chronic course, some studies have described patients with RA-ILD that died after acute exacerbations of ILD, similar to patients with IPF [12]. Histopathological studies revealed that patients with CTD-UIP had good prognosis compared to patients with IPF/UIP and had similar prognosis to patients with CTD-NSIP [35–37]. However, the prognosis for patients with RA-UIP was worse than those of patients with other CTD-UIP and patients with RA-NSIP [35–37]. In addition, some previous studies have reported that patients with RA-UIP had a better prognosis than those with IPF/UIP [36]; however, a comparable number of other studies have reported that both conditions had similarly poor prognoses [37]. On the other hand, although chronic fibrosing ILD is the main histopathological pattern of RA-ILD, it is often difficult to differentiate, based on only a single pattern, from the other histopathological types of IIPs.

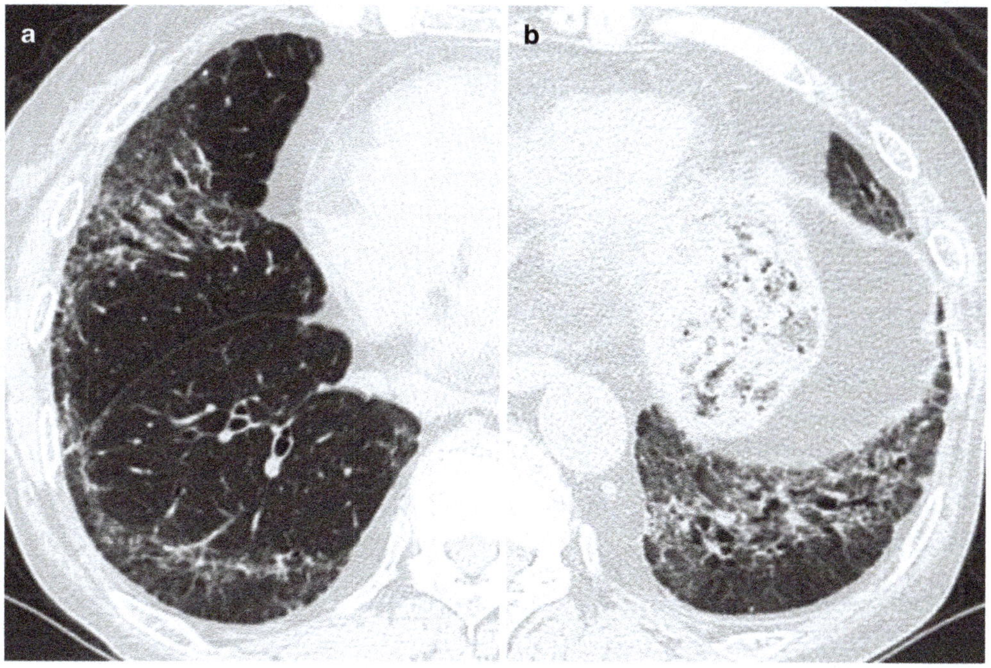

Fig. 8.6 62-year-old woman with antisynthetase syndrome (CT NSIP pattern). (**a**, **b**) HRCT (lower lung zone) images show diffuse areas of reticular opacities with GGO and with traction bronchiectasis predominantly seen in periphery and along bronchovascular bundles. Subpleural lung parenchyma is relatively sparing. CT pattern corresponds to NSIP pattern

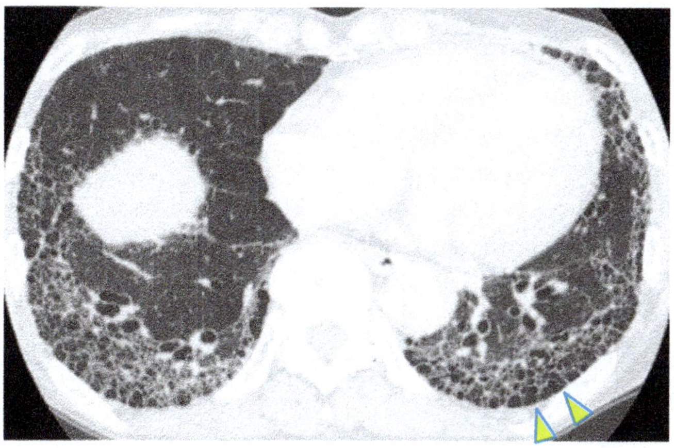

Fig. 8.7 64-year-old woman with mixed connective tissue disease. Thin-section CT (lower lung zone) shows diffuse areas of reticular opacities with airspace enlargement and traction bronchiectasis in subpleural region and also reveals architectural distortions and decrease of normal lung areas. In subpleural region of left basal zone, aircysts which share the wall each other are arranged in a line (like "honeycombing," arrowheads). CT pattern corresponds "UIP" pattern; however, areas of GGO are also seen, and spread pattern of abnormal opacities is homogenously (bilateral symmetry), which may present coexistent of NSIP pattern

8.3.2 CT Characteristics of RA-ILD

Chest radiography features of RA-ILD, in the early stage, include linear and reticular opacities, mainly in the lower lung fields. As the disease progresses, the reticular patterns become coarser and more diffuse and may develop into honeycombing [3, 4].

Reportedly, in HRCT images, the major findings of RA-ILD include patterns of UIP, NSIP, bronchitis, and OP [38]. Reticular shadows with or without honeycombing are consistent with UIP. Centrilobular nodules ± airway lesions (such as bronchiectasis and bronchiolitis obliterans) and consolidation are consistent with OP and chronic eosinophilic pneumonia. New multiple GGOs, in addition to the reticular opacities, during the treatment course suggest acute exacerbation of ILD [39].

RA-ILD with UIP pattern shows linear and reticular opacities, mainly in the subpleural area in the lower lung zones. As the lesions progress, the reticular patterns become coarser and more diffuse and may develop into honeycombing (Fig. 8.8). Generally, as the UIP patterns found in the images are similar to those found in IPF/UIP, it is considered difficult to make a differential diagnosis between the two conditions. On the other hand, a recent report suggested that a definite CT UIP pattern in RA-ILD was highly specific and moderately sensitive in predicting a histopathological UIP pattern. Thus, CT might be useful for accurately identifying UIP patterns in patients with RA [40]. It was reported that intralobular reticular opacities reflected fibrosis and correlated with prognosis in patients with a histological diagnosis of UIP and a clinical diagnosis of IPF [41]. Similarly, intralobular reticular opacities were identified as a prognostic imaging factor in patients with RA-UIP [36].

Accumulations of multiple cystic air-filled structures may be commonly identified as honeycombing on CT images. However, in some patients, traction bronchiectasis in fibroproliferative lesions, airspace enlargement with fibrosis [42, 43], pre-existing smoking-related lesions (emphysema) with

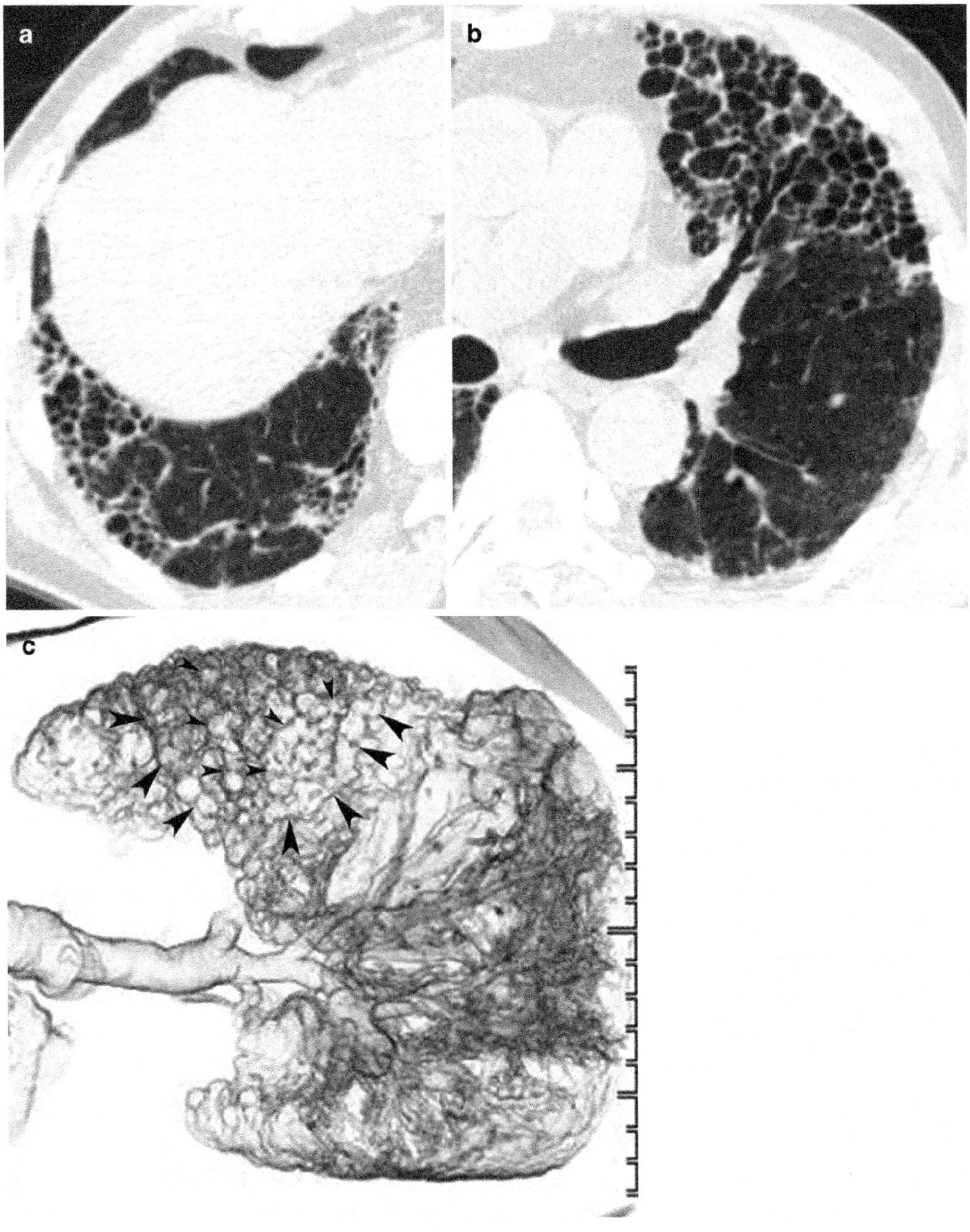

Fig. 8.8 63-year-old man with RA showing CT UIP pattern. (**a**) On HRCT images intralobular reticular opacities suggesting fibroproliferative changes are patchy distributed in the right lung base. Although it seems honeycombing, there are mainly reticular opacities and ground-glass opacities (GGOs) with small airspace enlargement and traction bronchiolectasis, which are forming aggregation of multiple small aircystic lesions. (**b**) In the left middle lung zone, GGOs and fine reticular opacities are seen from proximal to subpleural parenchyma. In lingular segment, there is aggregation of small aircysts of about a few millimeters to 1 cm which share the walls of each other to the pleural surface. In particular, the peripheral region may be suggestive of "honeycombing." On the other hand, traction bronchiolectasis is seen from the central side, but small cysts from the inner layer seem to also see the tangential image of this extension. (**c**) MIP image at middle lung zone: the multicystic changes of the inner zonal part (except under the pleura) seen in (**b**) can be confirmed to have continuity from the central side to periphery (large and small arrowheads), which correspond to traction bronchiectasis

fibrosis of the surrounding area may resemble honeycombing in some patients (Figs. 8.4 and 8.8c). Therefore, a finding of multiple air-filled cystic lesions should be interpreted with caution [26, 27]. On the other hand, it is important to know that even if microscopic honeycombing is present histologically, recognition of the presence of honeycombing on CT is often difficult because of differentiation of spatial resolution. Further, for example, when there is a mucus retention in honeycomb cysts, cysts may disappear on CT, and only areas of GGO may be seen (Fig. 8.9).

RA-ILD with NSIP pattern shows reticular opacities with traction bronchiectasis, GGO, and consolidation along peribronchovascular bundles or in subpleural area in the bilateral lower lung zones, presenting with image similar to those of idiopathic NSIP (Fig. 8.10).

In patients with RA, the NSIP and UIP patterns often overlap. The characteristic CT findings are relatively extensive GGOs, superimposed on areas of reticular opacities with/without traction bronchiectasis or honeycombing. Anatomically, parenchymal architectural distortions and lung volume reductions occur in patients with advanced conditions, and CT images show an intermingling of reticular opacities, traction bronchiectasis, and honeycombing [4].

RA-ILD with OP pattern is characterized by patchy parenchymal opacities, such as consolidations and GGOs (Fig. 8.11), which may migrate over time (called "wandering pneumo-

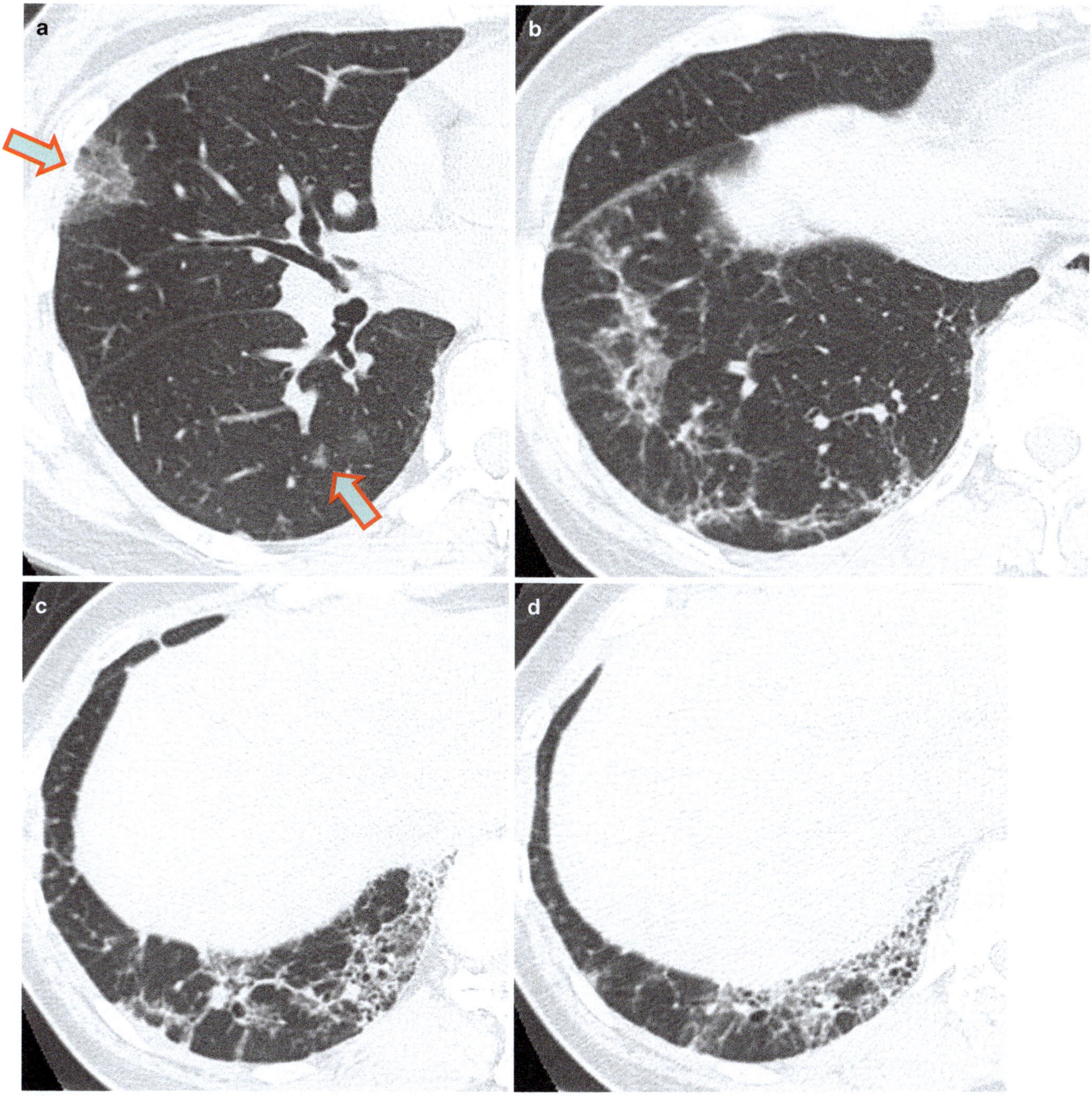

Fig. 8.9 50-year-old woman with RA-ILD. (**a**) HRCT (middle lung zone) shows patchy areas of GGO (arrows) which corresponds to OP pattern. (**b**) HRCT (basal lung zone) shows perilobular distribution of irregular linear/reticular opacities, GGO with traction bronchiectasis, and architectural distortion, but subpleural areas are sparing. (**c**, **d**) Subpleural irregular linear/reticular opacities and areas with GGO are seen. Coexisting fibroproliferative changes, such as traction bronchiolectasis and focal volume loss, and subpleural small cystic changes are also seen. No definite honeycombing on HRCT is visible; however, spatial disease distribution and temporal disease severity are nonuniform impression. (**e–g**) Low power views of pathologic specimen from the right basal segment (HE, original mag. ×2). (**e**) The specimen shows chronic fibrosing interstitial pneumonia with microscopic honeycombing (UIP pattern) and lymphoid follicles with germinal center. Note marked irregular fibrosis in a peripheral and subpleural distribution transitioning to normal lung tissues (so-called abrupt change). Although the basic pathology fits best to UIP pattern, presence of marked lymphoid hyperplasia and airway disease is often a clue finding in the patient with CTD, such as RA or SjS. (**f**) Multicystic areas with lymphoid follicules are shown. (**g**) Interstitial fibrosis and lymphoid follicules are visible. Note mucin retention in dilated airspaces (mucinosis)

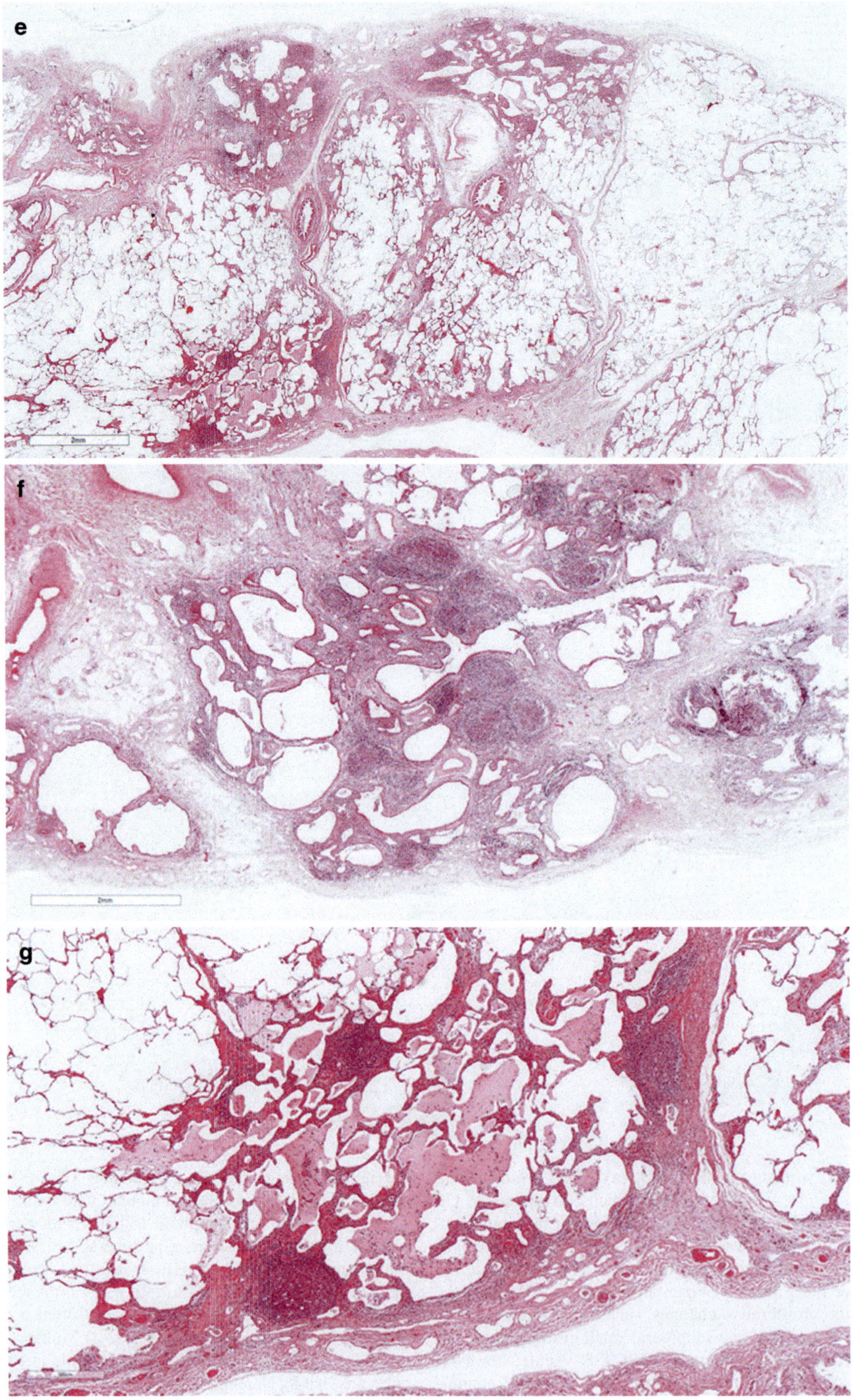

Fig. 8.9 (continued)

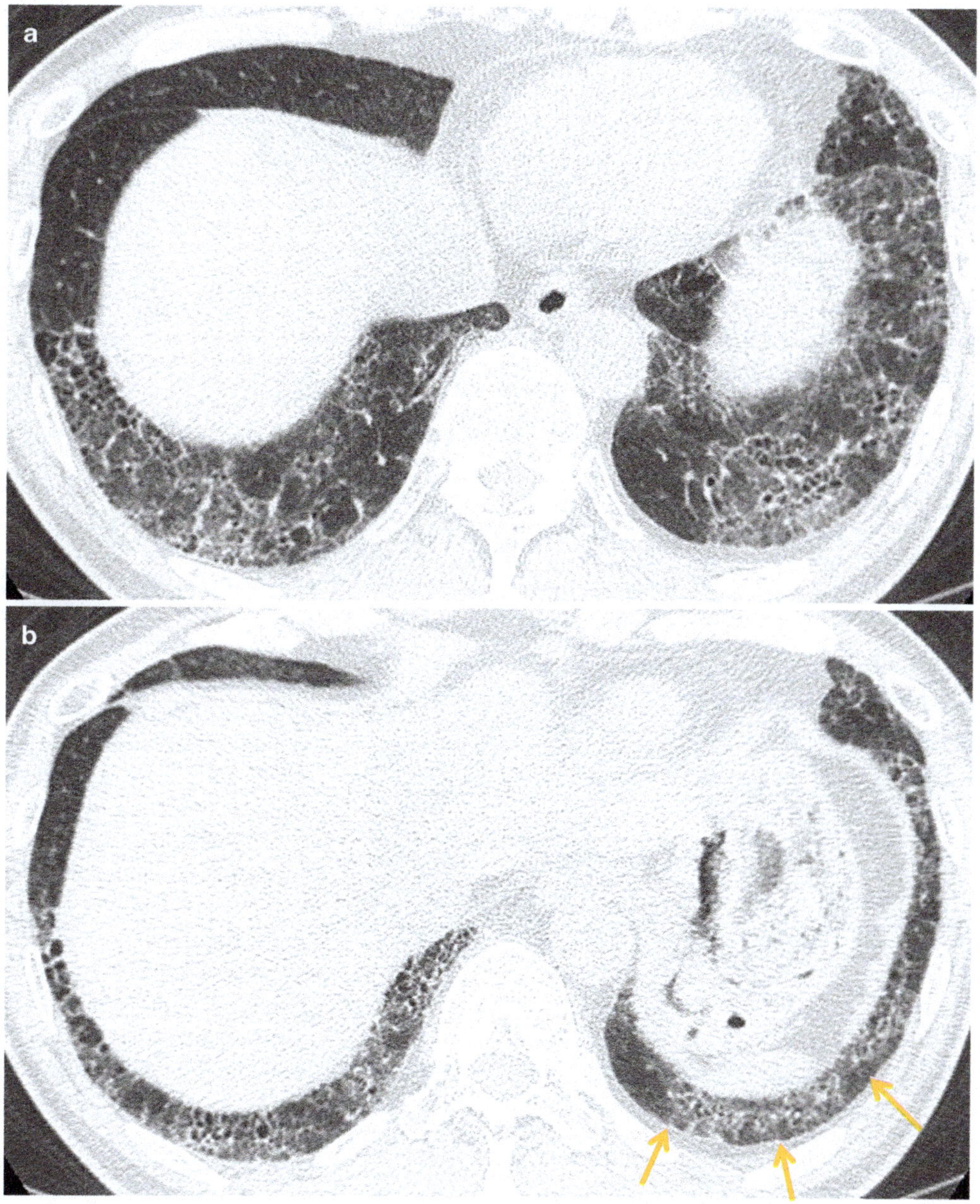

Fig. 8.10 64-year-old man with RA-ILD (NSIP pattern). (**a**) Thin-section CT shows diffuse areas of reticular opacities with GGO predominantly in bilateral peripheral lung parenchyma. Note extent areas of GGO > areas of reticular opacities. (**b**) At bottom of lung, subpleural areas are relatively spared (arrows), and reticular opacities with GGO are present around bronchioles (2–3 mm distant from pleura)

nia") [44, 45]. Although not always present, OP pattern may exhibit the reversed CT halo sign [46] (Fig. 8.12), and sometimes the features may overlap with those typical of the NSIP pattern (called "NSIP with OP pattern") (Fig. 8.13). Importantly, this pattern should always be considered in the differential diagnosis of lung infections and drug adverse reactions.

Several case reports have described patients with RA that developed upper lobe fibrosis associated with cavitation. On images, these features resembled tuberculosis [47, 48] or pleuroparenchymal elastofibrosis (PPFE) [49] (Fig. 8.14). However, this complication is quite rare.

8.3.3 CT Findings of Airway Impairments in RA

RA is often complicated with airway lesions, like bronchiectasis or follicular or constrictive bronchiolitis [33]. In a study of 34 patients with RA that had respiratory symptoms, HRCT images frequently displayed peribronchial wall thickening (85%) and bronchial dilatation (62%), but honeycombing was only detected in three patients (9%) [50]. Constrictive bronchiolitis (bronchiolitis obliterans [BO]) occurs due to inflammation and fibrosis in the bronchiolar walls. It results in narrowing or obliteration of the bronchiolar lumen. The

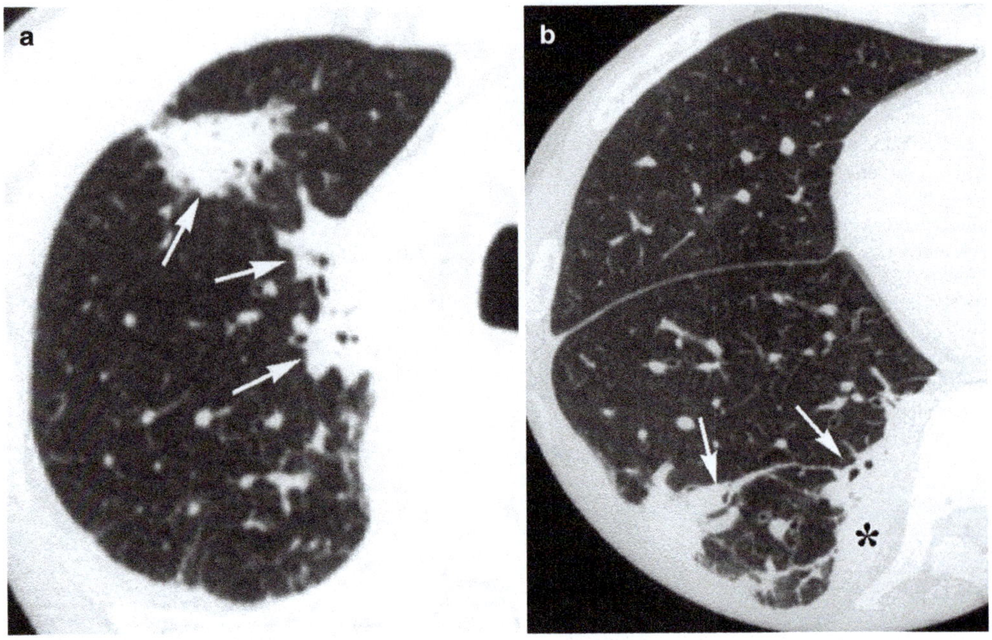

Fig. 8.11 54-year-old-man with RA showing OP pattern and pleuritis. (**a**) On HRCT image (upper lung zone), patchy areas of consolidation with airbronchogram are seen in periphery of the right lung S3. (**b**) In lung base section, pleural thickening, collapse of subpleural lung (arrows), and small amount of pleural effusion (asterisk) are also seen

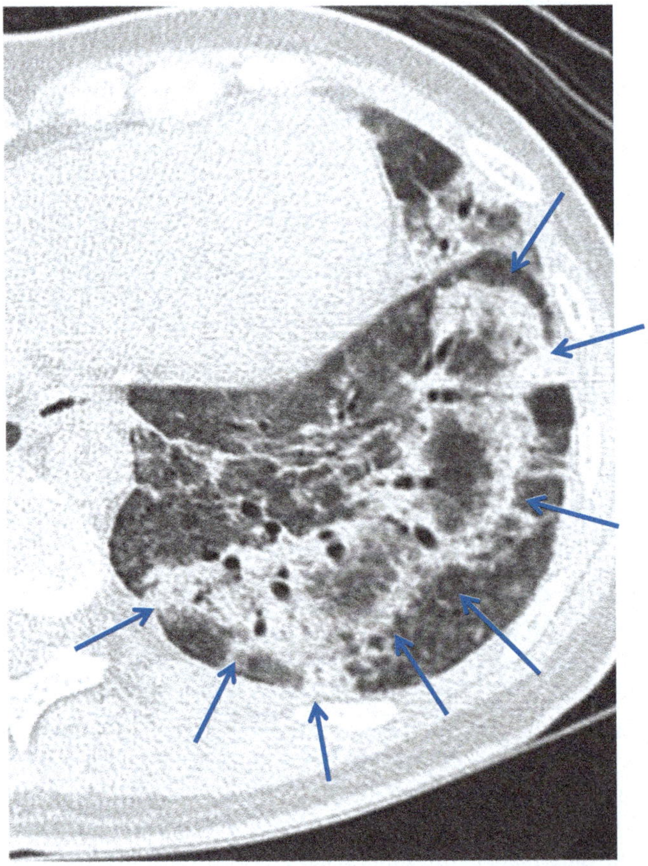

Fig. 8.12 50-year-old woman idiopathic NSIP with OP. HRCT (through left basal segment) shows consolidation distributing along airway (arrows) with mild bronchial dilatation, but lung distortion nor traction is less represented. Central areas surrounded by consolidation show GGO (like "reveresd CT-halo sign"). Histopathologically, there was coexistence of cellular and fibrotic NSIP and OP (NSIP with OP or fibrosing OP)

most common causes are childhood infections and hematopoietic stem cell, lung, or heart-lung transplantation. Among the CTDs, BO is most commonly observed in RA and occasionally in SjS, SLE, and SSc.

The HRCT features characteristic of BO consist of areas of decreased attenuation and vascularity (mosaic perfusion pattern) on inspiratory scans (Fig. 8.15) and air trapping on expiratory scans. These features enhance hypoattenuation areas and make it easier to visualize this condition [3–8]. Other CT findings include bronchiectasis and bronchiolectasis, peribronchial wall thickening, small centrilobular nodules, and branching structures [3–8] (Fig. 8.16).

8.3.4 Peripheral Aircystic Lesions Coexisting in RA-ILD

As previously described, airway lesions are frequently observed in patients with RA-ILD. However, several important points remain unclear. First, it is not clear what mechanisms cause the formation of air-filled cystic lesions (hereafter, "aircystic lesions," which is like honeycombing), which are often observed in RA-ILD. Second, it is not clear what role airway lesions play in the development of aircystic structures. Recently, these points have been discussed from new perspectives, based on assessments of histopathological and HRCT findings [51] (see Chap. 7).

In those discussions, the formation of aircystic lesions was suggested to arise from chronic, persistent intralobular airway inflammation, which could disrupt the bronchiolar walls and pulmonary alveoli; the result would be the formation of aircysts in the intralobular area (Fig. 8.17). Therefore,

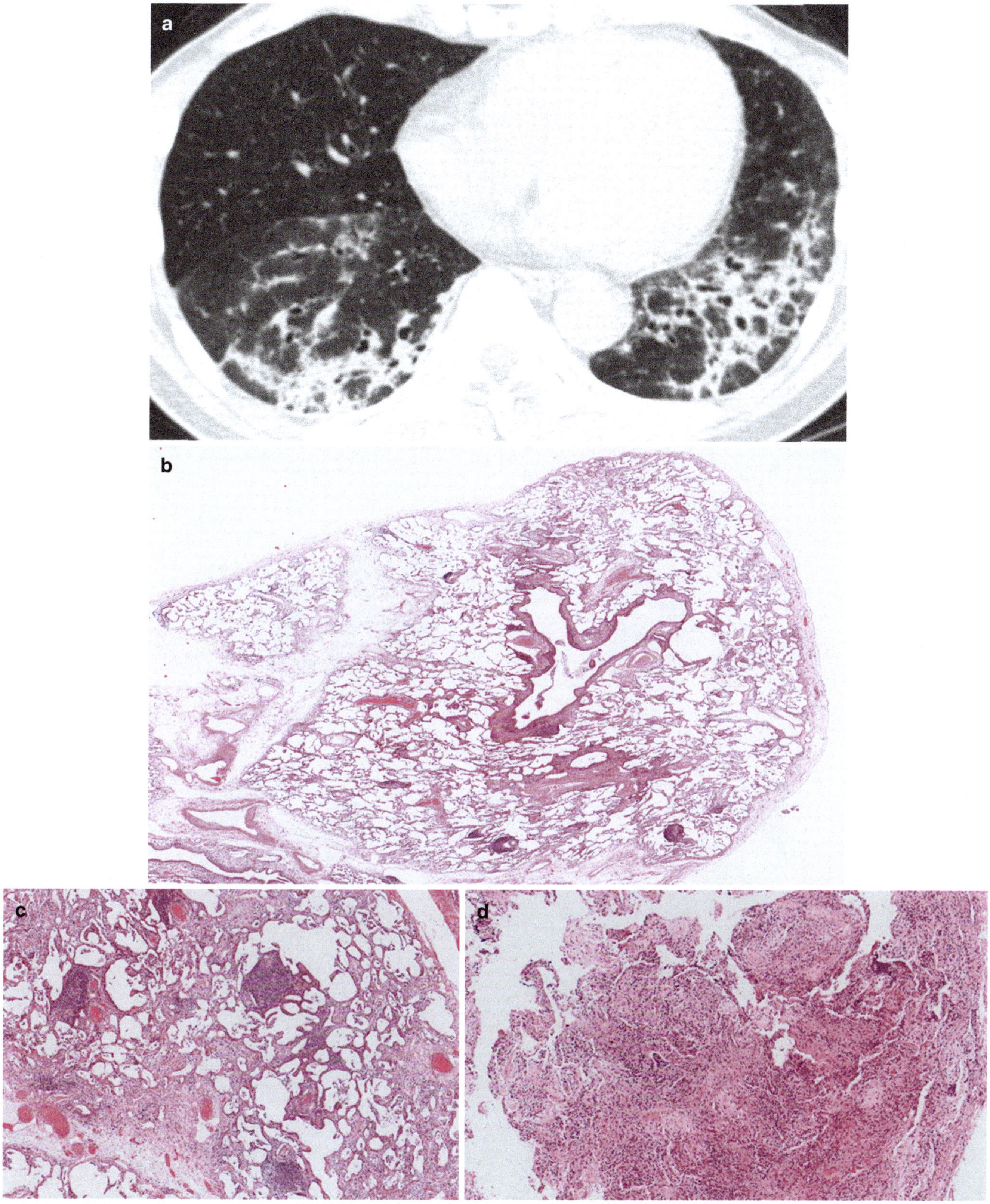

Fig. 8.13 56-year-old woman with RA showing NSIP with OP pattern. (**a**) On HRCT image of lower lung zone, decrease in lung volume and architectural structure distortion are recognized predominantly in bilateral lung basilar zones. GGOs and band-shaped irregular consolidation with traction bronchiectasis infiltrate nonsegmentally. Subpleural areas are partly spared, and also an airway centric distribution pattern is shown. (**b–d**) Low power views of pathologic specimen from the right basal segment (HE). Pathologically, cellular and fibrotic NSIP pattern was the main finding (**b**), and there were mixed various findings, including diffuse lymphocytic hyperplasia (**c**), follicular bronchiolitis, and OP (**d**). Note NSIP pattern of fibrosis showing diffuse involvement compared with Fig. 8.9e (UIP pattern)

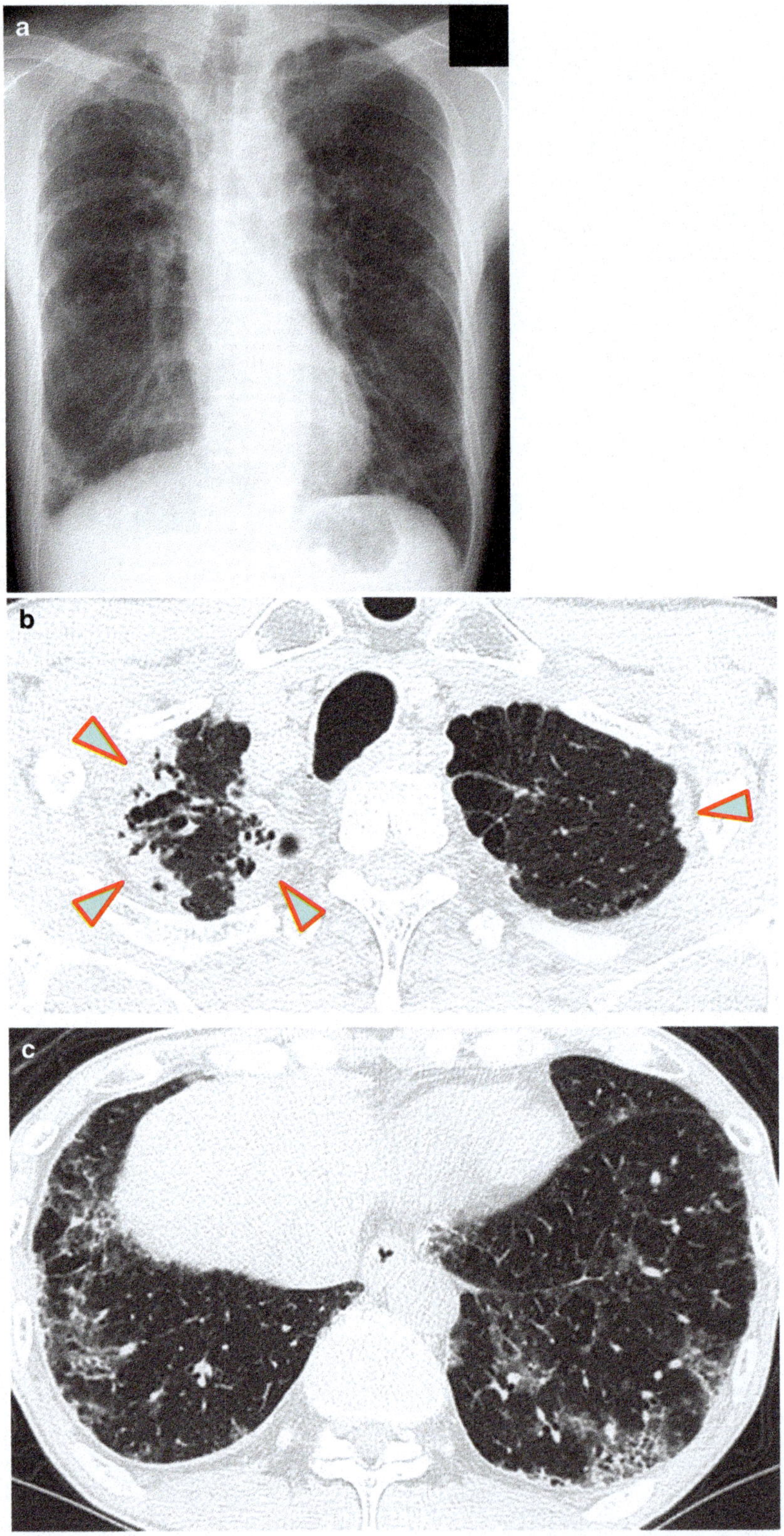

Fig. 8.14 60-year-old man with RA-ILD (unclassifiable ILD). (**a**) Chest radiograph shows upper lobe shrinkage caused by irregular-shaped linear opacities and pleural thickening-like changes in lung apex. Furthermore, irregular linear/reticular opacities and GGO area are also seen predominantly in periphery of middle to lower lung zone. (**b**) HRCT through the upper lobes shows pleuroparenchymal opacities (irregular-shaped consolidation with/without traction bronchiectasis, arrowheads) and distortion of the underlying lung parenchyma. (**c**) In the lower lung zones, scattered irregular-shaped areas of reticular opacities and GGO with bronchiolar dilatation are seen, but pleural-based irregular opacities are less prominently than upper lobes. The CT pattern is considered to be unclassifiable ILD pattern because of presence of NSIP with OP like opacities, bronchial impairments, and PPFE-like change

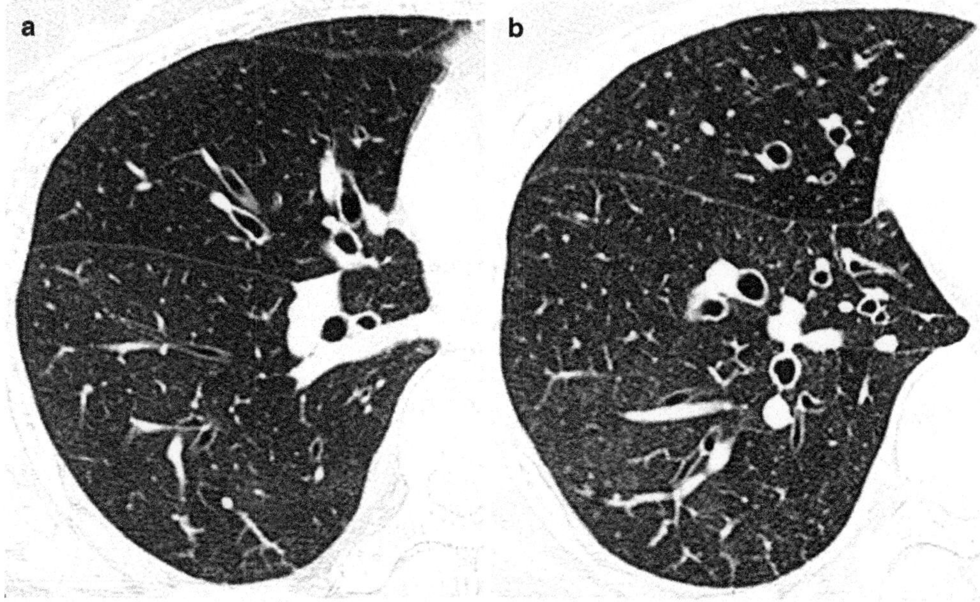

Fig. 8.15 55-year-old woman with RA, histopathologically showing acute lung injury pattern with clinically BO. (**a**, **b**) On HRCT of the lower right lung zone, low-attenuation areas and high-attenuation areas are mixed geographically, and a mosaic attenuation pattern is present. Bronchial dilatations are seen from the relatively proximal branch, and the bronchial wall is somewhat conspicuous. In the periphery, intralobular branching structures are seen, and the peripheral lung fields show hypoattenuation. Histopathologically, acute to subacute fibrotic lesions (acute lung injury or subacute interstitial pneumonia pattern) around the airway are conspicuous, and moderate constrictive bronchiolitis partly confirmed, which was considered to be clinically obstructive bronchiolitis (BO)

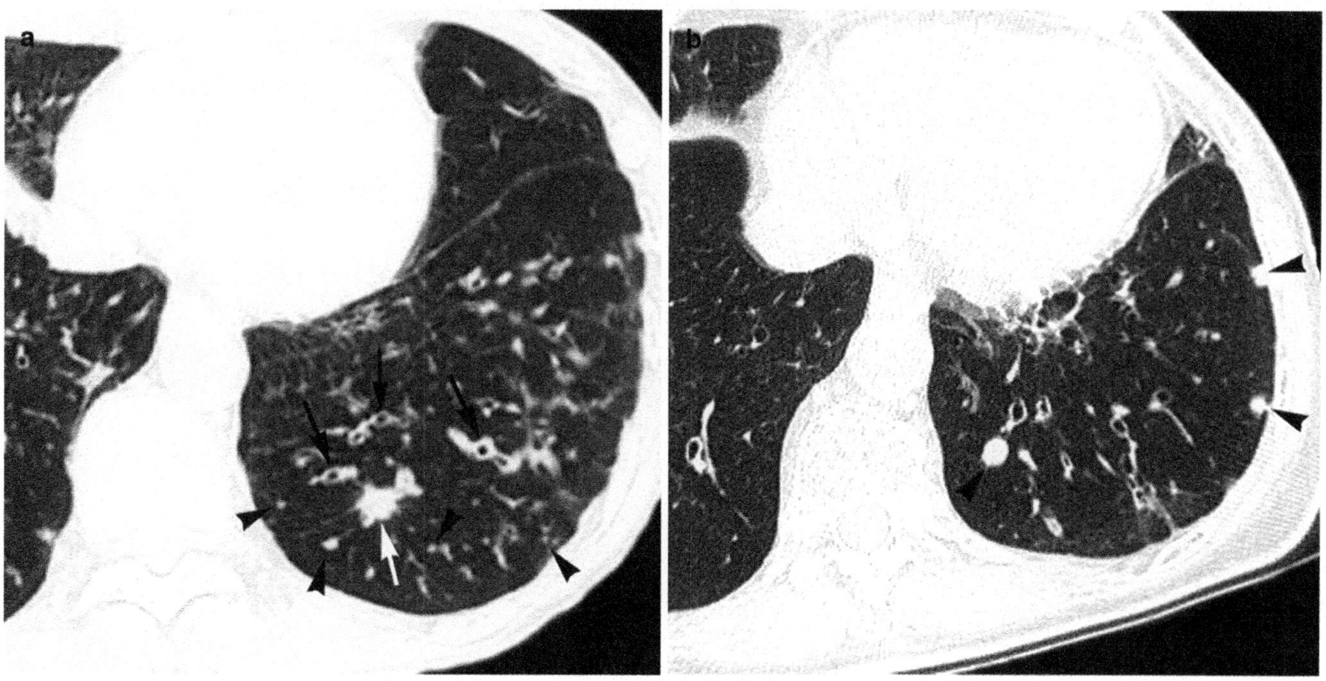

Fig. 8.16 65-year-old woman with RA and airway lesions. (**a**, **b**) HRCT images (left lung basal zone) show bronchial dilatation and peribronchial wall thickening (black arrows) superimposed on hypoattenuation areas of lung parenchyma suggestive of hyperinflation. Multiple subpleural small nodules (rheumatoid necrobiotic nodule) and intralobular nodules (peribronchiolar inflammatory nodules) are also seen (arrowheads)

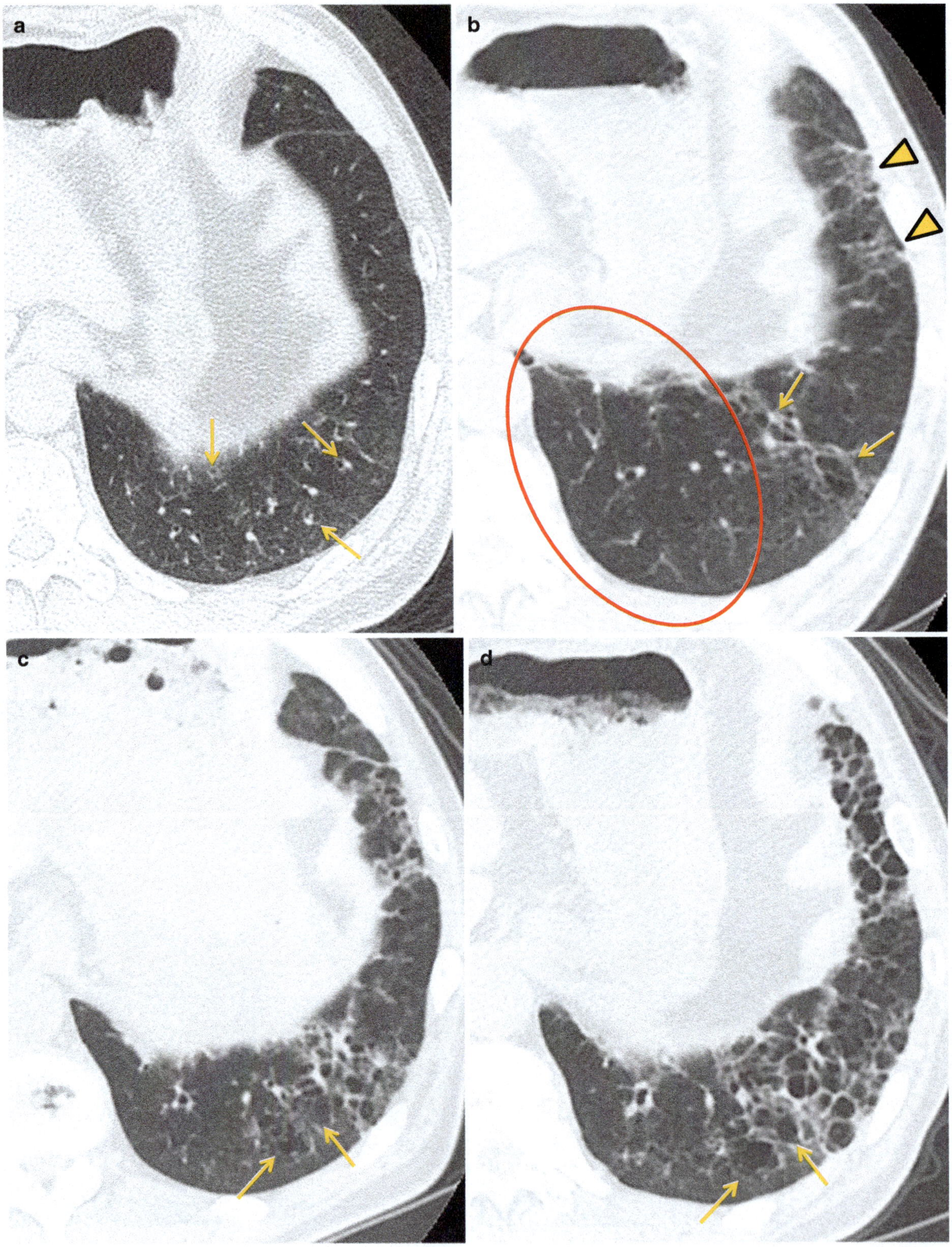

Fig. 8.17 61-year-old man with RA-ILD with UIP pattern. (**a**) Initial HRCT of left basal zone (6.5 years before obtaining image **d**) shows slight bronchiolar dilatation and milder peribronchiolar thickening (arrowheads). (**b**) HRCT (5.5 years before) shows irregular linear opacities and cystic change along bronchovascular sheaths (arrows) and intralobular reticular opacities (arrowheds). Note areas of increase in lung volume due to emphysematous change (red circle), compared with previous CT. (**c**) HRCT (3 years before) shows reticular opacities with aircystic changes and architectural distortion. These lesions seem to cause from respiratory tract changes and appear to progress around the airway. Note focal areas likely to be emphysema/airway enlargement (arrows). (**d**) HRCT (current) shows aggregate of aircysts like honeycombing, but some of them seem to be emphysema/airway enlargement with fibrosis (arrows). Furthermore, with referring to the time course of theses lesions, neighboring some aggregates of aircysts seems to be also related to bronchiolar or airway enlargement and fibrotic change

this mechanism is likely to be different from the mechanisms that give rise to honeycombing in IPF/UIP. Namely, among the cases that were identified as UIP pattern in RA-ILD, some aircystic lesions that developed from inflammatory mechanisms may have been confused with honeycomb structures in the microscopic examinations or interpretations of HRCT images. This mistake could result in a diagnosis of a refractory lesion or a poor prognosis. Undoubtedly, this topic represents an important future theme in discussions regarding RA-ILD treatments.

8.3.5 Acute Exacerbation in CTD-ILD and in RA-ILD

Acute exacerbations are defined based on consensus criteria for acute exacerbations in IPF, which have been recently revised [52]. Acute exacerbation is defined as an acute, clinically significant, respiratory deterioration characterized by evidence of new widespread alveolar abnormality. Acute exacerbations are increasingly recognized as a rare complication of CTD-ILD [11, 53–55]. Histopathologically, acute exacerbations commonly show DAD, acute lung injury (ALI), or OP pattern, superimposed on underlying chronic interstitial fibrosis. The revised diagnostic criteria (2016 version) of acute exacerbation of IPF [52] are (a) previous or concurrent diagnosis of IPF, (b) acute worsening or development of dyspnea typically <1 month duration, (c) CT with new GGO and/or consolidation superimposed on a background pattern consistent with UIP pattern, and (d) deterioration not fully explained by cardiac failure or fluid overload. Acute exacerbation of CTD-ILD will be diagnosed based on these same criteria (replace "IPF" with "CTD-ILD"). Acute exacerbations of CTD-ILD occur most frequently in patients with RA (Figs. 8.18 and 8.19). These patients have a worse outcome and a higher risk of early mortality than patients with RA-NSIP [53]. In a case-control study, acute exacerbation of RA was associated with a mortality of 64% [12]. On the other hand,

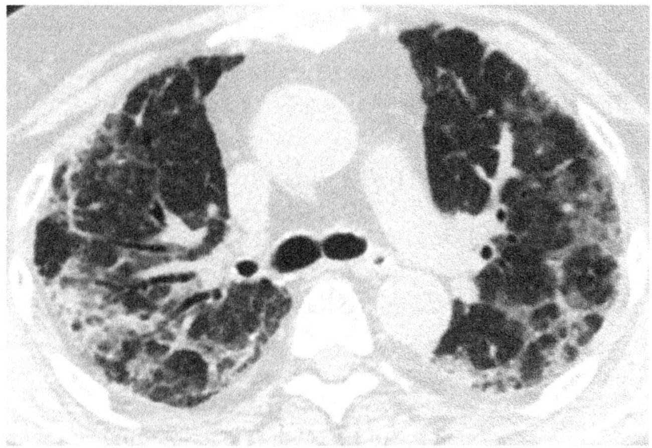

Fig. 8.18 70-year-old woman with RA and lung injury caused by methotrexate. HRCT through the upper lung field shows geographically distributed mixed areas of GGO and consolidation with bronchial dilatation. CT pattern is considered to be acute lung injury or DAD pattern. Drug adverse reaction was considered, and abnormal opacities have disappeared by discontinuation of methotrexate. This case was not acute exacerbation of RA-ILD, but diagnosed as methotrexate-related ILD

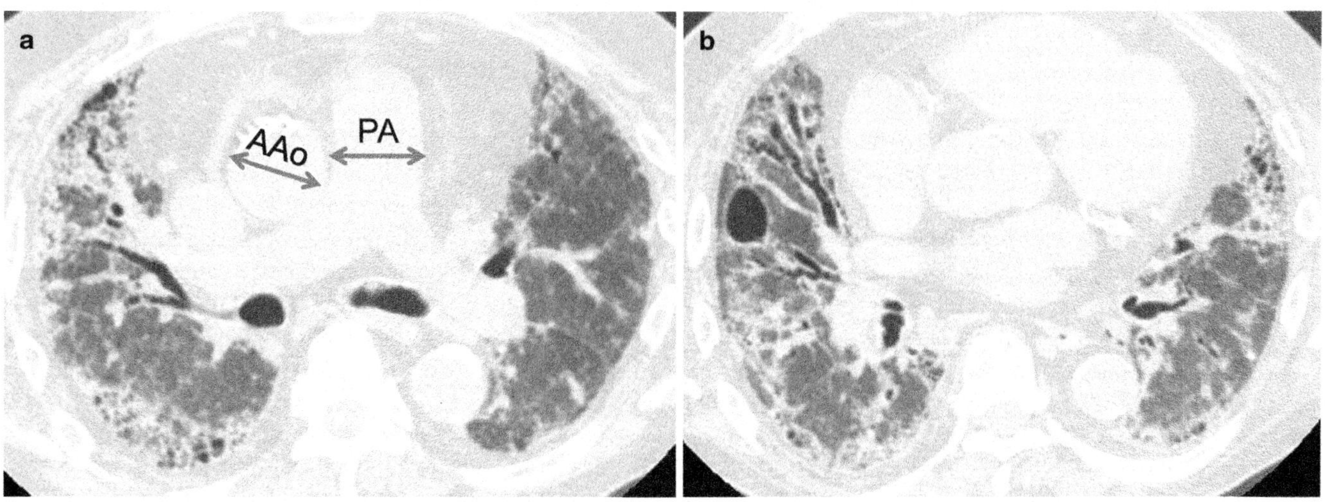

Fig. 8.19 Acute exacerbation of RA-ILD. (**a**, **b**) The patient undergoing follow-up as RA-ILD at outpatient department for 3 years had suddenly symptoms of severe dyspnea and cough. Although no cardiac failure, fluid overload, nor other causes of deterioration were found. Thin-section CT images (2 weeks after onset) show diffuse areas of GGO with irregular, varicoid bronchial dilatation and air-cysts superimposed on reticular opacities (chronic fibrosis) and marked lung volume decrease (ALI/DAD pattern). Furthermore PA trunk dilatation (PA/AAo diameter ratio > 1.0, suspicious of pulmonary hypertension) is also seen. Unfortunately the patient died. Abbreviations: *AAo* diameter of ascending aorta, *PA* diameter of pulmonary arterial trunk

although lesions in joints and muscles in patients with RA other than infectious diseases and ILD can be relentless and progressive, it is seldom directly responsible for the death of an individual.

Among clinical factors, visual scoring system based on HRCT findings (particularly the extent of GGO with traction bronchiectasis and honeycombing) has been shown to predict mortality in patients with acute exacerbations of IPF [56]. Thus, an HRCT scoring system may be also expected for predicting mortality in patients with RA.

8.4 Interstitial Pneumonia with Autoimmune Features: IPAF

8.4.1 Clinical Concept of IPAF

Patients with ILD may present with any features of systemic autoimmune diseases; therefore, the presence of CTD should be considered at all times. However, the condition often does not completely meet the criteria of the American College of Rheumatology (ACR) for each CTD. Consequently, it may not be possible to make a definitive diagnosis.

On the other hand, patients with CTD might present with the characteristic symptoms or signs of ILD, and often have concurrent ILD, but the ILD may precede the manifestation of systemic symptoms. In this situation, when lesions other than compromised lungs are ambiguous or absent, the condition will not meet the diagnostic criteria for CTD, and the patient might be diagnosed with ILD of unknown cause (i.e., suspected IIPs) [3, 4] (Fig. 8.20).

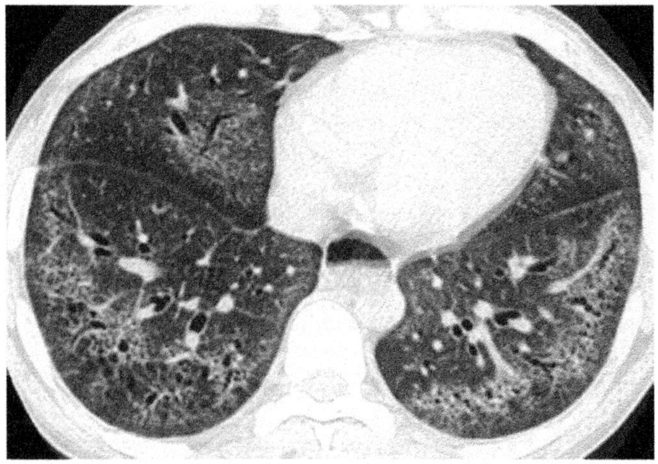

Fig. 8.20 66-year-old man with ILD (fibrotic NSIP) that precedes CTD (PM-DM). A patient had symptoms of breathlessness on exertion and dry cough referred to our hospital for complete examination and treatment. Thin-section CT (lower lung zone) shows diffuse areas of reticular opacities with GGO and with traction bronchiectasis and small aircysts (enlargement of airspace, but not honeycombing). Note distribution being predominantly peribronchovascular bundles and periphery, but sparing subpleural area. CT pattern corresponds to NSIP pattern, and histopathologic findings by surgical lung biopsy revealed fibrotic NSIP. After diagnosis the patient treated as idiopathic NSIP; however, clinical symptoms consistent with PM appeared and deteriorated in the course of about 2 years; further specific antibodies became positive and met the diagnostic criteria

As just described, some patients with IIPs might show symptoms, signs, or laboratory test results that are suggestive of CTD, but the findings do not meet all the CTD diagnostic criteria. In these cases, it has been proposed that the diagnosis should be termed undifferentiated CTD (UCTD) [15], lung-dominant CTD (LD-CTD) [16], or autoimmune-featured ILD (AIF-ILD) [17], based on the different classification criteria.

Recently, the ERS/ATS research statement [18] proposed that all ILDs with features "suggestive" of CTD should be collectively referred to as the term "interstitial pneumonia with autoimmune features (IPAF)." Thus, the term IPAF reflects a unification of terms, and its criteria are expected to promote multinational and multicenter research, which will provide new knowledge. However, it should be noted that this classification is intended to be expedient and should not be used as a definitive clinical diagnosis (Fig. 8.21).

According to this ERS/ATS statement, the criteria for the IPAF classification are defined as the presence of a combination of features from any two of the three following domains: the clinical domain, which includes specific extrathoracic features; the serological domain, which includes specific autoantibodies; and the morphological domain, which includes specific chest imaging, histopathological, or pulmonary physiological features [57].

8.4.2 CT Findings in IPAF

HRCT image patterns in the morphological domain of IPAF include NSIP, OP, NSIP with OP overlap (Fig. 8.22), and lymphoid interstitial pneumonia (LIP) [18]. All these patterns are commonly observed in cases of suspected CTD involvement. On the other hand, when the UIP pattern appears alone, it is not a strong indication of CTD; therefore, it was not included in the IPAF morphologic domain. However, when image findings show only the UIP pattern, IPAF cannot be excluded. As can be seen from the reports on LD-CTDs [58] and AIF-ILDs [17], the UIP patterns are abundantly present in diseases that show implications of CTD. When radiological or histological patterns are identified as UIP patterns, it is important to consider other categories in the clinical, serological, and morphological domains to confirm the presence of features that are unlikely to be present in IPF.

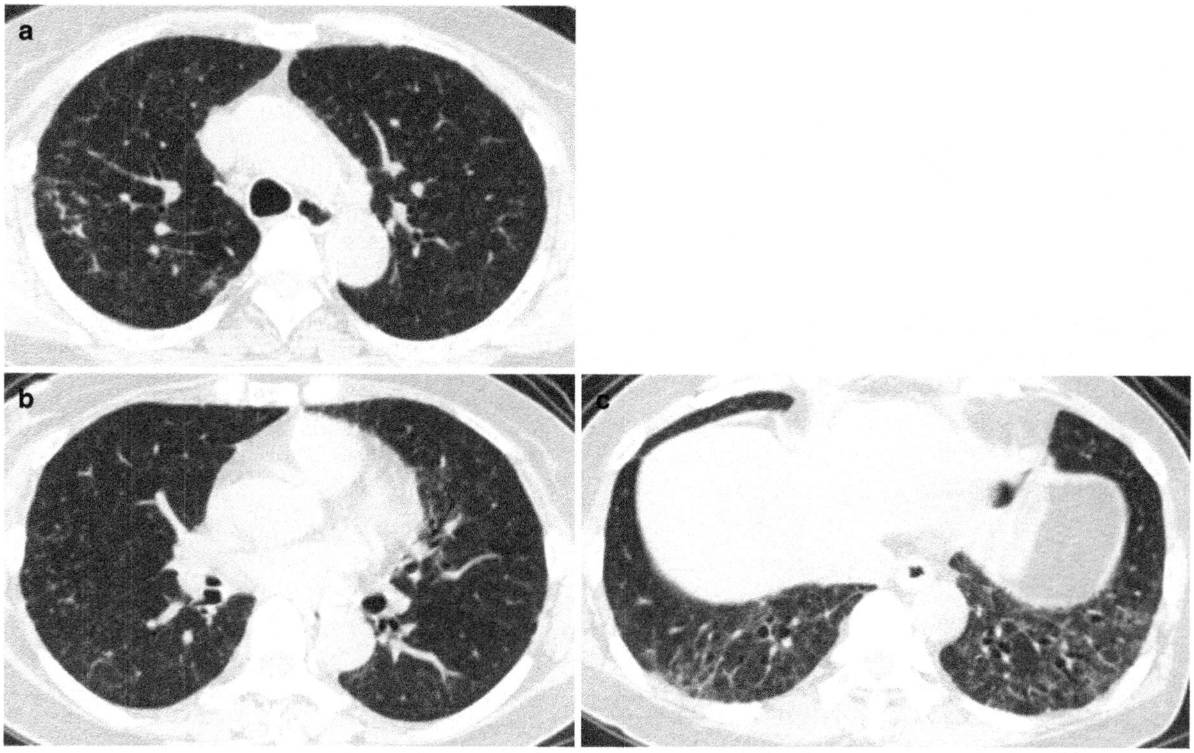

Fig. 8.21 ILD unknown cause (unclassifiable ILD met the classification criteria for IPAF). A 65-year-old woman, nonsmoker, having symptoms of productive cough and mild dyspnea from 5 years before was diagnosed as interstitial pneumonia by a nearby home-doctor, but left untreated. Cough and dyspnea worsened and she was referred to our hospital. No findings suggestive of autoimmune disease were observed. HRCT images at hospitalization (**a**–**c**): Diffuse areas of mosaic attenuation (air-trapping phenomenon) are recognized in all lung fields. In upper and middle lung zones (**a**, **b**), micronodular opacities and branching linear structures are seen in the peripheral lung parenchyma, and linear and reticular opacities with areas of ground-glass opacity (GGO) are also recognized. At the lung base (**c**), there are reticular opacities and GGOs along the peribronchovascular bundles accompanied by airway dilatation and a decrease in lung volume. In the IPF guideline 2011, it was categorized as the inconsistent with UIP pattern. Based on clinical and image findings, it was considered to be fibrosing NSIP with airway lesion or fibrosis around the peripheral airway. On HRCT findings, CTDs and chronic hypersensitivity pneumonia were suspected as secondary ILD. In histopathological findings, framework matches fibrosing NSIP, but prominent infiltration of lymphocytes with lymphoid follicles was observed, and thus lymphoproliferative diseases and rheumatoid arthritis or Sjögren's syndrome as CTD were suspected. Although HRCT and histopathological findings were strongly suggestive of secondary ILD, because of absence of characteristic clinical findings, it was finally categorized as "unclassifiable ILD" in MDD. On the disease behavior classification, the progress has been partially improved, the lesions remained and requires long-term follow-up observation

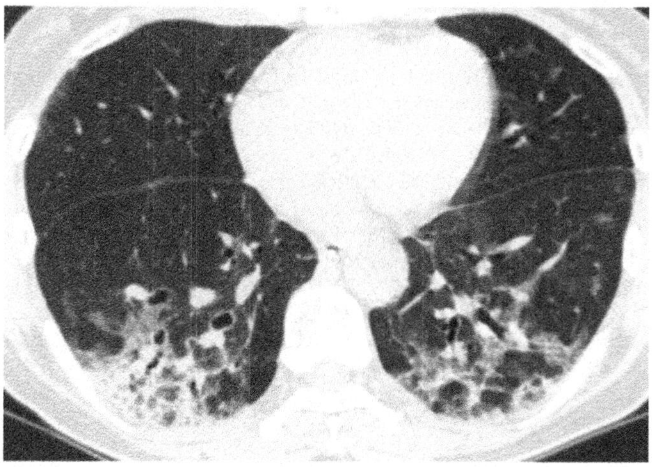

Fig. 8.22 NSIP with OP overlap ("fibrosing OP") pattern. A 60-year-old woman had met IPAF criteria, but later developed DM and met its diagnostic criteria. Thin-section CT (through lower lung zone) displays consolidation and GGO showing peribronchovascular (airway-centered) distribution. Linear and cord-like opacities are also seen within the opacification

8.4.3 CT Pattern and Prognostic Factors

One study suggested that approximately one-third (n = 144) of their initial cohort (n = 422) of patients with IIP, UCTD-ILD, or unclassifiable ILD met the IPAF criteria [59]. Indeed, earlier reports [14–17] had confirmed that autoimmune features were common in patients with IIP. Both morphological and serological domain criteria were satisfied in over three-quarters of patients with IPAF (including a significant subgroup, which satisfied the criteria for all three domains). Mortality in patients that meet IPAF criteria was marginally lower than in patients with IPF, but higher than in patients with CTD-ILD. Patients with IPAF that displayed non-UIP pattern had better prognosis than those that displayed UIP pattern, and those with IPAF/UIP had prognosis similar to those with IPF/UIP. Based on these observations, it can be concluded with confidence that, among patients that meet the IPAF criteria, the distinction between UIP and non-UIP pattern, whether detected on HRCT or histopathology, has major prognostic significance.

Another study (by a group similar to that mentioned above) [60] reported that, among 136 patients that met IPAF criteria, 70 patients (52%) were categorized into UIP pattern, 19 into possible UIP pattern, and 47 into inconsistent with UIP pattern, according to the IPF guideline. Approximately one-fourth of those subjects (27%, 37/136) showed NSIP pattern on CT. This frequency of patterns on CT images was similar to the frequencies reported in another study, which found that, among patients with LD-CTD, 57% showed UIP and 30% showed NSIP [58]. They concluded that IPAF most often presented with UIP pattern on CT, and it was associated with poor survival, when concomitant honeycombing or pulmonary artery enlargement was present [60].

Conclusion

Classification of radiological and histopathological patterns in CTD-ILDs (including RA-ILD) is based on the international statement of IIP classifications, which include UIP, NSIP, OP, OP variants, LIP/DLH, and others. In CTD-ILD, both CT and histopathological analyses most frequently reveal NSIP pattern, but patients with RA-ILD are more likely to show UIP pattern than NSIP pattern. In addition, airway impairment and pleural disease are well-known comorbidities in patients with RA, and these disorders often coexist. Acute exacerbation of ILD is known as a life-threatening event for patients with RA-ILD as with CTD-ILD. In patients with RA-ILD, the extent of reticular opacities and honeycombing, which correspond to fibroproliferative changes in lung parenchyma, and the presence of UIP pattern are prognostic factors. IPAF is currently the proposed term for ILD that possibly precedes CTD, and in the case of patients with IPAF, it is reported that the UIP pattern is detected more frequently than the NSIP pattern, contrary to expectations. This condition is notable, because the presence of IPAF may indicate a patient that will develop RA or another autoimmune disease in the future.

Acknowledgment The author greatly appreciate Dr. Masaki Okamoto and Dr. Shinjiro Kaieda, Department of Medicine, Division of Respirology, Neurology, and Rheumatology, Kurume University School of Medicine; and Dr. Mikiko Hashisako and Prof. Junya Fukuoka, Department of Pathology, Nagasaki University Graduate School of Biomedical Sciences for their helpful advices and valuable illustrations of radiologic and histologic findings.

References

1. American Thoracic Society/European Respiratory Society International Multidisciplinary Consensus Classification of the Idiopathic Interstitial Pneumonias. This joint statement of the American Thoracic Society (ATS), and the European Respiratory Society (ERS) was adopted by the ATS board of directors, June 2001 and by the ERS Executive Committee, June 2001. Am J Respir Crit Care Med. 2002;165:277–304.
2. Travis WD, Costabel U, Hansell DM, King TE, Ltnch DA, Nicholson AG, et al. An official American Thoracic Society/European Respiratory Society Statement: update of the international multidisciplinary classification of the idiopathic interstitial pneumonias. Am J Respir Crit Care Med. 2013;188:733–48.
3. Fujimoto K. Imaging diagnosis of secondary UIP: 1. Connective tissue diseases and its associated diseases. In: Sakai F, Johkoh T, Noma S, editors. Imaging diagnosis of idiopathic pulmonary fibrosis. Tokyo: Medical Science International; 2015. p. 163–82. (in Japanese).
4. Fujimoto K, Okamoto M. ABC of connective tissue diseases. In: Takahashi M, editor. Essential of diagnostic radiology, pearls in thoracic radiology. new ed. Tokyo: Medical View; 2014. p. 237–59. (in Japanese).
5. Kim EA, Lee KS, Johkoh T, Kim TS, Suh GY, Kwon OJ, Han J. Interstitial lung diseases associated with collagen vascular disease; radiologic and histopathologic findings. Radiographics. 2002;22:S151–65.
6. Lynch DA. Lung disease related to collagen vascular disease. J Thorac Imaging. 2009;24:299–309.
7. Capobianco J, Grimberg A, Thompson BM, Antunes VB, Jasinowodolinski D, Meirelles GS. Thoracic manifestations of collagen vascular diseases. Radiographics. 2012;32:33–50.
8. Wells A, Denton CP. Interstitial lung disease in connective tissue disease: mechanisms and management. Nat Rev Rheumatol. 2014;10:728–39.
9. Japan Intractable Diseases Information Center. http://www.nanbyou.or.jp/. Accessed 20 May 2017.
10. Marie I, Hachulla E, Cherin P, Sominique S, Hatron PY, Hellot MF, et al. Interstitial lung disease in polymyositis and dermatomyositis. Arthritis Rheum. 2002;47:614–22.
11. Park IN, Kim DS, Shim TS, Lim CM, Lee SD, Koh Y, et al. Acute exacerbation of interstitial pneumonia other than idiopathic pulmonary fibrosis. Chest. 2007;132:214–20.
12. Hozumi H, Nakamura Y, JOhkoh T, Sumikawa H, Colby TV, Kono M, et al. Acute exacerbation in rheumatoid arthritis-associated interstitial lung disease: a retrospective case control study. BMJ Open. 2013;3:e003132.
13. Tomiyama F, Watanabe R, Ishii T, Kamogawa Y, Fujita Y, Shirota K, et al. High prevalence of acute exacerbation of interstitial lung disease in Japanese patients with systemic sclerosis. Tohoku J Exp Med. 2016;239:297–305.
14. Fujimoto K, Muller NL, Johkoh T, Lee KS, Ichikado K, Taniguchi H, et al. Interstitial pneumonia as an initial presenting feature of collagen vascular disease: clinicopathologic and high-resolution CT findings in 28 patients. Radiology. 2006; 241(P): Suppl.
15. Kinder BW, Collard HR, Koth L, Daikh DI, Wolters PJ, Elicker B, et al. Idiopathic nonspecific interstitial pneumonia: lung manifestation of undifferentiated connective tissue disease? Am J Respire Crit Care Med. 2007;176:691–7.

16. Fisher A, West SG, Swigris JJ, Brown KK, du Bois RM. Connective tissue disease-associated interstitial lung disease: a call for clarification. Chest. 2010;138:251–6.
17. Vij R, Noth I, Strek ME. Autoimmune-featured interstitial lung disease: a distinct entity. Chest. 2011;140:1292–9.
18. Fisher A, Antoniou KM, Brown KK, et al. An official European Respiratory Society/American Thoracic Society research statement: interstitial pneumonia with autoimmune features. Eur Respir J. 2015;46:978–87.
19. Smith ML. Update on pulmonary fibrosis. Not all fibrosis is created equally. Arch Pathol Lab Med. 2016;140:221–9.
20. Fukuoka J, Leslie KO. Chronic diffuse lung diseases. In: Leslie KO, Wick MR, editors. Practical pulmonary pathology. A diagnostic approach. 2nd ed. Philadelphia: Elsevier Saunders; 2011. p. 213–76.
21. Kuranishi LT, Leslie KO, Ferreira RG, Coletta EA, Storreer KM, Soares MR, de Castro Pereira CA. Airway-centered interstitial fibrosis: etiology, clinical findings and prognosis. Respir Res. 2015;16:55.
22. Yousem SA, Dacic S. Idiopathic bronchiolocentric interstitial pneumonia. Mod Pathol. 2002;15:1148–53.
23. de Carvalho ME, Kairalla RA, Capelozzi VL, Deheinzelin D, do Nascimento Saldiva PH, de Carvalho CR. Centrilobular fibrosis: a novel histological pattern of idiopathic interstitial pneumonia. Pathol Res Pract. 2002;198:577–83.
24. Raghu G, Collard HR, Egan JJ, Martinez FJ, Behr J, Brown KK, et al. An official ATS/ERS/JRS/ALAT statement: idiopathic pulmonary fibrosis: evidence-based guidelines for diagnosis and management. Am J Respir Crit Care Med. 2011;183: 788–824.
25. Hansell DM, Bankier AA, MacMahon H, McLoud TC, Muller NL, Remy J. Fleischner society: glossary of terms for thoracic imaging. Radiology. 2008;246:697–722.
26. Watadani T, Sakai F, Johkoh T, Noma S, Akira M, Fujimoto K, et al. Interobserver valiability in the CT assessment of honeycombing in the lung. Radiology. 2013;266:936–44.
27. Sakai F, Noma S, Akira M, Johkoh T, Fujimoto K, Inoue Y, et al. CT atlas of honeycomb lung. Ann Jpn Respir Society. 2012;1: 537–40. (in Japanese).
28. Lynch DA, Sverzellati N, Travis WD, Brown KK, Colby TV, Galvin JR, et al. Diagnostic croteria for idiopathic pulmonary fibrosis: a Fleischner Society White Paper. Lancet Respir Med. 2017; Published Online, Nov. 29, 2017; http://dx.doi.org/10.1016/S2213-2600(17)30433-2.
29. Chung JH, Chawla A, Peljto AL, Cool CD, Groshong SD, Talbert JL, et al. CT scan findings of probable usual interstitial pneumonitis have a high predictive value for histologic usual interstitial pneumonitis. Chest. 2015;147:450–9.
30. Song JW, Do KH, Kim MY, Jang SJ, Colby TV, Kim DS. Pathologic and radiologic differences between idiopathic and collagen vascular disease-related usual interstitial pneumonia. Chest. 2009;136:23–30.
31. Tanoue LT. Pulmonary manifestations of rheumatoidarthritis. Clin Chest Med. 1998;19:667–85.
32. Jurik AG, Davidsen D, Graudal H. Prevalence of pulmonary involvement in rheumatoid arthritis and its relationship to some characteristics of the patients: a radiological and clinical study. Scand J Rheumatol. 1982;11:217–24.
33. Remy-Jardin M, Remy J, Cortet B, et al. Lung changes in rheumatoid arthritis: CT findings. Radiology. 1994;193:375–82.
34. Gabbay E, Tarala R, Will R, et al. Interstitial lung disease in recent-onset rheumatoid arthritis. Am J Respir Crit Care Med. 1997;156:528–35.
35. Kim EJ, Elicker BM, Maldonado F, Webb WR, Ryu JH, Uden V, et al. Usual interstitial pneumonia in rheumatoid arthritis-associated interstitial lung disease. Eur Respir J. 2010;35:1322–8.
36. Song JW, Lee HK, Lee CK, Chae EJ, Jang SJ, Colby TV, Kim DS. Clinical course and outcome of rheumatoid arthritis-related usual interstitial pneumonia. Sarcoidosis Vasc Diffuse Lung Dis. 2013;30:103–12.
37. Moua T, Martinez ACZ, Baqir M, Vassallo R, Limper AH, Ryu JH. Predictors of diagnosis and survival in idiopathic pulmonary fibrosis and connective tissue diseases-related usual interstitial pneumonia. Respir Res. 2014;15:154.
38. Tanaka N, Kim JS, Newell JD, Brown KK, Cool CD, Meehan R, et al. Rheumatoid arthritis-related lung diseases. CT findings. Radiology. 2004;232:81–91.
39. Akira M, Sakatani M, Hara H. Thin-section CT findings in rheumatoid arthriris-associated lung disease; CT pattern and their courses. J Comput Assist Tomogr. 1999;23:941–8.
40. Assayag D, Elicker BM, Urbania TH, Colby TV, Kang BH, et al. Reumatoid arthritis-associated interstitial lung disease: radiologic identification of usual interstitial pneumonia pattern. Radiology. 2014;270:583–8.
41. Sumikawa H, Johkoh T, Colby TV, Ichikado K, Suga M, Taniguchi H, Kondoh Y, Ogura T, Arakawa H, Fujimoto K, Inoue A, Mihara N, Honda O, Tomiyama N, Nakamura H, Muller NL. Computed tomography findings in pathological usual interstitial pneumonia: relationship to survival. Am J Respir Crit Care Med. 2008;177:433–9.
42. Kawabata Y, Hoshi E, Murai K, Ikeya T, Takahashi N, Saitou Y, et al. Smoking-related changes in the background lung of specimens resected for lung cancer: a semiquantitative study with correlation to postoperative course. Histopathology. 2008;53:707–14.
43. Yamada T, Nakanishi Y, Homma T, Uehara K, Mizutani T, Hoshi E, et al. Airspace enlargement with fibrosis shows characteristic histology and immunohistology different from usual interstitial pneumonia, nonspecific interstitial pneumonia and centrilobular emphysema. Pathol Int. 2013;63:206–13.
44. Haddock JAA, Hansell DM. The terminology and radiology of cryptogenic organizing pneumonia. Br J Radiol. 1992;65: 674–80.
45. Keane MA, Hansell DM, Hind CR. Wandering consolidation. Postgrad Med J. 1995;71:685–6.
46. Kim SJ, Lee KS, Ryu YH, Yoon YC, Choe KO, Kim TS, Sung KJ. Reversed halo sign on high-resolution CT of cryptogenic organizing pneumonia: diagnostic implications. AJR Am J Roentgenol. 2003;180:1251–4.
47. Petrie GR, Bloomfield P, Grant IWB, Crompton GK. Upper lobe fibrosis and cavitation in rheumatoid disease. Br J Dis Chest. 1980;74:263–7.
48. Yue CC, Park CH, Kushner I. Apical fibrocavitary lesions of the lung in rheumatoid arthritis. Report of two cases and review of the literature. Am J Med. 1986;81:741–6.
49. Watanabe K. Pleuroparenchymal fibroelastosis: its clinical characteristics. Curr Res Med Rev. 2013;9:229–37.
50. Terasaki H, Fujimoto K, Hayabuchi N, Ogoh Y, Fukuda T, Muller NL. Respiratory symptoms in rheumatoid arthritis: relaton between high resolution CT findings and functional impairment. Radiat Med. 2004;22:179–85.
51. Takemura T. Pathology of chronic interstitial pneumonia and honeycombing. In: Sakai F, Johkoh T, Noma S, editors. Imaging diagnosis of idiopathic pulmonary fibrosis. Tokyo: Medical Science International; 2015. p. 25–56. (in Japanese).
52. Collard HR, Ryerson CJ, Corte TJ, Jenkins G, Kondoh Y, Lederer DJ, et al. Acute exacerbation of idiopathic pulmonary fibrosis. An

international working group report. Am J Respir Crit Care Med. 2016;194:265–75.
53. Parambil JG, Myers JL, Ryu JH. Diffuse alveolar damage. Uncommon manifestation of pulmonary involvement in patients with connective tissue diseases. Chest. 2006;130:553–8.
54. Suda T, Kaida Y, Nakamura Y, Enomoto N, Fujisawa T, Imokawa S, et al. Acute exacerbation of interstitial pneumonia associated with collagen vascular disease. Respir Med. 2009;103:846–53.
55. Toyoda Y, Hanibuchi M, Kishi J, Kawano H, Morizumi S, Sato S, et al. Clinical features and outcome of acute exacerbation of interstitial pneumonia associated with connective tissue disease. J Med Investig. 2016;63:294–9.
56. Fujimoto K, Taniguchi H, Johkoh T, Kondoh Y, Ichikado K, SumiKawa H, et al. Acute exacerbation of idiopathic pulmonary fibrosis: high-resolution CT scores predict mortality. Eur Radiol. 2012;22:83–92.
57. Luppi F, Wells AU. Interstitial pneumonia with autoimmune features (IPAF): a work in progress. Eur Repir J. 2016;47:1622–4.
58. Omote N, Taniguch H, Kondoh Y, Watanabe N, Sakamoto K, Kimura T, et al. Lung-dominant connective tissue disease. Clinical, radiologic, and histologic features. Chest. 2015;148:1438–46.
59. Oldhan JM, Adequnsoye A, Valenzi E, Lee C, Witt L, Chen L, et al. Characterisation of patients with interstitial pneumonia with autoimmune features. Eur Respir J. 2016;47:1767–75.
60. Chung JH, Montner SM, Adequnsoye A, Lee C, Oldham JM, Husain AN, et al. CT findings, radiologic-pathologic correlation, and imaging predictors of survival for patients with interstitial pneumonia with autoimmune features. AJR. 2017;208:1–8.

Therapeutic Strategies for Interstitial Lung Diseases in Rheumatoid Arthritis

9

Takafumi Suda

Abstract

Pulmonary involvement is common in rheumatoid arthritis (RA) and affects all components of the lung. Interstitial lung disease (ILD) is the most predominant pulmonary manifestation and has been identified as the main cause of morbidity and mortality in RA. There are distinct histological and/or radiological subtypes in RA-associated ILD (RA-ILD) with different clinical phenotypes and natural courses. An optimal treatment for RA-ILD has not yet been established, because there have been no randomized controlled trials on RA-ILD. Current therapeutic regimens typically include corticosteroids with or without immunosuppressive drugs; however, supporting evidence is limited by the small numbers of patients and uncontrolled study designs. Several novel agents, such as rituximab, pirfenidone, and nintedanib, are currently under investigation. Furthermore, optimal treatments may differ depending on the histological and/or radiological subtypes of RA-ILD. In order to address these issues, prospective controlled studies with a large number of RA-ILD patients are urgently needed. In this chapter, the treatment of RA-ILD will be described by overviewing recent studies in this field, and the best available evidence to inform a treatment rationale will be provided.

Keywords

Rheumatoid arthritis • Interstitial lung disease • Interstitial pneumonia • Treatment • Therapy

9.1 Introduction

Rheumatoid arthritis (RA) is primarily characterized by destructive inflammatory arthritis; however, a large proportion of RA patients present extra-articular manifestations involving the skin, eyes, heart, and lungs [1]. Pulmonary involvement is common, affecting all components of the lung, such as the airways, parenchyma, pleura, and pulmonary vasculature. Of these, interstitial lung disease (ILD) is the most predominant manifestation. As described in Chaps. 6–8, RA-associated ILD (RA-ILD) comprises a number of disorders with distinct histological and/or radiological patterns, such as usual interstitial pneumonia (UIP), nonspecific interstitial pneumonia (NSIP), and organizing pneumonia (OP). The prognosis of RA-ILD was recently reported to be poor in several large longitudinal studies, with a mean survival of only 3 years from the diagnosis of ILD [2, 3]. Thus, RA-ILD is associated with high morbidity and mortality [4]. However, an optimal treatment for RA-ILD has not yet been established because there have been no randomized clinical trials on RA-ILD. In this chapter, the treatment of RA-ILD will be described by overviewing recent studies in this field, and the best available evidence to inform a treatment rationale will be provided. Since acute forms of RA-ILD are discussed in Chaps. 12–13, this chapter will focus primarily on chronic forms of RA-ILD.

9.2 Indication for Treatment

There is no evidence for the indication of treatment for RA-ILD. In addition, the natural history of RA-ILD remains poorly defined, and consensus therapy has not yet been

T. Suda, M.D., Ph.D.
Second Division, Department of Internal Medicine, Hamamatsu University School of Medicine, Hamamatsu, Shizuoka, Japan
e-mail: suda@hama-med.ac.jp

T. Gono et al. (eds.), *Lung Disease Associated with Rheumatoid Arthritis*, https://doi.org/10.1007/978-981-10-6750-1_9

established. Under these conditions, treatments specifically for RA-ILD are empirically introduced in the clinical setting. Due to the absence of evidence for therapy and its potential adverse effects, the decision to treat needs to be made based on the balance between its benefits and the burden of the disease in each patient. Disease progression and its severity are the two main determinants that need to be considered when deciding to treat. Treatment is typically initiated in RA-ILD patients who show a progressive course with respiratory symptoms, while asymptomatic patients are generally just monitored. It is important to carefully follow-up RA-ILD patients, even asymptomatic ones, at optimal intervals with imaging (chest radiographs and/or HRCT) and pulmonary function tests (PFTs). Age is another factor to consider, and treatment is more likely to be beneficial in younger patients.

9.3 Pharmacological Treatment

One of the main issues associated with the pharmacological treatment of RA-ILD is whether the treatment needs to be changed depending on pathological and/or radiological patterns. Similar to IIPs, RA-ILD with the histological and/or radiological UIP pattern has been shown to have a markedly poorer prognosis than that with other patterns, such as the NSIP and OP patterns [5–7]. In IIPs, patients with the UIP pattern are treated with antifibrotic drugs, including pirfenidone and nintedanib, while those with the NSIP or OP pattern are administered corticosteroids [8]. Several studies have suggested that the response to therapy correlated with histological patterns in RA-ILD [5, 6, 9]. RA-ILD with the NSIP pattern had more favorable responses to therapy than that with the UIP pattern, resulting in a better prognosis [5, 6, 9]. Moreover, patients with the OP pattern typically showed rapid improvements in response to corticosteroid therapy with a complete recovery [10, 11]. These findings suggest that therapeutic strategies differ with histological and/or radiological patterns in RA-ILD. However, since there has been no convincing evidence to support this, treatments for RA-ILD will be described as a whole in this chapter, regardless of histological or radiological patterns. In practice, treatments for RA-ILD are empirically selected because of limited evidence, and current therapeutic regimens generally include corticosteroids with or without immunosuppressive drugs, such as cyclophosphamide, azathioprine, cyclosporine, and mycophenolate mofetil (MMF).

9.3.1 Corticosteroids

Corticosteroids are generally used as first-line agents for RA-ILD. Several uncontrolled studies reported that corticosteroids improved symptoms, radiological findings, and pulmonary function in RA-ILD patients [12–14]. Initial doses of oral prednisolone are typically recommended at 0.5–0.75 mg/kg/day. If a clinical response is achieved, the dose of corticosteroids administered is gradually tapered. Immunosuppressive drugs are often added when patients fail to respond to corticosteroids or side effects occur. In RA-ILD patients with a rapidly deteriorating respiratory status, called acute exacerbation [15], pulsed intravenous methylprednisolone (1.0 g/day for 3 days) is typically administered.

9.3.2 Cyclophosphamide

Cyclophosphamide belongs to a group of alkylating drugs that exert immunosuppressive effects on lymphocytes and neutrophils. It has been widely used in the treatment of autoimmune diseases, such as granulomatosis with polyangiitis (GPA), microscopic polyangiitis (MPA), and systemic lupus erythematosus (SLE). Regarding ILD, although no clinical benefit of cyclophosphamide has been defined in IPF [16, 17], randomized, controlled trials (Scleroderma Lung Study I) showed a significant improvement in pulmonary function in patients with scleroderma-associated ILD (SSc-ILD) receiving oral cyclophosphamide [18]. However, not all studies have confirmed this finding. A recent systematic review and meta-analysis of randomized clinical trials and prospective observational studies on SSc-ILD concluded that cyclophosphamide does not result in clinically significant improvements in pulmonary function [19]. Cyclophosphamide is administered either orally or intravenously. The oral regimen is 1–2 mg/kg/day, while the intravenous pulse regimen is 500–1000 mg/m^2 every 2–4 weeks (intermittent pulse intravenous cyclophosphamide therapy, IVCY). In RA-ILD, Chan et al. reported that cyclophosphamide was mainly used for advanced RA-ILD patients with the UIP pattern, albeit with limited efficacy data [20]. A recent study by Schupp et al. showed that IVCY stabilized pulmonary function in seven patients with RA-ILD [21]. More recently, Ota et al. investigated the effects of immunosuppressive therapy in 17 RA-ILD patients who showed acute or subacute exacerbation [22]. Of these, nine patients received cyclophosphamide (four oral and five IVCY), and this drug improved their prognosis together with improvements in pulmonary function as well as radiological findings.

9.3.3 Azathioprine

Azathioprine is a cytotoxic drug with immunosuppressive activity that inhibits a broad range of inflammatory cells, such as lymphocytes and macrophages. It is widely utilized in the treatment of chronic inflammatory diseases, including inflammatory bowel diseases as well as RA. Administered doses of azathioprine are typically 2–3 mg/kg/day with a low initial dose (50 mg/day). A few studies have examined the efficacy of azathioprine for RA-ILD. Cohen et al. reported that azathioprine induced a significant sustained improvement in pulmonary function as well as the clinical status of RA-ILD [23]. Rojas-Serrano et al. recently showed that the administration of high doses of corticosteroids (1 mg/kg/day) and disease-modifying antirheumatic drugs (DMARDs) significantly increased forced vital capacity (FVC) in 40 patients with RA-ILD [24]. Of these, 22 patients (55%) were given azathioprine.

9.3.4 MMF

MMF is an immunosuppressive drug that diminishes the proliferation of T cells and B cells by inhibiting the purine synthesis pathway. This drug has also been shown to exert an antifibrotic effect by repressing the proliferation and function of fibroblasts and smooth muscle cells [25]. MMF was initially used for organ transplantation and has become increasingly utilized in the treatment of autoimmune diseases, including Behçet's disease, SLE, and SSc. In connective tissue-associated ILD (CTD-ILD), mainly SSc-ILD, MMF has been shown to stabilize or improve pulmonary function and also to be safe and tolerated well [26–28]. Scleroderma Lung Study II (SLC II) recently showed that a treatment with MMF for 2 years resulted in significant improvements in pulmonary function over the course of 2 years, which were similar to those achieved with cyclophosphamide for 1 year [29]. In addition, MMF was tolerated better and associated with less toxicity than cyclophosphamide. Thus, MMF may be preferentially used in the treatment of SSc-ILD because of its better tolerability and weaker toxicity. The dose of MMF for autoimmune diseases is typically 500–2000 mg/day orally. Limited information is available on the use of MMF in RA-ILD. Among 125 CTD-ILD patients treated with MMF, including 18 RA-ILD patients, Fischer et al. reported slight increases in %FVC [28]. Saketkoo et al. demonstrated symptomatic improvements and the stabilization of or improvement in pulmonary function in RA-ILD patients treated with MMF and concluded that MMF is more useful than other immunosuppressive drugs because of its safety and antifibrotic properties [27, 30]. However, reported evidence of its use in RA-ILD remains very limited.

9.3.5 Calcineurin Inhibitors

Calcineurin inhibitors suppress the effects of calcineurin, a protein phosphatase involved in the activation of T cells. They inhibit the immune system by preventing interleukin-2 (IL-2) production by T cells. Among these inhibitors, cyclosporine and tacrolimus were widely used for transplantation, autoimmune diseases, and atopic dermatitis.

Cyclosporine has been used in the treatment of several types of ILD. In IPF, a small prospective trial revealed a slight reduction in the FVC decline in patients treated with cyclosporine; however, this was not conclusive due to the limited patient number [31]. Several studies have shown that the early administration of cyclosporine resulted in better survival for polymyositis/dermatomyositis-associated ILD (PM/DM-ILD) [32, 33]. The initial dose of cyclosporine is 2–4 mg/kg/day, which is adjusted based on trough levels (100–150 ng/mL) as well as the area under curve (AUC). A few studies have examined the efficacy of cyclosporine for RA-ILD [34–36]. Two case reports demonstrated the effectiveness of cyclosporine for RA-ILD patients who were corticosteroid resistant or failed to continue high-dose corticosteroids because of adverse effects [34, 36].

Tacrolimus is a more potent inhibitor of calcineurin than cyclosporine in vitro (50–100 times) and is reported to exert an antifibrotic effect in bleomycin-induced lung fibrosis [37]. In PM/DM-ILD, tacrolimus has been shown to improve prognoses, even in cases refractory to conventional therapy [38–42]. Tacrolimus is typically administered at an initial dose of 0.075 mg/kg/day in order to achieve a plasma trough concentration of 5–10 ng/mL. Limited information is currently available on the use of tacrolimus for RA-ILD patients. Ochi et al. reported a case of RA-ILD that was successfully treated with tacrolimus in combination with corticosteroids [43]. On the other hand, rheumatologists have become aware of tacrolimus-induced ILD [44–46]. Sakaki et al. investigated the characteristics of tacrolimus-induced ILD in the database of the Japanese Pharmaceuticals and Medical Devices Agency (PMDA) and found that its prevalence was 3% in all cases of tacrolimus-related adverse events [46]. Tacrolimus-induced ILD was associated with relatively high mortality, with two thirds of RA patients having preexisting ILD.

9.3.6 Methotrexate

Methotrexate (MTX) is an antifolate drug that inhibits the activation of folic acid in the body. MTX was first developed as an anticancer drug, but has become one of the most effective and widely used medications for the treatment of RA. MTX is known to cause drug-induced pneumonitis. A recent meta-analysis demonstrated that the risk of lung disease was significantly higher in RA patients treated with MTX than in those treated with other DMARDs and biologic agents [47]. In 64 RA patients with asymptomatic preclinical ILD, MTX was shown to significantly increase the risk of the progression of ILD [48].

Thus, MTX is not typically administered for the treatment of RA-ILD because of its pulmonary toxicity.

9.3.7 Rituximab

Rituximab is a chimeric monoclonal antibody against CD20, which is widely expressed on B cells, and eliminates B cells from the body. It was originally used to treat B cell lymphoma and has been shown to be effective for autoimmune diseases, such as refractory RA, GPA, and MPA. Several studies have indicated the efficacy of rituximab for CTD-ILD [49, 50]. In SSc-ILD, accumulating evidence supports the therapeutic use of B cell depletion with rituximab [51–55]. A recent multicenter, open-labeled study revealed the beneficial effects of rituximab on pulmonary function as well as skin fibrosis in 51 patients with SSc-ILD [56]. In contrast, a small retrospective study by Chartland et al. failed to demonstrate the usefulness of rituximab in 24 patients with CTD-ILD [57]. Rituximab has potential for therapeutic use for RA-ILD. Hartung et al. reported a case of RA-ILD that had not responded to conventional immunosuppressive therapy, but was successfully treated with rituximab [58]. A case of severe RA-ILD with pneumothorax was rescued with rituximab [59]. Kabia et al. examined the safety and efficacy of rituximab in 53 patients with RA-ILD and found that most patients treated with rituximab remained stable over a prolonged follow-up without severe adverse events [60]. In the 2016 Annual Meeting of the American College of Rheumatology (ACR), Druce et al. reported 5-year mortality rates in patients with RA-ILD starting either rituximab or anti-TNF drugs as their first biologic therapy for RA [61]. Among 353 patients with RA-ILD, 310 received anti-TNF drugs, while 43 were treated with rituximab. Strikingly, the mortality rate of rituximab-treated patients was approximately half that of anti-TNF drug-treated patients. Although concrete conclusions cannot be reached based solely on Druce's findings, the administration of rituximab appears to be associated with a favorable prognosis in patients with RA-ILD. Future prospective studies on a large population of RA-ILD patients will elucidate this issue. Similar to other biologic agents, concerns have been expressed about the pulmonary toxicity of rituximab. However, rituximab-induced pulmonary toxicity is rare [62].

9.3.8 Antitumor Necrosis Factor Drugs

Tumor necrosis factor (TNF) is a proinflammatory cytokine that is involved in a number of inflammatory disorders, such as RA, inflammatory bowel diseases, and psoriasis. Anti-TNF drugs, such as a monoclonal antibody for TNF or TNF receptor-fusion protein, have been licensed for autoimmune diseases. They have shown great efficacy in improving the articular manifestations of RA. The therapeutic potential of anti-TNF drugs has been reported in the treatment of RA-ILD [63–66]. Infliximab was shown to induce the stabilization of or improvements in pulmonary function in RA-ILD [63–65]. Etanercept improved respiratory symptoms, pulmonary function, and radiological findings in RA-ILD [66]. However, evidence for the use of anti-TNF drugs in the treatment of RA-ILD is limited to case reports or small case series. Moreover, concerns have recently been raised regarding the pulmonary toxicity of anti-TNF drugs. Panopoulos et al. described the new onset or exacerbation of preexisting ILD with high mortality in 144 RA patients among randomized controlled trials [67]. Perez-Alvarez et al. showed that ILD was induced or exacerbated in 122 RA patients who had a poor prognosis [68]. Patients with preexisting ILD had markedly higher mortality rates. Horai et al. documented 11 RA patients that developed ILD in association with the use of etanercept, 6 of whom had preexisting ILD. Therefore, caution is advised when administering anti-TNF drugs to RA patients with preexisting ILD. Thus, no consensus on or evidence for the use of anti-TNF drugs for RA-ILD has yet been established.

9.3.9 Tocilizumab

Tocilizumab is a humanized monoclonal antibody against the interleukin-6 receptor (IL-6R), which is used in the treatment of RA and systemic juvenile idiopathic arthritis. A single case report demonstrated that tocilizumab improved RA-ILD [69]. However, other reports described the development or exacerbation of ILD in RA patients treated with tocilizumab [70–73]. A recent retrospective, case-control study reviewed 395 RA patients receiving tocilizumab, including 78 patients with ILD [74]. Among patients with RA-ILD, six developed the acute exacerbation of ILD during the tocilizumab treatment. Higher arthritis activity was shown to be associated with the acute exacerbation of ILD.

9.3.10 Abatacept

Abatacept is a fusion protein that comprises cytotoxic T-lymphocyte-associated protein 4 and the Fc portion of immunoglobulin G1. It is used to treat autoimmune diseases, such as RA. Abatacept has been reported to have weak pulmonary toxicity [62]. For example, Nakashita et al. recently showed that none of the 16 RA-ILD patients receiving abatacept exhibited the aggravation of preexisting ILD, suggesting abatacept has a lower risk than other anti-TNF drugs [75]. However, another study by Curtis et al. found no significant difference in the risk of ILD between patients exposed to tocilizumab, rituximab, or abatacept than to anti-TNF drugs [73]. Few studies have investigated the efficacy of abatacept for RA-ILD. Mera-Varela et al. showed that abatacept stabilized pulmonary function in RA-ILD patients without adverse effects [76].

9.3.11 Other Agents

Pirfenidone is an oral antifibrotic drug with pleiotropic effects, including anti-inflammatory and antioxidative properties. It inhibits the proliferation of and collagen production by fibroblasts in vitro and in vivo. In IPF, several randomized controlled trials have revealed that pirfenidone reduces the decline of FVC [77–80]. Additionally, a pooled analysis suggested improved mortality with pirfenidone [81]. Besides IPF, the LOTTUS trial showed that pirfenidone was generally tolerated well by patients with SSc-ILD [82]; however, its efficacy currently remains unclear. Collectively, there is a biologically plausible mechanism for pirfenidone in RA-ILD, particularly the chronic fibrotic type. A randomized, double-blind, placebo-controlled phase 2 study to evaluate the safety and efficacy of pirfenidone in RA-ILD patients is currently underway (NCT02808871).

Nintedanib is an oral tyrosine kinase inhibitor that targets multiple growth factor receptors, such as vascular endothelial growth factor receptor (VEGFR), fibroblast growth factor receptor (FGFR), and platelet-derived growth factor receptor (PDGFR), all of which are involved in pulmonary fibrosis. Two randomized, double-blind, placebo-controlled phase 3 trials recently showed a significant reduction in the annual FVC decline in IPF [83]. In SSc-ILD, a randomized, double-blind, placebo-controlled trial to evaluate the safety and efficacy of nintedanib is now being conducted. Thus, although the efficacy of nintedanib for RA-ILD warrants investigation, no clinical trials have been conducted in this field to date. A randomized, double-blind, placebo-controlled phase 3 trial to examine the usefulness of nintedanib in patients with progressive fibrosing interstitial lung diseases, including RA-ILD, is currently preparing to open for participant recruitment (NCT02999178).

9.4 Non-pharmacological Treatment

The cessation of smoking is regarded as essential for smokers with RA-ILD. Smoking is not only a risk factor for the development of RA-ILD; it also aggravates the severity of articular disease as well as lung disease [84–86]. Supplement oxygen therapy needs to be considered for RA-ILD patients with severe respiratory failure, which attenuates their symptoms. Although supplement oxygen therapy has not been proven to improve the prognosis of RA-ILD, this therapy is likely to at least have a palliative role. In IPF, pulmonary rehabilitation improves walking distance, symptoms, and quality of life (QoL) [87, 88]; however, its benefits have not yet been defined for RA-ILD. In addition, joint disorders in RA-ILD patients may limit the introduction of pulmonary rehabilitation. Lung transplantation is a possible therapeutic option for patients with severe respiratory failure. Yazdani et al. recently compared survival and QoL after lung transplantation between RA-ILD and other ILDs, including IPF and SSc-ILD [89]. They demonstrated that RA-ILD patients had similar survival rates and improvements in QoL after transplantation to those of IPF patients, suggesting that lung transplantation needs to be considered for patients with end-stage RA-ILD. Vaccinations for pneumococcus and influenza are also recommended, particularly for RA-ILD patients receiving immunosuppressive therapy.

Conclusions

Clinicians have recently noted that RA-ILD causes significant morbidity and mortality in RA patients, and its prognosis is markedly worse than originally considered. However, the clinical characteristics of RA-ILD, including its natural course, have not been fully established. Moreover, no consensus treatment for RA-ILD has been defined. Therefore, this chapter summarized current knowledge on therapeutic strategies for RA-ILD. Nevertheless, many studies described in this chapter are limited by the small numbers of patients and uncontrolled study designs. Additionally, some of the evidence obtained is extrapolated from other CTD-ILD with uncertain comparability. Thus, prospective controlled studies with a large number of RA-ILD patients are urgently required for the development of efficacious therapies. As described, there are distinct histological and radiological subtypes in RA-ILD, which appear to have different clinical phenotypes and natural courses. One of the potentially interesting future directions is to clarify whether distinct therapeutic strategies need to be employed depending on the different histological and/or radiological patterns in RA-ILD. We hope that further investigations will address this issue.

References

1. Turesson C, O'Fallon WM, Crowson CS, Gabriel SE, Matteson EL. Extra-articular disease manifestations in rheumatoid arthritis: incidence trends and risk factors over 46 years. Ann Rheum Dis. 2003;62:722–7.
2. Koduri G, Norton S, Young A, Cox N, Davies P, Devlin J, et al. Interstitial lung disease has a poor prognosis in rheumatoid arthritis: results from an inception cohort. Rheumatology (Oxford). 2010;49:1483–9.
3. Bongartz T, Nannini C, Medina-Velasquez YF, Achenbach SJ, Crowson CS, Ryu JH, et al. Incidence and mortality of intersti-

tial lung disease in rheumatoid arthritis: a population-based study. Arthritis Rheum. 2010;62:1583–91.
4. Prete M, Racanelli V, Digiglio L, Vacca A, Dammacco F, Perosa F. Extra-articular manifestations of rheumatoid arthritis: an update. Autoimmun Rev. 2011;11:123–31.
5. Kim EJ, Elicker BM, Maldonado F, Webb WR, Ryu JH, Van Uden JH, et al. Usual interstitial pneumonia in rheumatoid arthritis-associated interstitial lung disease. Eur Respir J. 2010;35:1322–8.
6. Tsuchiya Y, Takayanagi N, Sugiura H, Miyahara Y, Tokunaga D, Kawabata Y, et al. Lung diseases directly associated with rheumatoid arthritis and their relationship to outcome. Eur Respir J. 2011;37:1411–7.
7. Kelly CA, Saravanan V, Nisar M, Arthanari S, Woodhead FA, Price-Forbes AN, et al. Rheumatoid arthritis-related interstitial lung disease: associations, prognostic factors and physiological and radiological characteristics—a large multicentre UK study. Rheumatology (Oxford). 2014;53:1676–82.
8. Raghu G, Rochwerg B, Zhang Y, Garcia CA, Azuma A, Behr J, et al. An official ATS/ERS/JRS/ALAT clinical practice guideline: treatment of idiopathic pulmonary fibrosis. An update of the 2011 clinical practice guideline. Am J Respir Crit Care Med. 2015;192:e3–19.
9. Lee HK, Kim DS, Yoo B, Seo JB, Rho JY, Colby TV, et al. Histopathologic pattern and clinical features of rheumatoid arthritis-associated interstitial lung disease. Chest. 2005;127:2019–27.
10. Mori S, Cho I, Koga Y, Sugimoto M. A simultaneous onset of organizing pneumonia and rheumatoid arthritis, along with a review of the literature. Mod Rheumatol. 2008;18:60–6.
11. Hoshino C, Satoh N, Narita M, Kikuchi A, Inoue M. Organising pneumonia as the first manifestation of rheumatoid arthritis. BMJ Case Rep 2011;2011.
12. Doctor L, Snider GL. Diffuse interstitial pulmonary fibrosis associated with arthritis, with comments on the definition of rheumatoid lung disease. Am Rev Respir Dis. 1962;85:413–22.
13. Walker WC, Wright V. Diffuse interstitial pulmonary fibrosis and rheumatoid arthritis. Ann Rheum Dis. 1969;28:252–9.
14. Anaya JM, Diethelm L, Ortiz LA, Gutierrez M, Citera G, Welsh RA, et al. Pulmonary involvement in rheumatoid arthritis. Semin Arthritis Rheum. 1995;24:242–54.
15. Hozumi H, Nakamura Y, Johkoh T, Sumikawa H, Colby TV, Kono M, et al. Acute exacerbation in rheumatoid arthritis-associated interstitial lung disease: a retrospective case control study. BMJ Open. 2013;3:e003132.
16. Johnson MA, Kwan S, Snell NJ, Nunn AJ, Darbyshire JH, Turner-Warwick M. Randomised controlled trial comparing prednisolone alone with cyclophosphamide and low dose prednisolone in combination in cryptogenic fibrosing alveolitis. Thorax. 1989;44:280–8.
17. Zisman DA, Lynch JP 3rd, Toews GB, Kazerooni EA, Flint A, Martinez FJ. Cyclophosphamide in the treatment of idiopathic pulmonary fibrosis: a prospective study in patients who failed to respond to corticosteroids. Chest. 2000;117:1619–26.
18. Tashkin DP, Elashoff R, Clements PJ, Goldin J, Roth MD, Furst DE, et al. Cyclophosphamide versus placebo in scleroderma lung disease. N Engl J Med. 2006;354:2655–66.
19. Nannini C, West CP, Erwin PJ, Matteson EL. Effects of cyclophosphamide on pulmonary function in patients with scleroderma and interstitial lung disease: a systematic review and meta-analysis of randomized controlled trials and observational prospective cohort studies. Arthritis Res Ther. 2008;10:R124.
20. Chan E, Chapman K, Kelly C. Interstitial lung disease in rheumatoid arthritis: a review. Arthritis Res Top Rev Ser. 2013;7:1–9.
21. Schupp JC, Kohler T, Muller-Quernheim J. Usefulness of cyclophosphamide pulse therapy in interstitial lung diseases. Respiration. 2016;91:296–301.
22. Ota M, Iwasaki Y, Harada H, Sasaki O, Nagafuchi Y, Nakachi S, et al. Efficacy of intensive immunosuppression in exacerbated rheumatoid arthritis-associated interstitial lung disease. Mod Rheumatol. 2017;27:22–8.
23. Cohen JM, Miller A, Spiera H. Interstitial pneumonitis complicating rheumatoid arthritis. Sustained remission with azathioprine therapy. Chest. 1977;72:521–4.
24. Rojas-Serrano J, Gonzalez-Velasquez E, Mejia M, Sanchez-Rodriguez A, Carrillo G. Interstitial lung disease related to rheumatoid arthritis: evolution after treatment. Reumatol Clin. 2012;8:68–71.
25. Roos N, Poulalhon N, Farge D, Madelaine I, Mauviel A, Verrecchia F. In vitro evidence for a direct antifibrotic role of the immunosuppressive drug mycophenolate mofetil. J Pharmacol Exp Ther. 2007;321:583–9.
26. Swigris JJ, Olson AL, Fischer A, Lynch DA, Cosgrove GP, Frankel SK, et al. Mycophenolate mofetil is safe, well tolerated, and preserves lung function in patients with connective tissue disease-related interstitial lung disease. Chest. 2006;130:30–6.
27. Saketkoo LA, Espinoza LR. Experience of mycophenolate mofetil in 10 patients with autoimmune-related interstitial lung disease demonstrates promising effects. Am J Med Sci. 2009;337:329–35.
28. Fischer A, Brown KK, Du Bois RM, Frankel SK, Cosgrove GP, Fernandez-Perez ER, et al. Mycophenolate mofetil improves lung function in connective tissue disease-associated interstitial lung disease. J Rheumatol. 2013;40:640–6.
29. Tashkin DP, Roth MD, Clements PJ, Furst DE, Khanna D, Kleerup EC, et al. Mycophenolate mofetil versus oral cyclophosphamide in scleroderma-related interstitial lung disease (SLS II): a randomised controlled, double-blind, parallel group trial. Lancet Respir Med. 2016;4:708–19.
30. Saketkoo LA, Espinoza LR. Rheumatoid arthritis interstitial lung disease: mycophenolate mofetil as an antifibrotic and disease-modifying antirheumatic drug. Arch Intern Med. 2008;168:1718–9.
31. Miyazaki Y, Azuma A, Inase N, Taniguchi H, Ogura T, Inoue E, et al. Cyclosporine A combined with low-dose corticosteroid treatment in patients with idiopathic pulmonary fibrosis. Respir Investig. 2015;53:288–95.
32. Takada K, Kishi J, Miyasaka N. Step-up versus primary intensive approach to the treatment of interstitial pneumonia associated with dermatomyositis/polymyositis: a retrospective study. Mod Rheumatol. 2007;17:123–30.
33. Go DJ, Park JK, Kang EH, Kwon HM, Lee YJ, Song YW, et al. Survival benefit associated with early cyclosporine treatment for dermatomyositis-associated interstitial lung disease. Rheumatol Int. 2016;36:125–31.
34. Puttick MP, Klinkhoff AV, Chalmers A, Ostrow DN. Treatment of progressive rheumatoid interstitial lung disease with cyclosporine. J Rheumatol. 1995;22:2163–5.
35. Ogawa D, Hashimoto H, Wada J, Ueno A, Yamasaki Y, Yamamura M, et al. Successful use of cyclosporin A for the treatment of acute interstitial pneumonitis associated with rheumatoid arthritis. Rheumatology (Oxford). 2000;39:1422–4.
36. Chang HK, Park W, Ryu DS. Successful treatment of progressive rheumatoid interstitial lung disease with cyclosporine: a case report. J Korean Med Sci. 2002;17:270–3.
37. Nagano J, Iyonaga K, Kawamura K, Yamashita A, Ichiyasu H, Okamoto T, et al. Use of tacrolimus, a potent antifibrotic agent, in bleomycin-induced lung fibrosis. Eur Respir J. 2006;27:460–9.
38. Oddis CV, Sciurba FC, Elmagd KA, Starzl TE. Tacrolimus in refractory polymyositis with interstitial lung disease. Lancet. 1999;353:1762–3.
39. Ochi S, Nanki T, Takada K, Suzuki F, Komano Y, Kubota T, et al. Favorable outcomes with tacrolimus in two patients with refractory interstitial lung disease associated with polymyositis/dermatomyositis. Clin Exp Rheumatol. 2005;23:707–10.
40. Ando M, Miyazaki E, Yamasue M, Sadamura Y, Ishii T, Takenaka R, et al. Successful treatment with tacrolimus of progressive inter-

stitial pneumonia associated with amyopathic dermatomyositis refractory to cyclosporine. Clin Rheumatol. 2010;29:443–5.
41. Ge Y, Zhou H, Shi J, Ye B, Peng Q, Lu X, et al. The efficacy of tacrolimus in patients with refractory dermatomyositis/polymyositis: a systematic review. Clin Rheumatol. 2015;34:2097–103.
42. Kurita T, Yasuda S, Oba K, Odani T, Kono M, Otomo K, et al. The efficacy of tacrolimus in patients with interstitial lung diseases complicated with polymyositis or dermatomyositis. Rheumatology (Oxford). 2015;54:1536.
43. Ochi S, Kubota T, Sugihara T, Ogawa J, Komano Y, Nonomura Y, et al. A case report of rheumatoid arthritis complicated with rapidly progressive interstitial pneumonia, multiple bullae and pneumomediastinum, which was successfully treated with tacrolimus. Nihon Rinsho Meneki Gakkai Kaishi. 2008;31:62–7.
44. Miwa Y, Isozaki T, Wakabayashi K, Odai T, Matsunawa M, Yajima N, et al. Tacrolimus-induced lung injury in a rheumatoid arthritis patient with interstitial pneumonitis. Mod Rheumatol. 2008;18:208–11.
45. Koike R, Tanaka M, Komano Y, Sakai F, Sugiyama H, Nanki T, et al. Tacrolimus-induced pulmonary injury in rheumatoid arthritis patients. Pulm Pharmacol Ther. 2011;24:401–6.
46. Sasaki T, Nakamura W, Inokuma S, Matsubara E. Characteristic features of tacrolimus-induced lung disease in rheumatoid arthritis patients. Clin Rheumatol. 2016;35:541–5.
47. Conway R, Low C, Coughlan RJ, O'Donnell MJ, Carey JJ. Methotrexate and lung disease in rheumatoid arthritis: a meta-analysis of randomized controlled trials. Arthritis Rheumatol. 2014;66:803–12.
48. Gochuico BR, Avila NA, Chow CK, Novero LJ, Wu HP, Ren P, et al. Progressive preclinical interstitial lung disease in rheumatoid arthritis. Arch Intern Med. 2008;168:159–66.
49. Lepri G, Avouac J, Airo P, Anguita Santos F, Bellando-Randone S, Blagojevic J, et al. Effects of rituximab in connective tissue disorders related interstitial lung disease. Clin Exp Rheumatol. 2016;34(Suppl 100):181–5.
50. Sharp C, McCabe M, Dodds N, Edey A, Mayers L, Adamali H, et al. Rituximab in autoimmune connective tissue disease-associated interstitial lung disease. Rheumatology (Oxford). 2016;55:1318–24.
51. McGonagle D, Tan AL, Madden J, Rawstron AC, Rehman A, Emery P, et al. Successful treatment of resistant scleroderma-associated interstitial lung disease with rituximab. Rheumatology (Oxford). 2008;47:552–3.
52. Daoussis D, Liossis SN, Tsamandas AC, Kalogeropoulou C, Kazantzi A, Sirinian C, et al. Experience with rituximab in scleroderma: results from a 1-year, proof-of-principle study. Rheumatology (Oxford). 2010;49:271–80.
53. Daoussis D, Liossis SN, Tsamandas AC, Kalogeropoulou C, Paliogianni F, Sirinian C, et al. Effect of long-term treatment with rituximab on pulmonary function and skin fibrosis in patients with diffuse systemic sclerosis. Clin Exp Rheumatol. 2012;30:S17–22.
54. Yoo WH. Successful treatment of steroid and cyclophosphamide-resistant diffuse scleroderma-associated interstitial lung disease with rituximab. Rheumatol Int. 2012;32:795–8.
55. Bosello SL, De Luca G, Rucco M, Berardi G, Falcione M, Danza FM, et al. Long-term efficacy of B cell depletion therapy on lung and skin involvement in diffuse systemic sclerosis. Semin Arthritis Rheum. 2015;44:428–36.
56. Daoussis D, Melissaropoulos K, Sakellaropoulos G, Antonopoulos I, Markatseli TE, Simopoulou T, et al. A multicenter, open-label, comparative study of B-cell depletion therapy with Rituximab for systemic sclerosis-associated interstitial lung disease. Semin Arthritis Rheum. 2017;46:625–31.
57. Chartrand S, Swigris JJ, Peykova L, Fischer A. Rituximab for the treatment of connective tissue disease-associated interstitial lung disease. Sarcoidosis Vasc Diffuse Lung Dis. 2016;32:296–304.
58. Hartung W, Maier J, Pfeifer M, Fleck M. Effective treatment of rheumatoid arthritis-associated interstitial lung disease by B-cell targeted therapy with rituximab. Case Reports Immunol. 2012;2012:272303.
59. Braun-Moscovici Y, Butbul-Aviel Y, Guralnik L, Toledano K, Markovits D, Rozin A, et al. Rituximab: rescue therapy in life-threatening complications or refractory autoimmune diseases: a single center experience. Rheumatol Int. 2013;33:1495–504.
60. Kabia A, Md Yusof M, Dass S, Vital E. Efficacy and safety of rituximab in rheumatoid arthritis patients with concomitant interstitial lung disease: 10-year experience at single centre. Rhematology. 2015;54(suppl 1).
61. Druce K, Iqbal K, Watson K, Symmons D, Hyrich KL, Kelly C. Mortality in patients with rheumatoid arthritis and interstitial lung disease treated with first line TNFi or rituximab therapies. Arthritis Rheumatol. 2016; Abstract No. 3065.
62. Hadjinicolaou AV, Nisar MK, Parfrey H, Chilvers ER, Ostor AJ. Non-infectious pulmonary toxicity of rituximab: a systematic review. Rheumatology (Oxford). 2012;51:653–62.
63. Vassallo R, Matteson E, Thomas CF Jr. Clinical response of rheumatoid arthritis-associated pulmonary fibrosis to tumor necrosis factor-alpha inhibition. Chest. 2002;122:1093–6.
64. Bargagli E, Galeazzi M, Rottoli P. Infliximab treatment in a patient with rheumatoid arthritis and pulmonary fibrosis. Eur Respir J. 2004;24:708.
65. Antoniou KM, Mamoulaki M, Malagari K, Kritikos HD, Bouros D, Siafakas NM, et al. Infliximab therapy in pulmonary fibrosis associated with collagen vascular disease. Clin Exp Rheumatol. 2007;25:23–8.
66. Wang Y, Xu SQ, Xu JH, Ding C. Treatment with etanercept in a patient with rheumatoid arthritis-associated interstitial lung disease. Clin Med Insights Case Rep. 2011;4:49–52.
67. Panopoulos ST, Sfikakis PP. Biological treatments and connective tissue disease associated interstitial lung disease. Curr Opin Pulm Med. 2011;17:362–7.
68. Perez-Alvarez R, Perez-de-Lis M, Diaz-Lagares C, Pego-Reigosa JM, Retamozo S, Bove A, et al. Interstitial lung disease induced or exacerbated by TNF-targeted therapies: analysis of 122 cases. Semin Arthritis Rheum. 2011;41:256–64.
69. Mohr M, Jacobi AM. Interstitial lung disease in rheumatoid arthritis: response to IL-6R blockade. Scand J Rheumatol. 2011;40:400–1.
70. Kawashiri SY, Kawakami A, Sakamoto N, Ishimatsu Y, Eguchi K. A fatal case of acute exacerbation of interstitial lung disease in a patient with rheumatoid arthritis during treatment with tocilizumab. Rheumatol Int. 2012;32:4023–6.
71. Wendling D, Vidon C, Godfrin-Valnet M, Rival G, Guillot X, Prati C. Exacerbation of combined pulmonary fibrosis and emphysema syndrome during tocilizumab therapy for rheumatoid arthritis. Joint Bone Spine. 2013;80:670–1.
72. Roubille C, Haraoui B. Interstitial lung diseases induced or exacerbated by DMARDS and biologic agents in rheumatoid arthritis: a systematic literature review. Semin Arthritis Rheum. 2014;43:613–26.
73. Curtis JR, Sarsour K, Napalkov P, Costa LA, Schulman KL. Incidence and complications of interstitial lung disease in users of tocilizumab, rituximab, abatacept and anti-tumor necrosis factor alpha agents, a retrospective cohort study. Arthritis Res Ther. 2015;17:319.
74. Akiyama M, Kaneko Y, Yamaoka K, Kondo H, Takeuchi T. Association of disease activity with acute exacerbation of interstitial lung disease during tocilizumab treatment in patients with rheumatoid arthritis: a retrospective, case-control study. Rheumatol Int. 2016;36:881–9.
75. Nakashita T, Ando K, Takahashi K, Motojima S. Possible effect of abatacept on the progression of interstitial lung disease in rheumatoid arthritis patients. Respir Invest. 2016;54:376–9.

76. Mera-Varela A, Perez-Pampin E. Abatacept therapy in rheumatoid arthritis with interstitial lung disease. J Clin Rheumatol. 2014;20:445–6.
77. Azuma A, Nukiwa T, Tsuboi E, Suga M, Abe S, Nakata K, et al. Double-blind, placebo-controlled trial of pirfenidone in patients with idiopathic pulmonary fibrosis. Am J Respir Crit Care Med. 2005;171:1040–7.
78. Taniguchi H, Ebina M, Kondoh Y, Ogura T, Azuma A, Suga M, et al. Pirfenidone in idiopathic pulmonary fibrosis. Eur Respir J. 2010;35:821–9.
79. Noble PW, Albera C, Bradford WZ, Costabel U, Glassberg MK, Kardatzke D, et al. Pirfenidone in patients with idiopathic pulmonary fibrosis (CAPACITY): two randomised trials. Lancet. 2011;377:1760–9.
80. King TE Jr, Bradford WZ, Castro-Bernardini S, Fagan EA, Glaspole I, Glassberg MK, et al. A phase 3 trial of pirfenidone in patients with idiopathic pulmonary fibrosis. N Engl J Med. 2014;370:2083–92.
81. Nathan SD, Albera C, Bradford WZ, Costabel U, Glaspole I, Glassberg MK, et al. Effect of pirfenidone on mortality: pooled analyses and meta-analyses of clinical trials in idiopathic pulmonary fibrosis. Lancet Respir Med. 2017;5:33–41.
82. Khanna D, Albera C, Fischer A, Khalidi N, Raghu G, Chung L, et al. An open-label, phase II study of the safety and tolerability of pirfenidone in patients with scleroderma-associated interstitial lung disease: the LOTUSS trial. J Rheumatol. 2016;43(9):1672.
83. Richeldi L, du Bois RM, Raghu G, Azuma A, Brown KK, Costabel U, et al. Efficacy and safety of nintedanib in idiopathic pulmonary fibrosis. N Engl J Med. 2014;370:2071–82.
84. Saag KG, Cerhan JR, Kolluri S, Ohashi K, Hunninghake GW, Schwartz DA. Cigarette smoking and rheumatoid arthritis severity. Ann Rheum Dis. 1997;56:463–9.
85. Luukkainen R, Saltyshev M, Pakkasela R, Nordqvist E, Huhtala H, Hakala M. Relationship of rheumatoid factor to lung diffusion capacity in smoking and non-smoking patients with rheumatoid arthritis. Scand J Rheumatol. 1995;24:119–20.
86. Zhu J, Zhou Y, Chen X, Li J. A metaanalysis of the increased risk of rheumatoid arthritis-related pulmonary disease as a result of serum anticitrullinated protein antibody positivity. J Rheumatol. 2014;41:1282–9.
87. Holland AE, Hill CJ, Conron M, Munro P, McDonald CF. Short term improvement in exercise capacity and symptoms following exercise training in interstitial lung disease. Thorax. 2008;63:549–54.
88. Nishiyama O, Kondoh Y, Kimura T, Kato K, Kataoka K, Ogawa T, et al. Effects of pulmonary rehabilitation in patients with idiopathic pulmonary fibrosis. Respirology. 2008;13:394–9.
89. Yazdani A, Singer LG, Strand V, Gelber AC, Williams L, Mittoo S. Survival and quality of life in rheumatoid arthritis-associated interstitial lung disease after lung transplantation. J Heart Lung Transplant. 2014;33:514–20.

Part IV

Diagnosis and Treatment of Acute Lung Disease in Rheumatoid Arthritis

Bacterial and Fungal Infections in Rheumatoid Arthritis

10

Yutaka Tsuchiya and Hironori Sagara

Abstract

The advent of novel therapeutics for rheumatoid arthritis (RA) has transformed articular improvement and systemic outcomes, but the number of respiratory infections has been increasing in the past decade. Important causes for the elevated susceptibility to bacterial and fungal respiratory infections are mainly due to immune dysregulation of RA, pulmonary comorbidities, and immunosuppressive treatments such as corticosteroids, methotrexate, and biological agents. Pneumonia is the most common infection, and fungal infection is also frequently seen in patients with RA. Respiratory infections in patients with RA are considered important factors that affect not only patient survival but also the development of RA itself. Thus, it is essential for clinicians to have sufficient knowledge of the characteristics of respiratory infections in these settings of RA. Because controlling respiratory infections improves the survival of patients with RA, proper diagnosis and prompt treatment of respiratory infections in these patients are necessary throughout their treatment period.

Keywords

Bacterial infection • Biological agents • Fungal infection • Interstitial lung disease *Pneumocystis jirovecii* pneumonia • Rheumatoid arthritis

10.1 Introduction

Patients with rheumatoid arthritis (RA) have long been recognized to suffer a greater burden of serious infection [1, 2]. Overall, documented serious infections occur twice as frequently in patients with RA as in matched non-RA controls [2, 3]. Among these infections, pneumonia is the most common and frequent infection when compared to those in non-RA cohorts [2]. Although the pathogenesis of respiratory infection in RA is not fully clear, multifactorial etiologies of RA are thought to be associated with the infection. In addition, while the advent of novel therapeutics for RA in the past decade has transformed systemic outcomes [4–7], the incidence of severe respiratory infection has been increasing in this setting [8–15].

This chapter focuses on the current evidence for the pathogenesis, diagnosis, and treatment of bacterial and fungal respiratory infections in RA. We also review the recent research on respiratory infections as a risk factor for the development of RA.

10.2 Risk Factors of Infection in RA

10.2.1 Immune Dysregulation of RA

Predisposition to infection in RA patients is thought to be inherent and, at the same time, to be a form of disease-related immune dysregulation. The main cause of this predisposition is

Y. Tsuchiya, M.D., Ph.D. (✉)
Department of Allergy and Respiratory Medicine, Showa University Koto Toyosu Hospital, Tokyo, Japan
e-mail: caeser@med.showa-u.ac.jp

H. Sagara, M.D., Ph.D.
Department of Medicine, Division of Respiratory Medicine and Allergology, Showa University, School of Medicine, Tokyo, Japan

T. Gono et al. (eds.), *Lung Disease Associated with Rheumatoid Arthritis*, https://doi.org/10.1007/978-981-10-6750-1_10

that patients with RA seem to have reduced capacity to generate new T lymphocytes, and their T-lymphocyte repertoire severely contracts over time [16]. This contraction in the T-cell repertoire is not limited to antigen-exposed memory T cells but also to naive T cells, which lead to defective immune responses to selected antigens [16] and previously unknown antigens [17]. Peripheral blood mononuclear cells from RA patients have shown decreased production of spontaneous and stimulated IgM-rheumatoid factor consequent to humoral immune defects without immunosuppressive treatment [18]. Also, specific genetic polymorphisms are in linkage with disequilibrium for defense against infection in patients with RA [19, 20].

10.2.2 Drugs for RA

The treatment for RA has developed rapidly and dramatically since methotrexate (MTX) or biological agents were first used, but serious infection has become a major issue for patients with RA.

Corticosteroid is useful in the treatment of early RA, but chronic steroid use is also associated with an increased risk of developing certain infectious diseases. Corticosteroid interferes with the phagocytosis of neutrophils and with intracellular sterilization and humoral immunodeficiency [21]. Stuck et al. reported that prednisone (PSL) >10 mg/day and a cumulative amount of PSL >700 mg are risk factors for infection in the presence of an underlying disease state [8]. In patients with RA, the infectious risk for those with PSL use is eight times higher (odds ratio [OR] = 8.0, 95% confidence interval [CI] 1.0–64.0) compared with nonsteroid use [22]. This predisposition is associated with a dose-related effect [2, 13], and the relationship is evident even with average daily dosages of ≤5 mg of PSL [23].

Low-dose MTX is now the most widely used of the first-line conventional synthetic disease-modifying antirheumatic drugs (csDMARDs) in the treatment of RA [24–26]. MTX decreases macrophage recruitment and function [27] and inhibits the production of potentially toxic metabolic compounds that accumulate in chronically inflamed tissues [28]. Even at low doses, MTX has been shown to have significant effects on neutrophil chemotaxis [29, 30]. In addition, MTX increases extracellular adenosine levels, which decrease the secretion of important inflammatory cytokines such as tumor necrosis factor (TNF)-α, interferon, and interleukin (IL)-6 [31, 32]. A nested case-control study including 23,733 RA patients conducted between 1980 and 2003 suggested an increased risk of pneumonia due to MTX (risk ratio [RR] = 1.16, 95% CI 1.02–1.33) [33]. In the database of systematic reviews regarding recent MTX treatment for RA, patients in the MTX group were more likely to have an infection compared with those in the placebo group (49% vs. 35%; RR = 1.3, 95% CI 1.0–1.6) [11], and the common infections were upper respiratory infections, bronchitis, and pneumonia. In contrast, some large prospective cohort studies showed no link between low-dose MTX and respiratory infection in RA patients [1, 2, 23, 33–36]. Infectious risk for other csDMARDs such as leflunomide [12], cyclophosphamide, and azathioprine was also reported [33], but the number of such reports is limited.

Biological agents are a new class of disease-modifying treatment options for RA that have been reported to show large clinical and radiographic improvements compared with traditional drugs [37–39]. Specific biological agents for RA include a soluble TNF receptor IgG Fc fusion protein (etanercept, ETN), several anti-TNF-α antibodies (infliximab, IFX; adalimumab, ADA; and golimumab), a pegylated antibody fragment (certolizumab pegol, CZP), and an anti-IL-6 receptor antibody (tocilizumab, TCZ). The anti-CD20 chimeric antibody rituximab is a B-cell-targeting agent, and a T-cell-targeting agent (abatacept) has been shown to be efficacious in the treatment of RA. All of these agents target cytokines or cells dysregulated in patients with RA. However, these targets are also key components of normal immune homeostasis and are involved in an array of normal physiologic responses. Therefore, blocking particular cytokines or cells might result in infections. The relationship between biological agents and infection is reported in various types of randomized controlled trials and meta-analyses. However, discordant results have been reported for these studies, with some studies detecting an association [40–43] and others not [23, 44–49]. Recent systematic reviews and a meta-analysis of the biological treatment of RA patients revealed that compared with csDMARDs, standard-dose biological agents (OR = 1.31, 95% CI 1.09–1.58) and high-dose biological agents (OR = 1.90, 95% CI 1.50–2.39) were associated with an increased risk of serious infections but low-dose biological agents (OR = 0.93, 95% CI 0.65–1.33) were not [14]. Of note, anti-IL-6 receptor antibody TCZ inhibits the elevation of C-reactive protein, which makes it difficult to diagnose acute infection. Clinicians should not use C-reactive protein alone as index of infection during treatment with this agent.

It is interesting that some large cohort studies revealed that infectious risk was conversely suppressed by some csDMARDs [2, 34]. The mechanism for reducing infection is not clear but may be related to a beneficial effect of controlling RA inflammation and counterbalancing the potential immunosuppressive effects of RA treatments, thus resulting in a net neutral effect on infections and improvement of activities of daily living. Ni Mhuircheartaigh et al. showed in a population-based inception cohort study with RA patients that the overall rate of serious infections declined from 9.6 per 100 patient-years in the prebiologics era cohort (1955–1994) to 6.6 per 100 patient-years in the biologic era cohort (1995–2007), although there was an increase in the rate of serious infections in patients who received biological agents [50]. Further longitudinal prospective studies are needed to prove the influence of RA treatment on infection.

10.2.3 Pulmonary Involvements Associated with RA

In patients with RA, lung diseases directly associated with RA (RA-LD) are important risk factors for respiratory infections. RA-LD includes interstitial lung diseases (ILD) such as usual interstitial pneumonia (Fig. 10.1), nonspecific interstitial pneumonia, organizing pneumonia, and diffuse alveolar damage; airway diseases such as bronchiectasis and bronchiolitis (Fig. 10.2); pleuritis; pulmonary vascular disease; and rheumatoid nodules. ILD is a common form of pulmonary involvement in RA. Olson et al. reported that the prevalence of clinically significant RA-ILD is approximately 6.8% in women and 9.8% in men [51]. Bongartz et al. reported a large cohort of RA patients whose estimated prevalence of ILD was between 4 and 7.9% with 10-, 20-, and 30-year cumulative incidences of 3.5%, 6.3%, and 7.7%, respectively [52]. The exact prevalence of airway disease in RA varies with the diagnostic modalities used. When pulmonary function testing is done, the prevalence of airway disease in RA ranges from 8 to 36% [53–55]. However, when more sensitive tests such as high-resolution computed tomography are performed, the majority of studies recently suggest approximately 35–41% of RA subjects have clinical or subclinical airway disease [55, 56]. In addition, RA patients without a smoking history are likely to have pulmonary emphysema [57]. In one population-based incidence cohort that included 603 patients with RA, the risk of developing obstructive lung disease was higher among male patients, current or former smokers, and individuals with more severe RA [58]. Takayanagi et al. reported in a large cohort study of respiratory infection in RA patients that 92% of the bacterial infections overlapped with underlying chronic lung diseases such as ILD, bronchiectasis, or pulmonary emphysema (Fig. 10.1) [59].

Owing to these involvements and reduced pulmonary function, serious respiratory infections may result in acute respiratory decompensation and higher rates of mortality. Thus, clinicians should pay attention to these clinical settings that potentially increase the risk of respiratory infections and carefully observe these patients throughout their treatment period.

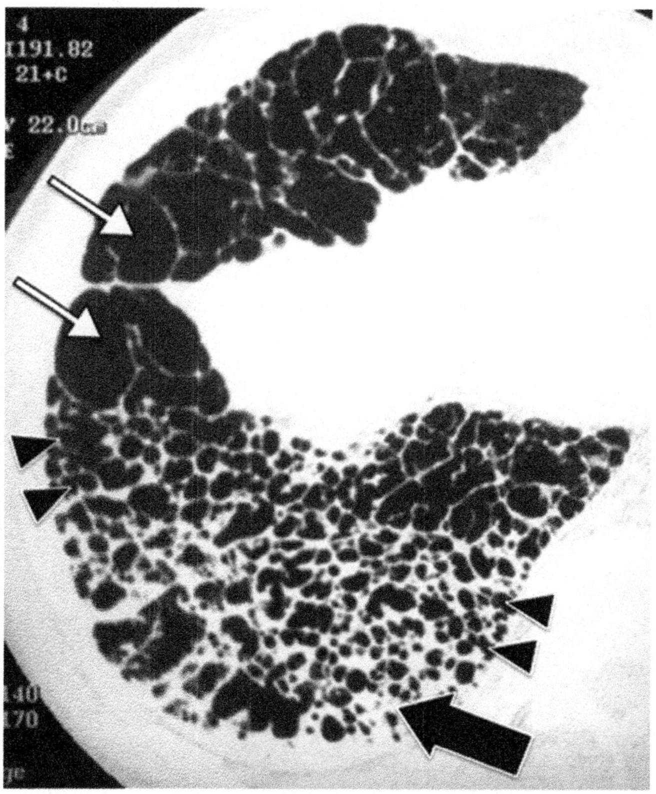

Fig. 10.1 Pneumonia with combined pulmonary fibrosis and emphysema in rheumatoid arthritis. Computed tomography image obtained through the lower lobe of the right lung in a 59-year-old man with pneumonia shows consolidation (thick black arrow) overlapping honeycombing (arrowheads) and emphysema (thin white arrows)

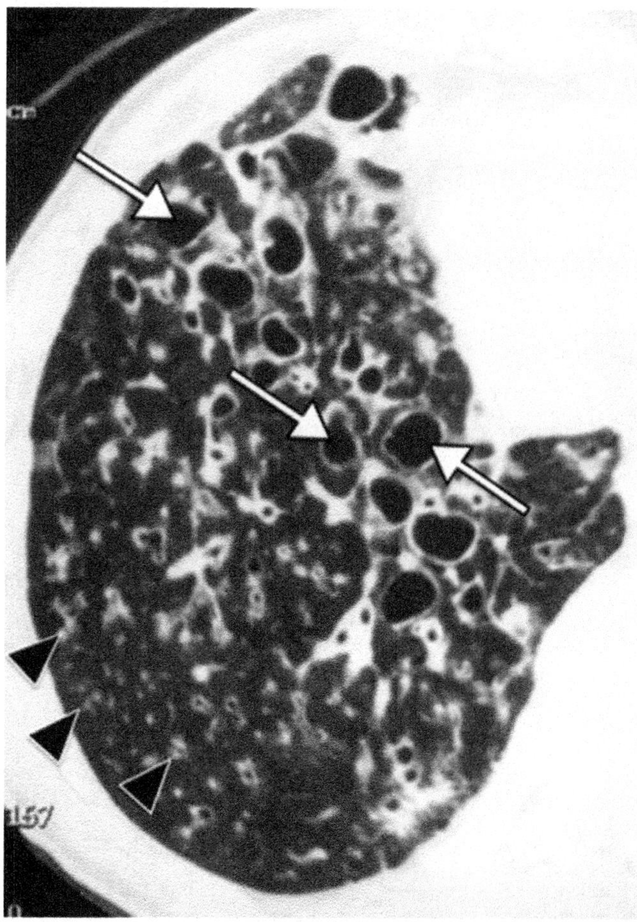

Fig. 10.2 Cystic bronchiectasis in rheumatoid arthritis. Computed tomography image obtained through the lower lobe of the right lung in a 60-year-old woman shows cystic bronchiectasis (thin arrows) with small clusters of centrilobular nodules or tree-in-bud appearance (arrowheads) suggesting bronchiolitis

10.3 Bacterial Infections

10.3.1 Pneumonia

10.3.1.1 Epidemiology

Pneumonia is the most common and frequent infection among patients with RA [2]. A nested case-control analysis of hospitalized infection based on 1993 RA cases and 9965 controls revealed the rate of pneumonia in the RA patients to be 2.3 times higher than that in the non-RA cohorts [2]. However, in patients with community-acquired pneumonia (CAP), the comorbidity of RA is an independent risk factor for CAP (OR = 1.84; 95% CI 1.62–2.10) [60]. The incidence densities of pneumonia in patients with RA receiving anti-rheumatic agents are shown in Table 10.1, which indicates that 5.3–34.4 per 1000 patient-years are developing pneumonia [2, 23, 50, 61–63]. The potential risk factors for pneumonia in RA patients are prolonged duration, high disease activity, and extensive disability of RA [23]. In the IORRA (Institute of Rheumatology, Rheumatoid Arthritis) cohort of 7926 Japanese patients with RA enrolled between 2000 and 2007 (before the introduction of biologics), pneumonia (12.1%) was the major cause of death following malignancies (24.2%). In the recent biologic era, a large cohort of 2683 patients with RA who had been exposed to biological agents showed pneumonia to be the most frequent cause of death (21.2%), and the standardized mortality ratio of pneumonia was 4.19 (95% CI 1.81–8.25) [64]. These epidemio-

Table 10.1 Incidence density of pneumonia, lower respiratory tract infection, *Pneumocystis jirovecii* pneumonia, and other fungal infections in patients with rheumatoid arthritis

Respiratory infection	Reference	Country	Year	n	Incidence: per 1000 person-years	Setting
Pneumonia	[50]	USA	1955–1994	609	31	Retrospective cohort study, corticosteroid, 46%; MTX, 18%; other csDMARDs, 73%; biological agents, 0.2%
			1995–2007	464	19.9	Corticosteroid, 90%, MTX, 73%; other csDMARDs, 98%; biological agents, 29%
	[62]	Canada	1992–2010	86,039	17.4	Population-based retrospective cohort study; PSL, 52%; MTX, 17.6%; other csDMARDs, 25.4%; at least one biological agent, 0.7%
	[2]	USA, Canada	1999–2006	24,530	8.4	Retrospective cohort study, corticosteroid, 46.9%; at least one csDMARD, 62%; at least one biological agent, 24%
	[61]	German	2001–2003	601	5.3	Prospective cohort study, csDMARDs
				346	24.6	IFX
				512	12.4	ETN
	[23]	USA	2001–2004	16,788	17	Prospective cohort study, PSL, 38.1%; MTX, 54.5%; other csDMARDs, 37.9%; at least one biological agent, 54%
	[63]	Japan	2008–2010	7901	34.4	PMS, TCZ
Lower respiratory tract infection	[61]	German	2001–2003	601	14.0	Prospective cohort study, csDMARDs
				346	46.1	IFX
				512	39.3	ETN
Pneumocystis jirovecii pneumonia	[94]	USA	1996–2007	Unknown	0.006–0.04	Population-based retrospective cohort study, drug, and prophylaxis unknown
	[96]	Japan	2005–2009	561	9.3	Retrospective cohort study, biological agents without prophylaxis
			2009–2010	214	0	Biological agents with prophylaxis
	[95]	USA, Europe	2005–2011	2965	0.1	RCTs, CZP, prophylaxis unknown
	[63]	Japan	2008–2010	7901	3.7	PMS, TCZ, prophylaxis unknown
Pulmonary aspergillosis	[95]	USA, Europe	2005–2011	2965	0.3	RCTs, CZP
Histoplasmosis	[95]	USA, Europe	2005–2011	2965	0.1	RCTs, CZP
	[136]	USA	2002–2005	10,050	0.3	RCT, open-label trials, and PMS, ADA

MTX methotrexate, *csDMARDs* conventional synthetic disease-modifying antirheumatic drugs, *IFX* infliximab, *ETN* etanercept, *PSL* prednisone, *PMS* postmarketing surveillance, *TCZ* tocilizumab, *RCT* randomized controlled trial, *CZP* certolizumab pegol, *ADA* adalimumab

logic studies suggest that pneumonia is a major complication and cause of death in patients with RA.

10.3.1.2 Diagnosis

Respiratory infections (e.g., bacterial, viral, fungal, and mycobacterial infections) and noninfectious diseases (e.g., drug-induced pneumonitis, malignancy, and RA-LDs) should be considered and carefully evaluated when RA patients have respiratory symptoms. Also, if infection overlaps on existing ILD or airway disease, it becomes more difficult to evaluate the infection (Fig. 10.1). Patients with pneumonia should be investigated for specific pathogens that would significantly alter standard (empirical) management decisions when the presence of specific pathogens is suspected on the basis of clinical and epidemiologic clues. Because patients with RA are at increased risk of dying from pneumonia compared to the general population [65], pneumococci, which are considered one of the main causative pathogens of pneumonia, should be checked with rapid antigen detection tests for *Streptococcus pneumoniae*. Also, as the risk of developing legionella pneumonia was reported to be higher especially among anti-TNF-treated patients in RA [66], that pathogen also needs to be screened for with rapid antigen detection tests for *Legionella pneumophila*. Also, influenza tests should be conducted during the influenza season. Computed tomography imaging can yield clues for diagnosis, but it cannot always identify specific pathogens. A microbial investigation with bronchoscopic bronchoalveolar lavage, protected specimen brushing, or transthoracic lung aspiration is needed for all CAP patients presenting with antimicrobial treatment failure [67, 68]. Nonresponsive patients may be considered to have concomitant or subsequent extrapulmonary infection, such as intravascular catheter, urinary, abdominal, and skin infections, or other noninfectious pulmonary diseases such as the above.

10.3.1.3 Prophylaxis

Vaccination is the primary measure used to reduce the onset of and prevent pneumonia. In general, as *Streptococcus pneumoniae* is the most important etiology in CAP, pneumococcal vaccination is justified for use in RA patients. In addition, because secondary bacterial pneumonia is an important complication after influenza, European League Against Rheumatism (EULAR) recommendations for vaccination in patients with RA recommend pneumococcal and influenza vaccinations during stable disease [69, 70]. However, under immunosuppressant treatments, can normal immunoreactions be induced by these vaccinations? Studies have shown that pneumococcal and influenza vaccinations are safe and produce an antibody response despite immunosuppressive medication in patients with RA [71, 72]. The exception is rituximab, which inhibits immunogenicity induced by pneumococcal [73] and influenza vaccinations [74].

10.3.1.4 Treatment

In general, causative organisms that should be considered in RA patients are similar bacteria, such as *Streptococcus pneumoniae*, *Haemophilus influenzae*, *Staphylococcus aureus*, *Moraxella* species, *Klebsiella pneumonia*, and *Pseudomonas aeruginosa*, and atypical pathogens, such as *Mycoplasma pneumoniae*, *Legionella pneumophila*, and *Chlamydophila pneumoniae*. Although few guidelines on the management of pneumonia in RA patients exist, the Japanese Respiratory Society (JRS) has recently elucidated its consensus statements and recommendations for the treatment of pneumonia treated with biological agents (Fig. 10.3) [75]. In this recommendation, it is notable that because a high frequency of respiratory infection caused by *P. aeruginosa* has been reported in RA patients with bronchopulmonary involvements [44], the JRS recommends that the possibility of *P. aeruginosa* as the causative organism should be carefully considered when administering antibiotic agents. Also, when choosing antibiotic agents, the antibiotic therapy should cover legionellosis under treatment with TNF-α antagonists [66]. Moreover, all patients with pneumonia need to be screened with rapid antigen detection tests for influenza to consider antiviral therapy and to prevent in-hospital transmission during the endemic season.

10.3.2 Acute Exacerbation of Bronchiectasis

Bronchiectasis is frequently seen in patients with RA [61, 76, 77], and common sources of infection are bacteria such as *H. influenzae*, *S. pneumoniae*, and *P. aeruginosa* [78, 79] (Fig. 10.2). Five-year survival rates of patients with RA and bronchiectasis are reported to range from 68.8 to 87.1% [77, 80]. Takayanagi et al. [59] and Tsuchiya et al. [77] reported that acute exacerbation of bronchiectasis, which is the acute deterioration of lower respiratory tract infection without pneumonia, is a common cause of death in RA-bronchiectasis. Takayanagi et al. showed in a report on pulmonary infections in RA patients that *P. aeruginosa* was the etiology of all fatal cases of exacerbation of bronchiectasis [59]. From the perspective of these reports, TAZ/PIPC, antipseudomonal carbapenem (IPM/CS, MEPM, or DRPM), or quinolone (LVFX, CPFX, or PZFX) should be administered in such patients [75].

10.3.3 Other Bacterial Infections

Lung abscess and empyema are other types of respiratory infection that are occasionally observed in RA patients. *Streptococcus* species, anaerobes, and *Gemella* species are common pathogens. When diagnosing lung abscess, compatible clinical features such as fever, productive cough, bad breath, chills, or chest pain in conjunction with cavities seen on chest radiography are clues to the diagnosis. Tuberculosis,

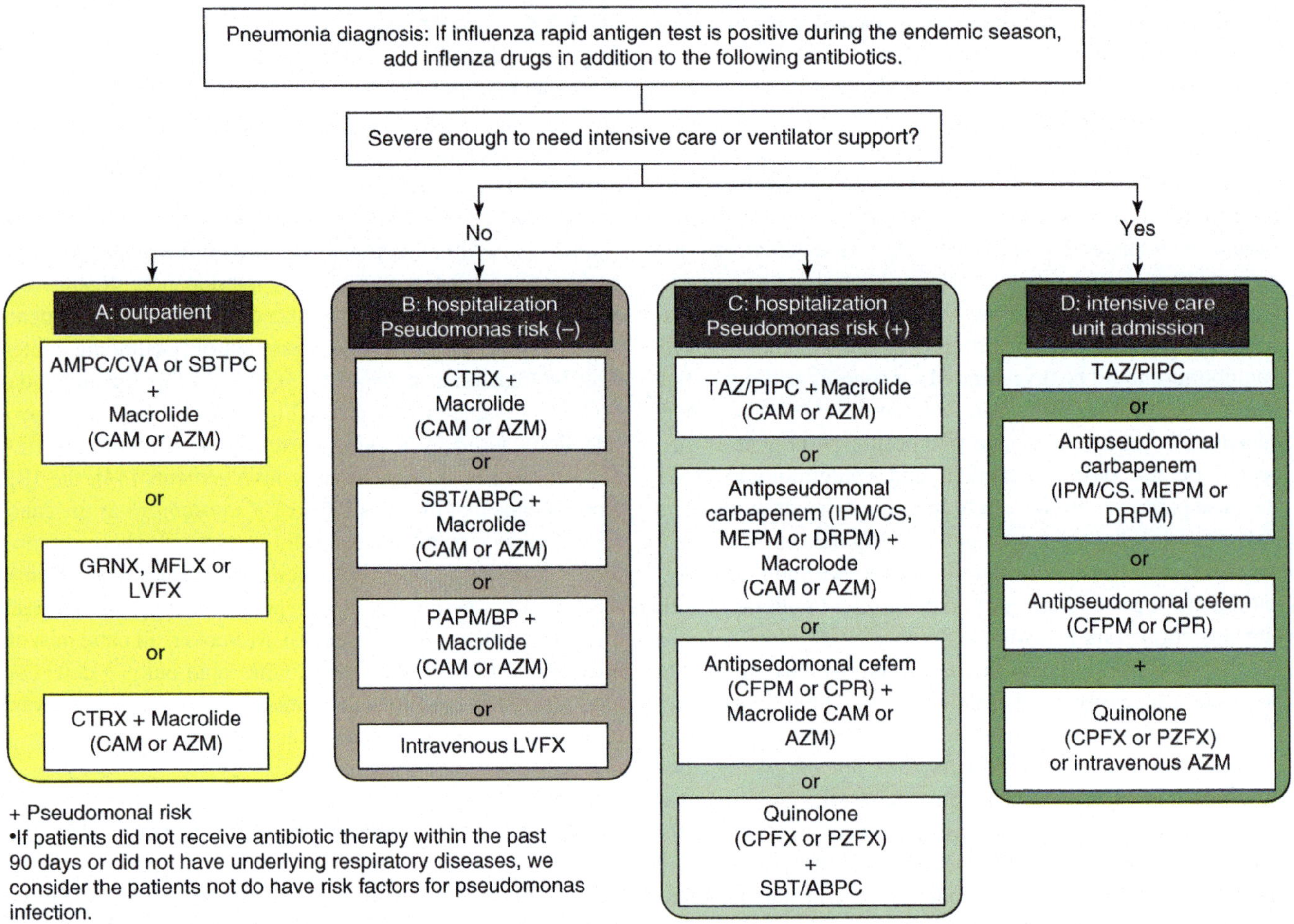

Fig. 10.3 2014 Japanese Respiratory Society recommendations for the treatment of pneumonia treated with biological agents. *AMPC/CVA* amoxicillin/clavulanate, *SBTPC* sultamicillin, *CAM* clarithromycin, *AZM* azithromycin, *GRNX* garenoxacin, *MFLX* moxifloxacin, *LVFX* levofloxacin, *CTRX* ceftriaxone, *SBT/ABPC* sulbactam/ampicillin, *PAPM/BP* panipenem/betamipron, *TAZ/PIPC* tazobactam/piperacillin, *IPM/CS* imipenem/cilastatin, *MEPM* meropenem, *DRPM* doripenem, *CFPM* cefepime, *CPR* cefpirome, *CPFX* ciprofloxacin, *PZFX* pazufloxacin

nocardiosis, pulmonary fungal infections, septic emboli, primary or metastatic lung cancer, or RA nodulosis should be carefully ruled out. When diagnosing empyema, thoracentesis is needed for staining, culture, and determination of pH and leukocyte counts of pleural effusion. Differential diagnoses of empyema are RA pleuritis, tuberculous pleuritis, and carcinomatous pleurisy. The antimicrobial therapy of first choice for lung abscess and empyema is SBT/ABPC. In addition, *Klebsiella* species and *P. aeruginosa* should also be considered if patients have underlying respiratory diseases, diabetes mellitus, or alcoholism. In these settings, TAZ/PIPC or antipseudomonal carbapenem (IPM/CS, MEPM, or DRPM) should be administered [75]. Insertion of chest drainage is needed for empyema with higher risk of poor outcome [81]. In patients who do not respond to treatment or in whom disease recurs, organisms should be obtained by bronchoscopy or needle aspiration, and *Nocardia* and *Actinomyces* species should be carefully eliminated as sources of infection.

10.4 Fungal Infections

Fungal infections are common opportunistic infections and potentially life-threatening complications for patients with RA. As described above, multifactorial etiologies, mainly immunosuppressive agents, make RA patients vulnerable to fungal infections such as *Pneumocystis jirovecii* pneumonia (PCP) and other pulmonary fungal infections.

10.4.1 *Pneumocystis jirovecii* Pneumonia

10.4.1.1 Epidemiology

Pneumocystis jirovecii is one of the most significant opportunistic fungal pathogens in RA. PCP occurring in adults was originally considered to be mostly due to a reactivation of latent childhood infection of *P. jirovecii*. However, several authors recently pointed out that new acquisition and carriage of *P. jirovecii* from a hospital environment and person-to-person transmission are also important etiologies of *P. jirovecii* infection in immunocompromised adults [82]. As *P. jirovecii* organisms predominantly colonize in elderly individuals with RA [83], immunosuppressant treatments are thought to have an important role as igniters of PCP in such carriers. Systemic corticosteroid therapy has been identified as a risk factor of PCP in patients with RA [84, 85]. Even low or moderate doses of corticosteroids can increase the risk of PCP in these patient populations [84–88]. PCP also sometimes occurs early in the course of MTX therapy in RA patients [89, 90]. The risk factors of RA-PCP under MTX therapy are lymphopenia and the combined use of corticosteroid [90]. The risk of PCP with MTX therapy increases in a dose-dependent manner, but PCP can also occur during low-dose MTX therapy without corticosteroid [83, 86]. With regard to biological agents, postmarketing surveillance reports in Japan indicated a high incidence of PCP in RA patients receiving IFX (0.4% of 5000 patients) [91], ETN (0.2% of 7091 patients) [92], and ADA (0.3% of 3000 patients) [93]. These data are more than ten times higher than the reported incidence of this infection in data from Western studies of these agents [91, 94, 95]. This disparity may be due to differences in race or geographic regions. The incidence densities of PCP in patients with RA are shown in Table 10.1. The risk factors of RA-PCP under biological agents are age ≥ 65 years, pulmonary comorbidities such as ILD or bronchiectasis, and corticosteroid use [96]. In addition, decreased serum albumin and IgG levels at the onset of PCP were also identified as risk factors in IFX-treated patients with RA [85], although these laboratory findings are not specific to this infection. Compared to PCP with HIV, RA-PCP has fewer pneumocystis organisms burden but more intense inflammation pathologically [97, 98]. In HIV patients, the main pathology of PCP is pulmonary injury due to a relative decrease in CD4+ lymphocytes in the lung, which leads to suppression of cell-mediated immunity. Contrastingly, in RA patients, although changes in the T-cell repertoire and its homeostatic balance lead to reduced clearance of pneumocystis organisms, immune function is still maintained. Therefore, the host inflammatory response in RA-PCP may induce a more intense reaction than that in HIV-PCP, thus contributing to severe lung injury. The mortality rate of RA-PCP (14.2–50%) has been reported to be higher than that of HIV-PCP [86, 97]. However, accurate diagnosis and prompt treatment by attending physicians who have prior experience with PCP can improve the prognosis of the patients [85, 99].

10.4.1.2 Diagnosis

Because RA-PCP commonly manifests with an acute and fulminant clinical course, delay in the diagnosis of PCP can be fatal. Physical examination typically reveals tachypnea, tachycardia, and normal findings on lung auscultation. Microscopic examinations for trophic forms or cysts of *P. jirovecii* are useful. However, because RA-PCP has fewer parasitic organisms, this lower organism burden results in a lower diagnostic yield of induced sputum and bronchoalveolar lavage fluid to confirm PCP as compared with HIV-PCP. Polymerase chain reaction (PCR), which detects pneumocystis nucleic acids, has been shown to have greater sensitivity (87.2%) and specificity (92.2%) in non-HIV-PCP [100]. To differentiate colonization from PCP, an elevated serum (1 → 3)-β-D-glucan level is useful in patients whose *P. jirovecii* is detected only by PCR. However, because of the lower parasitic burden in the lungs, specific and standardized cutoff values for clinical infection in RA patients are necessary for early and accurate diagnosis [101]. Lactate dehydrogenase and KL-6 levels are commonly elevated, but drug-induced pneumonitis and RA-ILD need to be differentiated in this situation. Chest X-ray is not sensitive in the early phase of PCP. Reflecting a host hyperinflammatory response similar to that of MTX pneumonitis, the computed tomography pattern of RA-PCP is analogous to MTX pneumonitis and is occasionally difficult to discriminate [97].

10.4.1.3 Prophylaxis

The most effective and most commonly used agent for prophylaxis is trimethoprim/sulfamethoxazole (TMP/SMX). However, patients prophylactically treated with TMP/SMX sometimes face serious adverse events such as rash, anaphylaxis, hematotoxicity, and hepatotoxicity. Utsunomiya et al. recently performed a non-blinded, randomized controlled trial to seek an effective prophylaxis regimen for PCP and revealed that half of the recommended dose of TMP/SMX daily was suggested to be feasible and optimal for the prophylaxis of PCP in patients with systemic rheumatic diseases [102]. Other preventive agents include aerosolized pentamidine, dapsone, and atovaquone. These agents, which are used as alternative prophylactic agents for TMP/SMX, have fewer adverse events but also a lower prophylactic effect compared with TMP/SMX [103–105]. Significant toxicities generally evolve within the first month of therapy; nevertheless, patients receive immunosuppressant treatments and small doses of prophylactic agents. In HIV-infected adults, prophylaxis for PCP is recommended if the patients have a past history of PCP, CD4+ counts of <200 cells/mm^3, or oral candidiasis [106]. Unfortunately, however, there are no clinically useful biologic markers to guide the initiation and termination of prophylaxis for RA-PCP. Katsuyama et al. recently showed that RA patients with two or three risk factors for PCP including older age (≥65 years), use of corticosteroid, and coexisting pulmonary disease benefited from primary prophylaxis [96]. Since many RA patients require the lifelong use of multiple antirheumatic drugs and have coexisting pulmonary diseases in practice, these patients are generally subject to PCP prophylaxis. However, severe adverse events due to prophylactic agent occasionally result in discontinuation of PCP prophylaxis. Therefore, it is not practical to administer and continue prophylaxis for all of these RA patients throughout anti-RA therapy. Thus, the requirements for PCP prophylaxis in RA patients should be taken into careful consideration based on a risk-benefit assessment performed before starting and throughout anti-RA therapy.

10.4.1.4 Treatment

The agent of first choice for PCP treatment is TMP/SMX [107]. Although TMP/SMX is highly effective, adverse effects may be experienced. One of the alternate drugs of choice for PCP is pentamidine, which is comparable to TMP/SMX in efficacy and frequency of adverse reactions [108] but has side effects such as hypotension, hypoglycemia, and renal toxicity. Atovaquone is less effective than TMP/SMX but can be safely used as an alternate choice instead of TMP/SMX in moderate and mild cases [109]. The recommended doses of these agents were derived from studies on efficacy and tolerance performed on HIV-positive patients. To date, there is no consensus on how many doses and for how long these drugs should be administered in RA-PCP. Because the burden of pneumocystis organisms is lower in the lungs of patients with RA-PCP, prospective randomized, controlled treatment trials should be performed to determine appropriate doses and durations of these agents in RA-PCP.

Because RA patients have a strong inflammatory response to pneumocystis organisms, it is reasonable that corticosteroid may play a beneficial role in the treatment of RA-PCP. It is recommended that patients with hypoxemia on room air (PaO_2 < 70 mmHg or alveolar-arterial O_2 gradient >35 mmHg) be administered adjunctive corticosteroid at an early stage of the disease [110]. Kameda et al. revealed in a retrospective, multicenter study including 24 patients with RA-PCP that 23 patients were administered moderate- to high-dose corticosteroid with TMP/SMX and the overall mortality rate was favorable at 4.2% [111]. Of note, the good outcome in this study was accomplished despite the fact that more than one-third of the patients could not complete the recommended dose of TMP/SMX therapy because of serious adverse effects. This result may indicate that RA-PCP is an aspect of hyperinflammation induced by pneumocystis organisms rather than infection.

10.4.2 Other Fungal Infections

Other fungal infections occasionally observed in RA patients include aspergillosis, candidiasis, cryptococcosis, histoplasmosis, coccidioidomycosis, and others. Ge et al. recently evaluated the risk factors of invasive pulmonary fungal infection in 2186 patients with connective tissue disease. They identified interstitial pneumonia, antimicrobial drug therapy, and maximum PSL dose of 30 mg per day within 3 months prior to the infection as risk factors for invasive pulmonary fungal infection [112]. The use of a TNF-α antagonist leads to a defective cellular immune response and subsequently to interference of granuloma formation and maintenance [113] against several fungi. Kourbeti et al. reviewed the association between biological agents and opportunistic infections in a meta-analysis of 3915 RA patients. There were nine invasive fungal infections, in which eight cases were treated with biological agents: five cases of invasive aspergillosis, two of histoplasmosis, and one of coccidioidomycosis. The study indicated that biological agents did not statistically increase the risk of invasive fungal infections [37]. In contrast, Tsiodras et al. reviewed invasive fungal infections associated with biological agents in which TNF-α antagonists were associated with invasive fungal infections [114]. The most common pattern of infection was pneumonia, and the most prevalent invasive fungal infections were histoplasmosis, candidiasis, and aspergillosis. They also stated that cryptococcosis, histoplasmosis, and coccidioidomycosis have all been associated with TNF-α antagonists, which indicates that anti-TNF treatments should be started cautiously in patients living in or visiting regions with endemic mycoses. In a large series of granulomatous infections, the risk for patients receiving IFX was significantly higher than that for patients receiving ETN (239 vs. 74 per 100,000 patients, $P < 0.001$), and this higher risk persisted when individual fungal infections, such as candidiasis, histoplasmosis, and coccidioidomycosis, were considered [115].

Post-licensure surveillance in the USA suggests that acute life-threatening histoplasmosis may complicate immunotherapy with TNF-α antagonists, particularly IFX. However, all patients with histoplasmosis resided in an area endemic for histoplasmosis, and all of them were receiving other immunosuppressant therapy such as corticosteroid concomitantly. Thus, there are limitations when analyzing diseases such as histoplasmosis and coccidioidomycosis that are endemic to specific geographic regions [116].

Reports of serious cryptococcal pneumonia have recently accumulated in patients with RA [114, 117–120]. These studies showed that chronic kidney disease and administration of corticosteroid [118] or biological agents [114, 118–120] were risk factors for cryptococcal pneumonia in RA.

TNF-α also appears to have a central role in neutrophil recruitment into the lungs in response to *Aspergillus fumigatus* [121] and in enhancing leukocyte killing of *A. fumigatus* [122]. According to Tsiodras et al., of the 281 patients who developed fungal infections associated with TNF-α antagonists, 64 were infected with *Aspergillus* species [114]. Among these 64 patients, 48 (75%) had received IFX, 14 (21%) ETN, and 2 (4%) ADA.

Because the published information on pulmonary fungal infections in RA patients is limited, it is still not clear whether

RA patients predispose to pulmonary fungal infections other than PCP. To date, however, considering the pharmacological actions of corticosteroid or biological agents, great caution should be exercised in patients with RA receiving antirheumatic agents. Surveillance of pulmonary fungal infections in RA patients with antirheumatic therapy is needed through well-organized prospective patient registries.

10.5 Pulmonary Infection as a Risk Factor for the Onset of RA

Recently, accumulating data suggest that RA may be triggered by microorganisms [76] (Fig. 10.4), in particular certain species of bacteria such as *Prevotella* species [123] and *Porphyromonas gingivalis* [124, 125]. Of note, culture-independent methodologies have led to the identification of these specific bacterial communities in the lung [126, 127]. Bacteria-specific mechanisms are known to influence the development of innate and adaptive immunity at mucosal surfaces [128, 129], and they also likely play a role in the development of autoimmunity through mechanisms such as bacteria-induced autoantibody generation and immune regulatory effects [130–132]. *P. gingivalis* contains citrullinated fibrinogen and α-enolase [124, 133, 134]. Antibodies to these citrullinated proteins are identified in the preclinical period of RA [135], suggesting a potential mechanism by which a certain bacterial species may lead to RA-related autoimmunity in the lung, and this mechanism may be contributed to by these pulmonary infections consequent to the

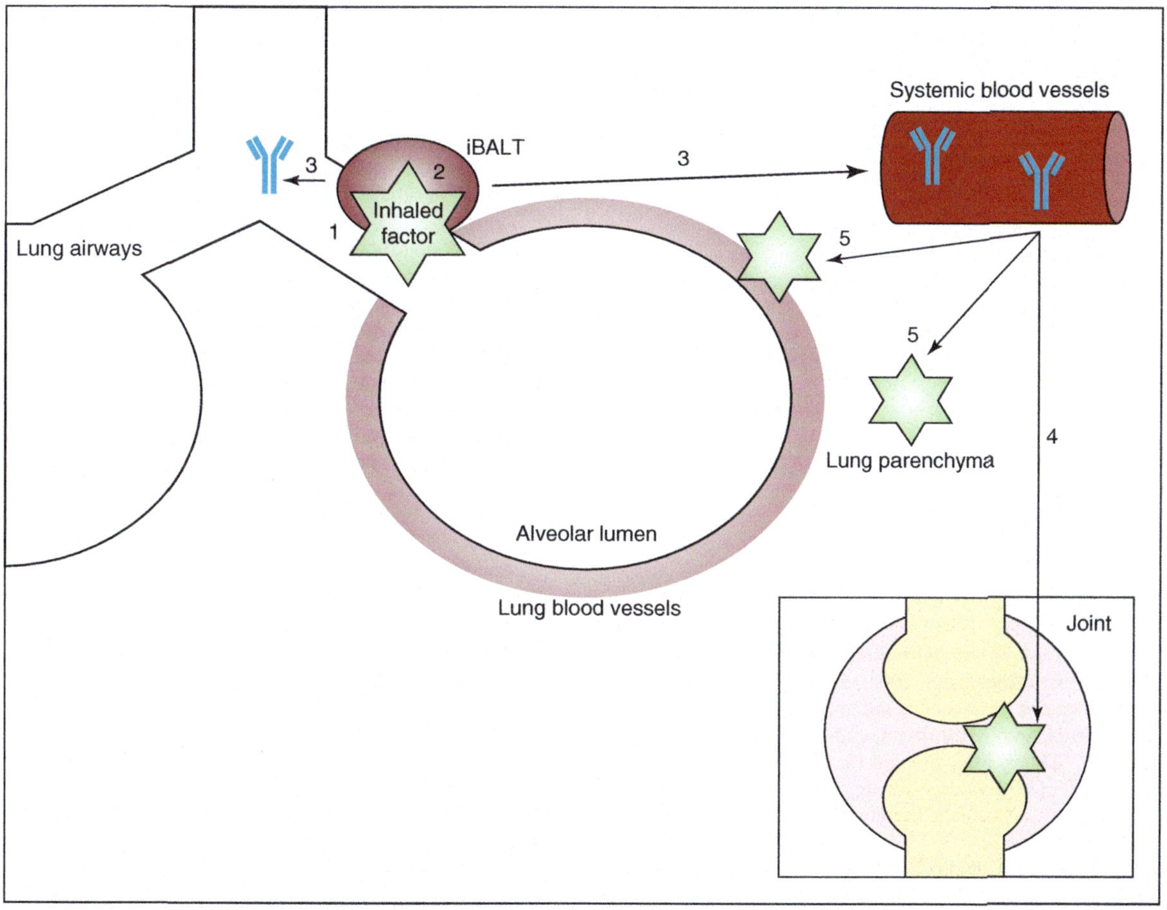

Fig. 10.4 Model for the role of the lung in RA pathogenesis. A hypothetical model for the involvement of the lung in RA is depicted in which an inhaled environmental factor interacts with the host immune system at the airway mucosa (1). This results in a local inflammatory immune reaction and induction of immune activity such as iBALT (2). iBALT can result in local generation of autoantibodies in the lung, but this can also transition to systemic autoimmunity through interactions with regional lymphatics (3). Over time, systemic RA-related autoantibodies can transition to joint inflammation classifiable as RA through currently unknown mechanisms, but possibilities include circulating immune complexes depositing in the joints or epitope spreading to include joint-specific antigens (4). During the preclinical or later stages of RA, symptomatic or worsening lung disease may develop via persistent exposure to inhaled antigens and ongoing airway inflammation that may also spread to the parenchyma (5), and iBALT may participate in local lung tissue damage (5), or circulating autoantibodies and other inflammatory factors may target the lung parenchyma (5). *Ab* antibody, *iBALT* inducible bronchus-associated lymphoid tissue, *RA* rheumatoid arthritis. Adapted from Demoruelle et al. [76]

development of RA. Infectious agents might not trigger RA in all cases but only in a certain subset of the cases, or disease onset may arise from an unfortunate combination of infection with other factors. Further studies are needed to define the mechanistic role of respiratory infections in the development of RA.

Conclusion

In patients with RA, respiratory infections are considered important factors that affect not only the development of RA itself but also patient survival. Although aggressive treatment with csDMARDs or biological agents early in the disease course can reduce the disease activity of RA and improve patient quality of life, they hold a higher risk of bacterial or fungal respiratory infections. Thus, it is essential for clinicians to have sufficient knowledge of the characteristics of respiratory infections in these settings of RA. Because controlling respiratory infections improves the survival of patients with RA, proper diagnosis and prompt treatment of respiratory infections in these patients are needed throughout the patient's treatment period.

Acknowledgment The authors greatly appreciate the special comments received from Dr. Megumi Jinno and Dr. Takenori Okada, Department of Allergy and Respiratory Medicine, and from Dr. Tomoki Hayashi, Dr. Ryo Yanai, Dr. Yusuke Miwa, and Dr. Tsuyoshi Kasama, Department of Rheumatology, Showa University Koto Toyosu Hospital.

References

1. Doran MF, Crowson CS, Pond GR, O'Fallon WM, Gabriel SE. Predictors of infection in rheumatoid arthritis. Arthritis Rheum. 2002;46(9):2294–300.
2. Smitten AL, Choi HK, Hochberg MC, Suissa S, Simon TA, Testa MA, et al. The risk of hospitalized infection in patients with rheumatoid arthritis. J Rheumatol. 2008;35(3):387–93.
3. Furst DE. The risk of infections with biologic therapies for rheumatoid arthritis. Semin Arthritis Rheum. 2010;39(5):327–46.
4. Stoffer MA, Schoels MM, Smolen JS, Aletaha D, Breedveld FC, Burmester G, et al. Evidence for treating rheumatoid arthritis to target: results of a systematic literature search update. Ann Rheum Dis. 2016;75(1):16–22.
5. Nam JL, Ramiro S, Gaujoux-Viala C, Takase K, Leon-Garcia M, Emery P, et al. Efficacy of biological disease-modifying antirheumatic drugs: a systematic literature review informing the 2013 update of the EULAR recommendations for the management of rheumatoid arthritis. Ann Rheum Dis. 2014;73(3):516–28.
6. Smolen JS, Aletaha D. Rheumatoid arthritis therapy reappraisal: strategies, opportunities and challenges. Nat Rev Rheumatol. 2015;11(5):276–89.
7. Ramiro S, Gaujoux-Viala C, Nam JL, Smolen JS, Buch M, Gossec L, et al. Safety of synthetic and biological DMARDs: a systematic literature review informing the 2013 update of the EULAR recommendations for management of rheumatoid arthritis. Ann Rheum Dis. 2014;73(3):529–35.
8. Stuck AE, Minder CE, Frey FJ. Risk of infectious complications in patients taking glucocorticosteroids. Rev Infect Dis. 1989;11(6):954–63.
9. Bartels CM, Bell CL, Shinki K, Rosenthal A, Bridges AJ. Changing trends in serious extra-articular manifestations of rheumatoid arthritis among United State veterans over 20 years. Rheumatology. 2010;49(9):1670–5.
10. Greenberg JD, Reed G, Kremer JM, Tindall E, Kavanaugh A, Zheng C, et al. Association of methotrexate and tumour necrosis factor antagonists with risk of infectious outcomes including opportunistic infections in the CORRONA registry. Ann Rheum Dis. 2010;69(2):380–6.
11. Lopez-Olivo MA, Siddhanamatha HR, Shea B, Tugwell P, Wells GA, Suarez-Almazor ME. Methotrexate for treating rheumatoid arthritis. Cochrane Database Syst Rev. 2014;6:CD000957.
12. Yoo HG, Yu HM, Jun JB, Jeon HS, Yoo WH. Risk factors of severe infections in patients with rheumatoid arthritis treated with leflunomide. Mod Rheumatol. 2013;23(4):709–15.
13. Gaujoux-Viala C, Smolen JS, Landewe R, Dougados M, Kvien TK, Mola EM, et al. Current evidence for the management of rheumatoid arthritis with synthetic disease-modifying antirheumatic drugs: a systematic literature review informing the EULAR recommendations for the management of rheumatoid arthritis. Ann Rheum Dis. 2010;69(6):1004–9.
14. Singh JA, Cameron C, Noorbaloochi S, Cullis T, Tucker M, Christensen R, et al. Risk of serious infection in biological treatment of patients with rheumatoid arthritis: a systematic review and meta-analysis. Lancet. 2015;386(9990):258–65.
15. Geri G, Dadoun S, Bui T, Del Castillo Pinol N, Paternotte S, Dougados M, et al. Risk of infections in bronchiectasis during disease-modifying treatment and biologics for rheumatic diseases. BMC Infect Dis. 2011;11:304.
16. Wagner UG, Koetz K, Weyand CM, Goronzy JJ. Perturbation of the T cell repertoire in rheumatoid arthritis. Proc Natl Acad Sci U S A. 1998;95(24):14447–52.
17. Koetz K, Bryl E, Spickschen K, O'Fallon WM, Goronzy JJ, Weyand CM. T cell homeostasis in patients with rheumatoid arthritis. Proc Natl Acad Sci U S A. 2000;97(16):9203–8.
18. Boling EP, Ohishi T, Wahl SM, Misiti J, Wistar R Jr, Wilder RL. Humoral immune function in severe, active rheumatoid arthritis. Clin Immunol Immunopathol. 1987;43(2):185–94.
19. Haeney MR. The role of the complement cascade in sepsis. J Antimicrob Chemother. 1998;41(Suppl A):41–6.
20. Panoulas VF, Smith JP, Nightingale P, Kitas GD. Association of the TRAF1/C5 locus with increased mortality, particularly from malignancy or sepsis, in patients with rheumatoid arthritis. Arthritis Rheum. 2009;60(1):39–46.
21. Klein NC, Go CH, Cunha BA. Infections associated with steroid use. Infect Dis Clin N Am. 2001;15(2):423–32. viii
22. Saag KG, Koehnke R, Caldwell JR, Brasington R, Burmeister LF, Zimmerman B, et al. Low dose long-term corticosteroid therapy in rheumatoid arthritis: an analysis of serious adverse events. Am J Med. 1994;96(2):115–23.
23. Wolfe F, Caplan L, Michaud K. Treatment for rheumatoid arthritis and the risk of hospitalization for pneumonia: associations with prednisone, disease-modifying antirheumatic drugs, and anti-tumor necrosis factor therapy. Arthritis Rheum. 2006;54(2):628–34.
24. Jobanputra P, Wilson J, Douglas K, Burls A. A survey of British rheumatologists' DMARD preferences for rheumatoid arthritis. Rheumatology. 2004;43(2):206–10.
25. Mikuls TR, O'Dell J. The changing face of rheumatoid arthritis therapy: results of serial surveys. Arthritis Rheum. 2000;43(2):464–5.
26. Grijalva CG, Chung CP, Stein CM, Mitchel EF Jr, Griffin MR. Changing patterns of medication use in patients with

rheumatoid arthritis in a Medicaid population. Rheumatology. 2008;47(7):1061–4.
27. Phillips DC, Woollard KJ, Griffiths HR. The anti-inflammatory actions of methotrexate are critically dependent upon the production of reactive oxygen species. Br J Pharmacol. 2003;138(3):501–11.
28. Nesher G, Osborn TG, Moore TL. Effect of treatment with methotrexate, hydroxychloroquine, and prednisone on lymphocyte polyamine levels in rheumatoid arthritis: correlation with the clinical response and rheumatoid factor synthesis. Clin Exp Rheumatol. 1997;15(4):343–7.
29. Pickering LK, Ericsson CD, Kohl S. Effect of chemotherapeutic agents on metabolic and bactericidal activity of polymorphonuclear leukocytes. Cancer. 1978;42(4):1741–6.
30. Kraan MC, de Koster BM, Elferink JG, Post WJ, Breedveld FC, Tak PP. Inhibition of neutrophil migration soon after initiation of treatment with leflunomide or methotrexate in patients with rheumatoid arthritis: findings in a prospective, randomized, double-blind clinical trial in fifteen patients. Arthritis Rheum. 2000;43(7):1488–95.
31. Cronstein BN. Going with the flow: methotrexate, adenosine, and blood flow. Ann Rheum Dis. 2006;65(4):421–2.
32. Riksen NP, Barrera P, van den Broek PH, van Riel PL, Smits P, Rongen GA. Methotrexate modulates the kinetics of adenosine in humans in vivo. Ann Rheum Dis. 2006;65(4):465–70.
33. Bernatsky S, Hudson M, Suissa S. Anti-rheumatic drug use and risk of serious infections in rheumatoid arthritis. Rheumatology. 2007;46(7):1157–60.
34. Lacaille D, Guh DP, Abrahamowicz M, Anis AH, Esdaile JM. Use of nonbiologic disease-modifying antirheumatic drugs and risk of infection in patients with rheumatoid arthritis. Arthritis Rheum. 2008;59(8):1074–81.
35. Franklin J, Lunt M, Bunn D, Symmons D, Silman A. Risk and predictors of infection leading to hospitalisation in a large primary-care-derived cohort of patients with inflammatory polyarthritis. Ann Rheum Dis. 2007;66(3):308–12.
36. Coyne P, Hamilton J, Heycock C, Saravanan V, Coulson E, Kelly CA. Acute lower respiratory tract infections in patients with rheumatoid arthritis. J Rheumatol. 2007;34(9):1832–6.
37. Kourbeti IS, Ziakas PD, Mylonakis E. Biologic therapies in rheumatoid arthritis and the risk of opportunistic infections: a meta-analysis. Clin Infect Dis. 2014;58(12):1649–57.
38. Scott DL, Wolfe F, Huizinga TW. Rheumatoid arthritis. Lancet. 2010;376(9746):1094–108.
39. Tugwell P, Singh JA, Wells GA. Biologicals for rheumatoid arthritis. BMJ. 2011;343:d4027.
40. Bongartz T, Sutton AJ, Sweeting MJ, Buchan I, Matteson EL, Montori V. Anti-TNF antibody therapy in rheumatoid arthritis and the risk of serious infections and malignancies: systematic review and meta-analysis of rare harmful effects in randomized controlled trials. JAMA. 2006;295(19):2275–85.
41. Askling J, Fored CM, Brandt L, Baecklund E, Bertilsson L, Feltelius N, et al. Time-dependent increase in risk of hospitalisation with infection among Swedish RA patients treated with TNF antagonists. Ann Rheum Dis. 2007;66(10):1339–44.
42. Strangfeld A, Eveslage M, Schneider M, Bergerhausen HJ, Klopsch T, Zink A, et al. Treatment benefit or survival of the fittest: what drives the time-dependent decrease in serious infection rates under TNF inhibition and what does this imply for the individual patient? Ann Rheum Dis. 2011;70(11):1914–20.
43. Galloway JB, Hyrich KL, Mercer LK, Dixon WG, Fu B, Ustianowski AP, et al. Anti-TNF therapy is associated with an increased risk of serious infections in patients with rheumatoid arthritis especially in the first 6 months of treatment: updated results from the British Society for Rheumatology Biologics Register with special emphasis on risks in the elderly. Rheumatology. 2011;50(1):124–31.
44. Dixon WG, Symmons DP, Lunt M, Watson KD, Hyrich KL. British Society for Rheumatology Biologics Register Control Centre Consortium, et al. Serious infection following anti-tumor necrosis factor alpha therapy in patients with rheumatoid arthritis: lessons from interpreting data from observational studies. Arthritis Rheum. 2007;56(9):2896–904.
45. Schneeweiss S, Setoguchi S, Weinblatt ME, Katz JN, Avorn J, Sax PE, et al. Anti-tumor necrosis factor alpha therapy and the risk of serious bacterial infections in elderly patients with rheumatoid arthritis. Arthritis Rheum. 2007;56(6):1754–64.
46. Grijalva CG, Chen L, Delzell E, Baddley JW, Beukelman T, Winthrop KL, et al. Initiation of tumor necrosis factor-alpha antagonists and the risk of hospitalization for infection in patients with autoimmune diseases. JAMA. 2011;306(21):2331–9.
47. Leombruno JP, Einarson TR, Keystone EC. The safety of anti-tumour necrosis factor treatments in rheumatoid arthritis: meta and exposure-adjusted pooled analyses of serious adverse events. Ann Rheum Dis. 2009;68(7):1136–45.
48. Salliot C, Dougados M, Gossec L. Risk of serious infections during rituximab, abatacept and anakinra treatments for rheumatoid arthritis: meta-analyses of randomised placebo-controlled trials. Ann Rheum Dis. 2009;68(1):25–32.
49. Thompson AE, Rieder SW, Pope JE. Tumor necrosis factor therapy and the risk of serious infection and malignancy in patients with early rheumatoid arthritis: a meta-analysis of randomized controlled trials. Arthritis Rheum. 2011;63(6):1479–85.
50. Ni Mhuircheartaigh OM, Matteson EL, Green AB, Crowson CS. Trends in serious infections in rheumatoid arthritis. J Rheumatol. 2013;40(5):611–6.
51. Olson AL, Swigris JJ, Sprunger DB, Fischer A, Fernandez-Perez ER, Solomon J, et al. Rheumatoid arthritis-interstitial lung disease-associated mortality. Am J Respir Crit Care Med. 2011;183(3):372–8.
52. Bongartz T, Nannini C, Medina-Velasquez YF, Achenbach SJ, Crowson CS, Ryu JH, et al. Incidence and mortality of interstitial lung disease in rheumatoid arthritis: a population-based study. Arthritis Rheum. 2010;62(6):1583–91.
53. Mori S, Koga Y, Sugimoto M. Different risk factors between interstitial lung disease and airway disease in rheumatoid arthritis. Respir Med. 2012;106(11):1591–9.
54. Demoruelle MK, Weisman MH, Simonian PL, Lynch DA, Sachs PB, Pedraza IF, et al. Brief report: airways abnormalities and rheumatoid arthritis-related autoantibodies in subjects without arthritis: early injury or initiating site of autoimmunity? Arthritis Rheum. 2012;64(6):1756–61.
55. Wilsher M, Voight L, Milne D, Teh M, Good N, Kolbe J, et al. Prevalence of airway and parenchymal abnormalities in newly diagnosed rheumatoid arthritis. Respir Med. 2012;106(10):1441–6.
56. Mori S, Cho I, Koga Y, Sugimoto M. Comparison of pulmonary abnormalities on high-resolution computed tomography in patients with early versus longstanding rheumatoid arthritis. J Rheumatol. 2008;35:1513–21.
57. Cottin V, Cordier JF. Combined pulmonary fibrosis and emphysema in connective tissue disease. Curr Opin Pulm Med. 2012;18(5):418–27.
58. Nannini C, Medina-Velasquez YF, Achenbach SJ, Crowson CS, Ryu JH, Vassallo R, et al. Incidence and mortality of obstructive lung disease in rheumatoid arthritis: a population-based study. Arthritis Care Res (Hoboken). 2013;65(8):1243–50.
59. Takayanagi N, Tsuchiya Y, Tokunaga D, Miyahara Y, Yamaguchi S. Saito H, et al. [Pulmonary infections in patients with rheumatoid arthritis]. Nihon Kokyuki Gakkai Zasshi. 2007;45(6): 465–73.

60. Vinogradova Y, Hippisley-Cox J, Coupland C. Identification of new risk factors for pneumonia: population-based case-control study. Br J Gen Pract. 2009;59(567):e329–38.
61. Listing J, Strangfeld A, Kary S, Rau R, von Hinueber U, Stoyanova-Scholz M, et al. Infections in patients with rheumatoid arthritis treated with biologic agents. Arthritis Rheum. 2005;52(11):3403–12.
62. Widdifield J, Bernatsky S, Paterson JM, Gunraj N, Thorne JC, Pope J, et al. Serious infections in a population-based cohort of 86,039 seniors with rheumatoid arthritis. Arthritis Care Res (Hoboken). 2013;65(3):353–61.
63. Koike T, Harigai M, Inokuma S, Ishiguro N, Ryu J, Takeuchi T, et al. Effectiveness and safety of tocilizumab: postmarketing surveillance of 7901 patients with rheumatoid arthritis in Japan. J Rheumatol. 2014;41(1):15–23.
64. Nakajima A, Saito K, Kojima T, Amano K, Yoshio T, Fukuda W, et al. No increased mortality in patients with rheumatoid arthritis treated with biologics: results from the biologics register of six rheumatology institutes in Japan. Mod Rheumatol. 2013;23(5):945–52.
65. Wolfe F, Mitchell DM, Sibley JT, Fries JF, Bloch DA, Williams CA, et al. The mortality of rheumatoid arthritis. Arthritis Rheum. 1994;37(4):481–94.
66. Mariette X, Gottenberg JE, Ravaud P, Combe B. Registries in rheumatoid arthritis and autoimmune diseases: data from the French registries. Rheumatology. 2011;50(1):222–9.
67. Arancibia F, Ewig S, Martinez JA, Ruiz M, Bauer T, Marcos MA, et al. Antimicrobial treatment failures in patients with community-acquired pneumonia: causes and prognostic implications. Am J Respir Crit Care Med. 2000;162(1):154–60.
68. van der Eerden MM, Vlaspolder F, de Graaff CS, Groot T, Jansen HM, Boersma WG. Value of intensive diagnostic microbiological investigation in low- and high-risk patients with community-acquired pneumonia. Eur J Clin Microbiol Infect Dis. 2005;24(4):241–9.
69. Müller-Ladner C, Müller-Ladner U. Vaccination and inflammatory arthritis: overview of current vaccines and recommended uses in rheumatology. Curr Rheumatol Rep. 2013;15(6):330.
70. van Assen S, Elkayam O, Agmon-Levin N, Cervera R, Doran MF, Dougados M, et al. Vaccination in adult patients with auto-immune inflammatory rheumatic diseases: a systematic literature review for the European League Against Rheumatism evidence-based recommendations for vaccination in adult patients with auto-immune inflammatory rheumatic diseases. Autoimmun Rev. 2011;10(6):341–52.
71. van Assen S, Agmon-Levin N, Elkayam O, Cervera R, Doran MF, Dougados M, et al. EULAR recommendations for vaccination in adult patients with autoimmune inflammatory rheumatic diseases. Ann Rheum Dis. 2011;70(3):414–22.
72. Kapetanovic MC, Saxne T, Sjoholm A, Truedsson L, Jonsson G, Geborek P. Influence of methotrexate, TNF blockers and prednisolone on antibody responses to pneumococcal polysaccharide vaccine in patients with rheumatoid arthritis. Rheumatology. 2006;45(1):106–11.
73. Crnkic Kapetanovic M, Saxne T, Jonsson G, Truedsson L, Geborek P. Rituximab and abatacept but not tocilizumab impair antibody response to pneumococcal conjugate vaccine in patients with rheumatoid arthritis. Arthritis Res Ther. 2013;15(5):R171.
74. van Assen S, Holvast A, Benne CA, Posthumus MD, van Leeuwen MA, Voskuyl AE, et al. Humoral responses after influenza vaccination are severely reduced in patients with rheumatoid arthritis treated with rituximab. Arthritis Rheum. 2010;62(1):75–81.
75. Tokuda H, Harigai M, Kameda H, Tomono K, Takayanagi N, Watanabe A, et al. Consensus statements for medical practice: biological agents and lung disease [Abridged English translation by the Japanese Respiratory Society]. Respir Investig. 2017;55(3):229–51.
76. Demoruelle MK, Solomon JJ, Fischer A, Deane KD. The lung may play a role in the pathogenesis of rheumatoid arthritis. Int J Clin Rheumtol. 2014;9(3):295–309.
77. Tsuchiya Y, Takayanagi N, Sugiura H, Miyahara Y, Tokunaga D, Kawabata Y, et al. Lung diseases directly associated with rheumatoid arthritis and their relationship to outcome. Eur Respir J. 2011;37(6):1411–7.
78. King PT, Hutchinson PE, Johnson PD, Holmes PW, Freezer NJ, Holdsworth SR. Adaptive immunity to nontypeable Haemophilus influenzae. Am J Respir Crit Care Med. 2003;167(4):587–92.
79. Sadikot RT, Blackwell TS, Christman JW, Prince AS. Pathogen-host interactions in Pseudomonas aeruginosa pneumonia. Am J Respir Crit Care Med. 2005;171(11):1209–23.
80. Swinson DR, Symmons D, Suresh U, Jones M, Booth J. Decreased survival in patients with co-existent rheumatoid arthritis and bronchiectasis. Br J Rheumatol. 1997;36(6):689–91.
81. Colice GL, Curtis A, Deslauriers J, Heffner J, Light R, Littenberg B, et al. Medical and surgical treatment of parapneumonic effusions: an evidence-based guideline. Chest. 2000;118(4):1158–71.
82. Mori S, Sugimoto M. Pneumocystis jirovecii pneumonia in rheumatoid arthritis patients: risks and prophylaxis recommendations. Clin Med Insights Circ Respir Pulm Med. 2015;9(Suppl 1):29–40.
83. Mori S, Cho I, Ichiyasu H, Sugimoto M. Asymptomatic carriage of Pneumocystis jiroveci in elderly patients with rheumatoid arthritis in Japan: a possible association between colonization and development of Pneumocystis jiroveci pneumonia during low-dose MTX therapy. Mod Rheumatol. 2008;18(3):240–6.
84. Harigai M, Koike R, Miyasaka N. Pneumocystis Pneumonia under Anti-Tumor Necrosis Factor Therapy Study G. Pneumocystis pneumonia associated with infliximab in Japan. N Engl J Med. 2007;357(18):1874–6.
85. Komano Y, Harigai M, Koike R, Sugiyama H, Ogawa J, Saito K, et al. Pneumocystis jiroveci pneumonia in patients with rheumatoid arthritis treated with infliximab: a retrospective review and case-control study of 21 patients. Arthritis Rheum. 2009;61(3):305–12.
86. Iikuni N, Kitahama M, Ohta S, Okamoto H, Kamatani N, Nishinarita M. Evaluation of Pneumocystis pneumonia infection risk factors in patients with connective tissue disease. Mod Rheumatol. 2006;16(5):282–8.
87. Ogawa J, Harigai M, Nagasaka K, Nakamura T, Miyasaka N. Prediction of and prophylaxis against Pneumocystis pneumonia in patients with connective tissue diseases undergoing medium- or high-dose corticosteroid therapy. Mod Rheumatol. 2005;15(2):91–6.
88. Teichtahl AJ, Morrisroe K, Ciciriello S, Jennens I, Tadros S, Wicks I. Pneumocystis jirovecci pneumonia in connective tissue diseases: comparison with other immunocompromised patients. Semin Arthritis Rheum. 2015;45(1):86–90.
89. Okuda Y, Oyama T, Oyama H, Miyamoto T, Takasugi K. Pneumocystis carinii pneumonia associated with low dose methotrexate treatment for malignant rheumatoid arthritis. Ryumachi. 1995;35(4):699–704.
90. Roux N, Flipo RM, Cortet B, Lafitte JJ, Tonnel AB, Duquesnoy B, et al. Pneumocystis carinii pneumonia in rheumatoid arthritis patients treated with methotrexate. A report of two cases. Rev Rhum Engl Ed. 1996;63(6):453–6.
91. Takeuchi T, Tatsuki Y, Nogami Y, Ishiguro N, Tanaka Y, Yamanaka H, et al. Postmarketing surveillance of the safety profile of infliximab in 5000 Japanese patients with rheumatoid arthritis. Ann Rheum Dis. 2008;67(2):189–94.
92. Koike T, Harigai M, Inokuma S, Inoue K, Ishiguro N, Ryu J, et al. Postmarketing surveillance of the safety and effectiveness of etanercept in Japan. J Rheumatol. 2009;36(5):898–906.

93. Koike T, Harigai M, Ishiguro N, Inokuma S, Takei S, Takeuchi T, et al. Safety and effectiveness of adalimumab in Japanese rheumatoid arthritis patients: postmarketing surveillance report of the first 3,000 patients. Mod Rheumatol. 2012;22(4):498–508.
94. Louie GH, Wang Z, Ward MM. Trends in hospitalizations for Pneumocystis jiroveci pneumonia among patients with rheumatoid arthritis in the US: 1996–2007. Arthritis Rheum. 2010;62(12):3826–7.
95. Bykerk VP, Cush J, Winthrop K, Calabrese L, Lortholary O, de Longueville M, et al. Update on the safety profile of certolizumab pegol in rheumatoid arthritis: an integrated analysis from clinical trials. Ann Rheum Dis. 2015;74(1):96–103.
96. Katsuyama T, Saito K, Kubo S, Nawata M, Tanaka Y. Prophylaxis for Pneumocystis pneumonia in patients with rheumatoid arthritis treated with biologics, based on risk factors found in a retrospective study. Arthritis Res Ther. 2014;16(1):R43.
97. Tokuda H, Sakai F, Yamada H, Johkoh T, Imamura A, Dohi M, et al. Clinical and radiological features of Pneumocystis pneumonia in patients with rheumatoid arthritis, in comparison with methotrexate pneumonitis and Pneumocystis pneumonia in acquired immunodeficiency syndrome: a multicenter study. Internal Med. 2008;47(10):915–23.
98. Limper AH, Offord KP, Smith TF, Martin WJ 2nd. Pneumocystis carinii pneumonia. Differences in lung parasite number and inflammation in patients with and without AIDS. Am Rev Respir Dis. 1989;140(5):1204–9.
99. Ward MM, Donald F. Pneumocystis carinii pneumonia in patients with connective tissue diseases: the role of hospital experience in diagnosis and mortality. Arthritis Rheum. 1999;42(4):780–9.
100. Azoulay E, Bergeron A, Chevret S, Bele N, Schlemmer B, Menotti J. Polymerase chain reaction for diagnosing pneumocystis pneumonia in non-HIV immunocompromised patients with pulmonary infiltrates. Chest. 2009;135(3):655–61.
101. Reid AB, Chen SC, Worth LJ. Pneumocystis jirovecii pneumonia in non-HIV-infected patients: new risks and diagnostic tools. Curr Opin Infect Dis. 2011;24(6):534–44.
102. Utsunomiya M, Dobashi H, Odani T, Saito K, Yokogawa N, Nagasaka K, et al. Optimal regimens of sulfamethoxazole-trimethoprim for chemoprophylaxis of Pneumocystis pneumonia in patients with systemic rheumatic diseases: results from a non-blinded, randomized controlled trial. Arthritis Res Ther. 2017;19(1):7.
103. Schneider MM, Hoepelman AI, Eeftinck Schattenkerk JK, Nielsen TL, van der Graaf Y, Frissen JP, et al. A controlled trial of aerosolized pentamidine or trimethoprim-sulfamethoxazole as primary prophylaxis against Pneumocystis carinii pneumonia in patients with human immunodeficiency virus infection. The Dutch AIDS Treatment Group. N Engl J Med. 1992;327(26):1836–41.
104. Ioannidis JP, Cappelleri JC, Skolnik PR, Lau J, Sacks HS. A meta-analysis of the relative efficacy and toxicity of Pneumocystis carinii prophylactic regimens. Arch Intern Med. 1996;156(2):177–88.
105. Warnock AC, Rimland D. Comparison of trimethoprim-sulfamethoxazole, dapsone, and pentamidine in the prophylaxis of Pneumocystis carinii pneumonia. Pharmacotherapy. 1996;16(6):1030–8.
106. Hughes WT, Kuhn S, Chaudhary S, Feldman S, Verzosa M, Aur RJ, et al. Successful chemoprophylaxis for Pneumocystis carinii pneumonitis. N Engl J Med. 1977;297(26):1419–26.
107. Thomas CF Jr, Limper AH. Pneumocystis pneumonia. N Engl J Med. 2004;350(24):2487–98.
108. Wharton JM, Coleman DL, Wofsy CB, Luce JM, Blumenfeld W, Hadley WK, et al. Trimethoprim-sulfamethoxazole or pentamidine for Pneumocystis carinii pneumonia in the acquired immunodeficiency syndrome. A prospective randomized trial. Ann Intern Med. 1986;105(1):37–44.
109. Hughes W, Leoung G, Kramer F, Bozzette SA, Safrin S, Frame P, et al. Comparison of atovaquone (566C80) with trimethoprim-sulfamethoxazole to treat Pneumocystis carinii pneumonia in patients with AIDS. N Engl J Med. 1993;328(21):1521–7.
110. Consensus statement on the use of corticosteroids as adjunctive therapy for pneumocystis pneumonia in the acquired immunodeficiency syndrome. The National Institutes of Health-University of California Expert Panel for Corticosteroids as Adjunctive Therapy for Pneumocystis Pneumonia. N Engl J Med. 1990;323(21):1500–4.
111. Kameda H, Tokuda H, Sakai F, Johkoh T, Mori S, Yoshida Y, et al. Clinical and radiological features of acute-onset diffuse interstitial lung diseases in patients with rheumatoid arthritis receiving treatment with biological agents: importance of Pneumocystis pneumonia in Japan revealed by a multicenter study. Internal Med. 2011;50(4):305–13.
112. Ge HF, Liu XQ, Zhu YQ, Chen HQ, Chen GZ. Invasive pulmonary fungal infections in patients with connective tissue disease: a retrospective study from northern China. Braz J Med Biol Res. 2016;49(10):e5531.
113. Kindler V, Sappino AP, Grau GE, Piguet PF, Vassalli P. The inducing role of tumor necrosis factor in the development of bactericidal granulomas during BCG infection. Cell. 1989;56(5):731–40.
114. Tsiodras S, Samonis G, Boumpas DT, Kontoyiannis DP. Fungal infections complicating tumor necrosis factor alpha blockade therapy. Mayo Clin Proc. 2008;83(2):181–94.
115. Wallis RS, Broder MS, Wong JY, Hanson ME, Beenhouwer DO. Granulomatous infectious diseases associated with tumor necrosis factor antagonists. Clin Infect Dis. 2004;38(9):1261–5.
116. Lee JH, Slifman NR, Gershon SK, Edwards ET, Schwieterman WD, Siegel JN, et al. Life-threatening histoplasmosis complicating immunotherapy with tumor necrosis factor alpha antagonists infliximab and etanercept. Arthritis Rheum. 2002;46(10):2565–70.
117. Baddley JW, Winthrop KL, Chen L, Liu L, Grijalva CG, Delzell E, et al. Non-viral opportunistic infections in new users of tumour necrosis factor inhibitor therapy: results of the SAfety Assessment of Biologic ThERapy (SABER) study. Ann Rheum Dis. 2014;73(11):1942–8.
118. Liao TL, Chen YM, Chen DY. Risk factors for cryptococcal infection among patients with rheumatoid arthritis receiving different immunosuppressive medications. Clin Microbiol Infect. 2016;22(9):815.e1–3.
119. Hage CA, Wood KL, Winer-Muram HT, Wilson SJ, Sarosi G, Knox KS. Pulmonary cryptococcosis after initiation of anti-tumor necrosis factor-alpha therapy. Chest. 2003;124(6):2395–7.
120. Iwata T, Nagano T, Tomita M, Suehiro Y, Nakatsuka S, Kimura H, et al. Adalimumab-associated pulmonary cryptococcosis. Ann Thorac Cardiovasc Surg. 2011;17(4):390–3.
121. Schelenz S, Smith DA, Bancroft GJ. Cytokine and chemokine responses following pulmonary challenge with Aspergillus fumigatus: obligatory role of TNF-alpha and GM-CSF in neutrophil recruitment. Med Mycol. 1999;37(3):183–94.
122. Roilides E, Dimitriadou-Georgiadou A, Sein T, Kadiltsoglou I, Walsh TJ. Tumor necrosis factor alpha enhances antifungal activities of polymorphonuclear and mononuclear phagocytes against Aspergillus fumigatus. Infect Immun. 1998;66(12):5999–6003.
123. Silman AJ, Pearson JE. Epidemiology and genetics of rheumatoid arthritis. Arthritis Res. 2002;4(Suppl 3):S265–72.
124. Wegner N, Lundberg K, Kinloch A, Fisher B, Malmstrom V, Feldmann M, et al. Autoimmunity to specific citrullinated proteins gives the first clues to the etiology of rheumatoid arthritis. Immunol Rev. 2010;233(1):34–54.
125. Scher JU, Ubeda C, Equinda M, Khanin R, Buischi Y, Viale A, et al. Periodontal disease and the oral microbiota in new-onset rheumatoid arthritis. Arthritis Rheum. 2012;64(10):3083–94.

126. Erb-Downward JR, Thompson DL, Han MK, Freeman CM, McCloskey L, Schmidt LA, et al. Analysis of the lung microbiome in the "healthy" smoker and in COPD. PLoS One. 2011;6(2):e16384.
127. Goleva E, Jackson LP, Harris JK, Robertson CE, Sutherland ER, Hall CF, et al. The effects of airway microbiome on corticosteroid responsiveness in asthma. Am J Respir Crit Care Med. 2013;188(10):1193–201.
128. Dimmitt RA, Staley EM, Chuang G, Tanner SM, Soltau TD, Lorenz RG. Role of postnatal acquisition of the intestinal microbiome in the early development of immune function. J Pediatr Gastroenterol Nutr. 2010;51(3):262–73.
129. Stebbings SM, Taylor C, Tannock GW, Baird MA, Highton J. The immune response to autologous bacteroides in ankylosing spondylitis is characterized by reduced interleukin 10 production. J Rheumatol. 2009;36(4):797–800.
130. Proal AD, Albert PJ, Marshall TG. The human microbiome and autoimmunity. Curr Opin Rheumatol. 2013;25(2):234–40.
131. Yeoh N, Burton JP, Suppiah P, Reid G, Stebbings S. The role of the microbiome in rheumatic diseases. Curr Rheumatol Rep. 2013;15(3):314.
132. Horai R, Saijo S, Tanioka H, Nakae S, Sudo K, Okahara A, et al. Development of chronic inflammatory arthropathy resembling rheumatoid arthritis in interleukin 1 receptor antagonist-deficient mice. J Exp Med. 2000;191(2):313–20.
133. Lundberg K, Kinloch A, Fisher BA, Wegner N, Wait R, Charles P, et al. Antibodies to citrullinated alpha-enolase peptide 1 are specific for rheumatoid arthritis and cross-react with bacterial enolase. Arthritis Rheum. 2008;58(10):3009–19.
134. Wegner N, Wait R, Sroka A, Eick S, Nguyen KA, Lundberg K, et al. Peptidylarginine deiminase from Porphyromonas gingivalis citrullinates human fibrinogen and alpha-enolase: implications for autoimmunity in rheumatoid arthritis. Arthritis Rheum. 2010;62(9):2662–72.
135. Sokolove J, Bromberg R, Deane KD, Lahey LJ, Derber LA, Chandra PE, et al. Autoantibody epitope spreading in the preclinical phase predicts progression to rheumatoid arthritis. PLoS One. 2012;7(5):e35296.
136. Schiff MH, Burmester GR, Kent JD, et al. Safety analyses of adalimumab (HUMIRA) in global clinical trials and US postmarketing surveillance of patients with rheumatoid arthritis. Ann Rheum Dis. 2006;65(7):889–94.

Mycobacterium Infections in Rheumatoid Arthritis (Tuberculosis and Nontuberculous Mycobacteriosis)

11

Hiroshi Moro and Toshiaki Kikuchi

Abstract

Biological agents have had a tremendous effect in the management of rheumatoid arthritis (RA). However, subsequent infection is regarded as an emerging problem owing to the suppression of host immunity by these agents. Cellular immunity with T lymphocytes plays a crucial role in host defense against mycobacterial infections; hence, immunosuppression due to these biological agents may lead to tuberculosis (TB) and nontuberculous mycobacteria (NTM) infections. Therefore, pretreatment screening for TB and NTM infection and appropriate management are crucial. In general, the lungs are the major site of infection caused by mycobacteria, and the disease may typically have a chronic course. Thus, persistent respiratory symptoms and signs trigger suspicion of pulmonary TB or NTM infection, and chest radiography as well as sputum examination plays a major role in the diagnosis. In addition, promising diagnostic tools such as interferon-gamma release assay (IGRA), anti-MAC antibody measurement, and Xpert MTB/rifampin (RIF) assay are newly available. Further research is needed to verify these assays. As a rule, to avoid development of drug-resistant strains, treatment with multiple drugs for a relatively extensive duration is required for therapy.

Keywords

Tuberculosis • Nontuberculous mycobacteriosis • Biological agent

11.1 Introduction

The airway system is one of the sites of extra-articular involvement of rheumatoid arthritis (RA), and RA-associated lung diseases include interstitial disease, bronchiectasis, small airway obstruction, and pulmonary nodules, [1–3]. In addition, respiratory infection, related to RA itself or drug-induced immunosuppression, may occur. In the management of RA, newly available biological agents have had a tremendous effect, although the subsequent infection, with the suppression of host immunity, is regarded as an emerging problem. Especially tuberculosis (TB) and nontuberculous mycobacteria (NTM) infections should be considered in the differential diagnosis of pulmonary infection.

Predisposing factors for mycobacterial diseases include underlying lung disease and immunosuppressive drugs. Cellular immunity with T lymphocytes plays a crucial role in host defense against mycobacterial infections; hence, suppression of this immunity by biological agents may lead to development of mycobacterial infections, which is drawing much attention as an adverse event of RA treatment with biological agents, including antitumor necrosis factor (TNF)-alpha therapy; thus, pretreatment screening and appropriate management are crucial. In this chapter, the diagnosis and treatment of TB and NTM infections will be described while accounting for RA with biological agents.

H. Moro, M.D., Ph.D. • T. Kikuchi, M.D., Ph.D. (✉)
Department of Respiratory Medicine and Infectious Diseases, Graduate School of Medical and Dental Sciences, Niigata University, Niigata, Japan
e-mail: kikuchi@med.niigata-u.ac.jp

T. Gono et al. (eds.), *Lung Disease Associated with Rheumatoid Arthritis*, https://doi.org/10.1007/978-981-10-6750-1_11

11.2 Tuberculosis

11.2.1 Overview

TB is defined as an infection caused by *Mycobacterium tuberculosis* complex. TB is transmitted from person to person through the air from individuals with active pulmonary TB disease, particularly those who have cavity or whose sputum is smear positive. Transmission of TB is a serious public health concern. Inhalation of *M. tuberculosis* and deposition in the lungs lead to immediate clearance of the organism in most cases but establishment of infection in some cases [4]. Individuals who become infected with *M. tuberculosis* rarely develop active disease, and the innate and adaptive immune response of the host plays a crucial role in this phase. The defense mechanisms against TB infection include cellular immunity, with interferon gamma and other cytokines, and recognition of the *M. tuberculosis* molecules via toll-like receptors.

Not everyone infected with *M. tuberculosis* develops active TB disease; only 5–10% of infected hosts will develop primary or reactivation TB disease during their lives; primary TB is rapid progression to active disease immediately after infection, and reactivation TB is the onset of active disease many years following a period of latent infection. For the remaining 90–95% of infected hosts, the tubercle bacilli are contained in granulomas by host defenses, in most cases. Latent TB infection (LTBI) is characterized by the presence of immune responses to previously infected tubercle bacilli without clinical evidence of active TB disease [5, 6]. However, latent infection has the potential to develop into active TB infection. The clinical manifestations of active pulmonary TB are characterized by cough, sputum, fever, chest pain, dyspnea, hemoptysis, general malaise, and loss of appetite.

M. tuberculosis can spread from the lungs via blood or lymph, or invade directly, causing disease outside of the lungs (i.e., extrapulmonary TB). Extrapulmonary TB consists of foci outside of the lungs, including lymph nodes, bone, joint, urogenital system, central nerve system, and larynx. Additionally, extrapulmonary TB also includes miliary TB, which refers to clinical disease resulting from the hematogenous dissemination of *M. tuberculosis*. Miliary TB can develop as a result of progressive primary TB or reactivation TB with subsequent spread.

Known risk factors for progression from LTBI to reactivation TB include human immunodeficiency virus (HIV) infection, type 2 diabetes mellitus, excessive alcohol use, cigarette smoking, etc. [4]. Additionally, some studies revealed that RA itself has been associated with the development of TB [7–9]. In LTBI, granuloma formation not only plays an important part in controlling infection but also plays a role in containing the tubercle bacilli for its long-term survival in the host in the dormancy phase. Maintenance of the granuloma requires cytokines and chemokines, including TNF-alpha and INF-gamma. For this reason, administration of immunosuppressants (e.g., glucocorticoids, TNF-alpha inhibitors) may affect the formation and maintenance of granulomas, resulting in the recurrence of TB [10, 11]. Taken together, patients with RA are considered to have a higher incidence of TB that is caused by treatment with biological agents rather than other diseases. In this way, in prescribing biological agents for RA, we should always keep in mind LTBI, as it is critical to take appropriate action in that case.

11.2.2 Diagnosis

Clinical manifestations, especially persistent cough, history of prior TB infection, possible TB exposure, tuberculin skin test (TST), IGRA, and radiographic imaging, may help establish the diagnosis of TB [12]. A positive sputum smear for acid-fast bacilli (AFB) or a cavity on the chest radiograph indicates the infectiousness of the patient, and transmission precautions must be followed.

11.2.2.1 Radiographic Findings

Chest radiography is a useful tool for evaluating suspected pulmonary TB. Typically, reactivation pulmonary TB presents focal infiltration with or without cavity in upper lobe (apical or posterior segment) or the lower lobe (superior segment) [13, 14]. Other findings include small fibronodular lesions along with bronchi, lung mass (tuberculoma), hilar adenopathy, and pleural effusion; these findings may be present unilaterally or bilaterally. Chest computed tomography (CT) is more sensitive than chest radiography for detecting subtle change. Although the resolution provided by CT is not always required for diagnosis of pulmonary TB, it may be useful for differential diagnosis.

In miliary TB, the classic appearance on chest radiography is a faint, micronodular shadow that is randomly distributed throughout the lungs [15], reflecting nodular interstitial spread without significant alveolar involvement. High-resolution CT (HRCT) of the chest is more sensitive, which can detect numerous small nodules (2–3 mm) distributed throughout the lung [16].

11.2.2.2 Microbiological Evaluation

Diagnosis of TB is confirmed by detection of organisms from secretions or tissue samples. If pulmonary TB is suspected, a series of at least three sputum samples should be obtained for AFB smears. For patients with difficulty in producing sputum, it can be induced by inhalation of aerosolized hypertonic saline with a nebulizer. Additionally, other clinical specimens and tissues, including pharyngeal/laryngeal swab, pleural effusion, pus, urine, feces, and cerebrospinal fluid may be helpful for the diagnosis of extrapulmonary TB.

Microscopic detection of mycobacteria cannot distinguish *M. tuberculosis* from NTM, and nucleic acid amplification is helpful to identify the organisms in this context [4]. Culture technique is required for species identification and drug susceptibility testing, although it may require extended incubation times (2–6 weeks). Recently, an automated real-time polymerase chain reaction assay for multidrug-resistant *M. tuberculosis*, Xpert MTB/rifampin (RIF) assay, was developed. It is an important tool for rapid diagnosis of TB and presence of rifampin resistance [17].

11.2.2.3 IGRA

Diagnosis of LTBI has been conducted using the TST in the past, but it is rapidly being replaced by IGRAs lately. The IGRA measures levels of interferon gamma released in response to sensitized T-cell stimulation with TB-specific antigen [18], and it reveals good sensitivity and specificity. Additionally, the test results are not affected by prior Bacille de Calmette-Guérin (BCG) vaccination, unlike TST; hence, it is favorable in areas with high BCG vaccination rates. IGRAs are increasingly used for LTBI screening in RA patients who are initiating treatment with biological agents. Commercially available IGRAs include QuantiFERON® TB Gold (QFT) and T-SPOT-TB assays. In severely immunocompromised individuals, IGRAs may give false-negative results. The sensitivity of the T-SPOT assay appears to be higher than that of the QFT assay, because an adequate number of peripheral blood mononuclear cells are available in the T-SPOT assay, even in the presence of lymphocytopenia.

11.2.3 Treatment

The principal objective of TB management is to maximize the elimination of the causative organism in patients with TB. Basically, drug-susceptible TB can be treated by taking at least three drugs, with different modes of action, for 6–9 months, and it is nearly always curable if patients are treated appropriately. First-line anti-TB agents for treatment of drug-susceptible TB include isoniazid, rifampin, pyrazinamide, and ethambutol.

11.2.3.1 Active TB Disease

Initial treatment of active TB consists of four-drug combination therapy with isoniazid (5 mg/kg, maximum dose 300 mg), rifampin (10 mg/kg, maximum dose 600 mg), and pyrazinamide (1000–2000 mg) plus ethambutol (800–1600 mg) daily for 2 months (intensive phase), followed by a combination therapy of isoniazid and rifampin for 4 months (continuation phase), for a total of 6 months [19]. If pyrazinamide cannot be administered for some reason (e.g., liver dysfunction, hyperuricemia, or pregnancy), isoniazid, rifampin, and ethambutol are given for 2 months followed by extended continuation phase with isoniazid and rifampin for 7 months (9 months total), as an alternative regimen. To maintain optimum therapeutic effect, and to prevent emergence of drug resistance, maintaining drug compliance is crucial, and direct observed therapy (DOT) is helpful to achieve the purpose.

11.2.3.2 LTBI

LTBI has the potential to develop active TB disease in patients at greater risk. Therefore treatment of LTBI aims to reduce the possibility of reactivation and the number of potential sources of infection [20]. For treatment of LTBI, 9 months of self-administered isoniazid (300 mg/day or 5 mg/kg/day) is recommended. Daily rifampin for 4 months may be indicated where isoniazid cannot be used for some reason. Alternative regimen includes isoniazid and rifapentine once weekly for 3 months with DOT [21].

11.2.3.3 Special Consideration for RA Patients

A TB screening algorithm for RA patients using biologic agents is shown in Fig. 11.1. In the case of LTBI, treatment with anti-TB drugs for at least 1 month is required prior to the initiation of immunosuppressive agents. Methotrexate for RA should be discontinued while fever continues, but it can be restarted when stability is obtained. It has not been found that this drug has suppressive effects for protective immunity against TB. In patients with active TB disease, administration of biologic agents, including TNF inhibitors, should be temporarily stopped until resolution of infection and completion of anti-TB therapy.

As for the use of glucocorticoids, discontinuation of drugs in this class raises the concern about deterioration of RA. For this reason, consensus statements of Japan recommend continuing corticosteroid medication during treatment of TB disease. In addition, concomitant use of steroids is expected to have a favorable effect on controlling a paradoxical reaction of TB. If rifampin were prescribed, it is necessary to increase the dosage of steroids since the blood concentration of steroids decreases through drug interaction.

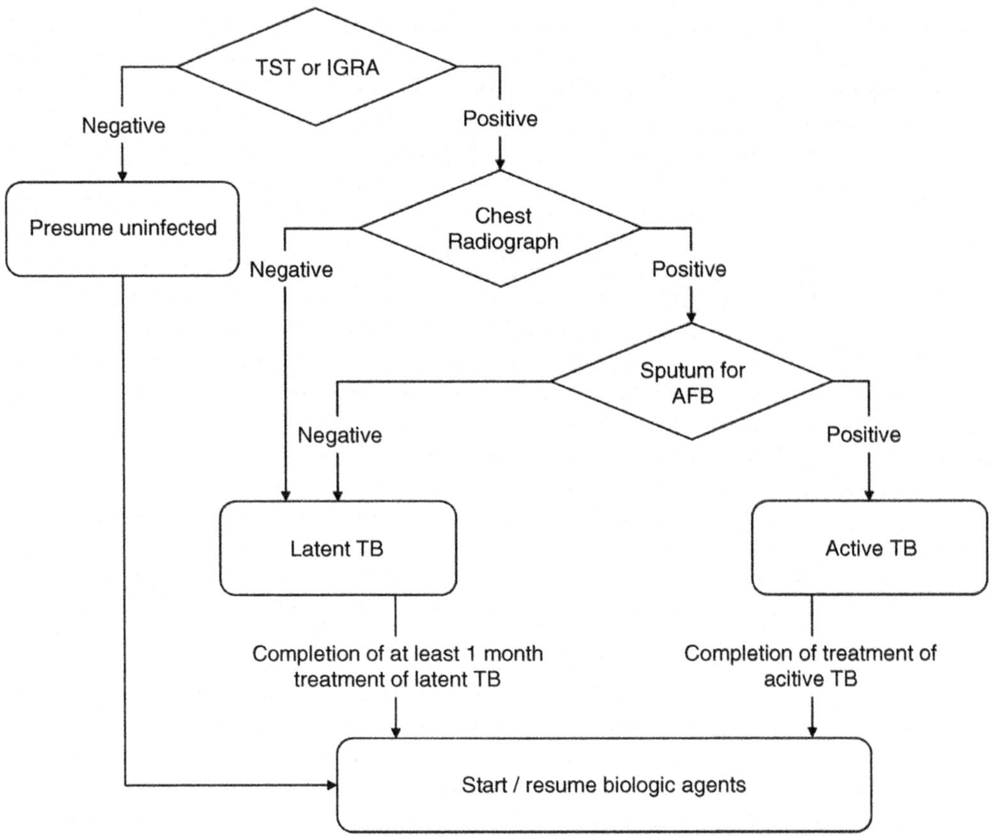

Fig. 11.1 TB screening algorithm for biologics. *TST* tuberculin skin test, *IGRA* interferon-gamma release assay, *AFB* acid-fast bacilli, *TB* tuberculosis

11.3 Nontuberculous Mycobacterium Infection

11.3.1 Overview

Nontuberculous mycobacteria are defined as mycobacteria except for *M. tuberculosis*. Unlike TB, NTM infection is acquired from the environment, not from a patient with active pulmonary disease, and therefore isolation of patients is unnecessary. The lungs are the major site of infection caused by NTM, and the clinical manifestations of pulmonary NTM infection are characterized by cough, sputum, malaise, bloody sputum, and dyspnea. Patients may describe weight loss, fatigue, and appetite loss, which reflect chronic inflammations. Common organisms include *M. avium*, *M. intracellulare*, *M. kansasii*, and *M. abscessus*; the first two organisms have similar characteristics and are collectively known as *M. avium intracellulare* complex (MAC).

Recent studies have determined that RA patients receiving anti-TNF-alpha therapy are at increased risk for NTM infection. In an epidemiological study performed in Asia, the incidence of NTM infection was 4.22 times greater in the RA group than in the non-RA group [22]. The adjusted hazard ratio of NTM infection for the RA group was 4.17 (95% confidence interval [CI]: 2.61–6.65). In addition, the other study in North America revealed that adjusted hazard ratio for NTM infection was 2.08 (95% CI: 1.84–2.32) in the RA group, relative to non-RA group [23]. Additionally, automated pharmacy records were reviewed for patients receiving anti-TNF-alpha therapy [24], and anti-TNF associated rates of NTM infection was 74 (95% CI: 37–111) per 100,000 person-years. Among anti-TNF users, compared with uninfected individuals, NTM case patients were more likely to have RA. This relatively frequent development of pulmonary NTM infection in RA patients may be associated with the preexisting structural abnormalities as extra-articular involvement by RA. Therefore, pretreatment screening and appropriate management of NTM infection is required and crucial in RA patients receiving anti-TNF-alpha therapy disease.

11.3.2 Diagnosis

11.3.2.1 Diagnostic Criteria

In 2007, the American Thoracic Society (ATS) and Infectious Diseases Society of America (IDSA) jointly established diagnostic criteria for NTM infection [25]. Diagnosis is based on characteristic radiographic findings and positive culture results from at least two separate expectorated sputum samples, and clinical manifestation is not necessary (Table 11.1).

Table 11.1 Clinical and microbiologic criteria for diagnosing nontuberculous mycobacterial lung disease

Clinical (both required)	
1.	Pulmonary symptoms, nodular or cavitary opacities on chest radiograph, or a high-resolution computed tomography scan that shows multifocal bronchiectasis with multiple small nodules
2.	Appropriate exclusion of other diagnoses
Microbiologic	
1.	Positive culture results from at least two separate expectorated sputum samples. If the results from the initial sputum samples are nondiagnostic, consider repeat sputum acid-fast bacilli (AFB) smears and cultures
2.	Positive culture result from at least one bronchial wash or lavage
3.	Transbronchial or other lung biopsy with mycobacterial histopathologic features (granulomatous inflammation or AFB) and positive culture for NTM or biopsy showing mycobacterial histopathologic features (granulomatous inflammation or AFB) and one or more sputum or bronchial washings that are culture positive for NTM

This criterion has some problem when applied to RA patients suspected having NTM infection. Of note, the image findings of airway disease complicated with RA are so similar to those of NTM infection on HRCT that they are difficult to differentiate. In addition, colonization of NTM in the airway is not so rare in RA patients; thus, NTM infection should be strictly diagnosed in accordance with diagnostic criteria in this setting. Prior to the administration of biological agents, HRCT should be performed, if possible, to evaluate the presence of airway disease. If NTM infection is suspected, multiple sputum examinations or sampling by bronchoscopy should be considered. Serological assay is promising in this context.

11.3.2.2 Radiographic Findings

Occasionally, early diagnosis of asymptomatic NTM infection may be suspected by chest radiography for screening purposes. The radiological findings of NTM infection vary depending on their species. Findings consistent with NTM infection in chest radiographs or HRCT include infiltration (usually nodular or reticular nodular), cavity, multifocal bronchiectasis, and/or multiple nodules [26]. Pleural exudate is rare, but reactive pleural thickening is often seen.

Pulmonary MAC disease consists of two types of diseases according to radiological findings: nodular bronchiectatic (NB) disease (Fig. 11.2) and fibrocavitary (Cav) disease (Fig. 11.3). NB disease accounts for most MAC disease and is common among middle-aged and older women who do not have a history of smoking. In Japan, approximately 80% patients with MAC lung disease have NB disease [27]. Nodules and bronchiectasis usually present in the right middle lobe and left lingular segment [28]. HRCT scans of the chest are particularly useful for diagnosing this pattern of MAC lung disease, as bronchiectasis and nodules cannot be easily discriminated from chest radiography [29]. Although the clinical course and prognosis of NB disease varies, the prognosis is relatively good. NB disease is also found in other NTM pathogens, including *M. abscessus*.

Cav disease is prevalent among elderly men with preexisting lung diseases, such as emphysema and obsolete TB. In general, Cav disease usually progress rapidly and is known to be a risk factor for poor prognosis. Therefore, early treatment intervention should be considered when diagnosing Cav disease. Cavities caused by these organisms tend to have thinner walls than those caused by TB [30, 31]. Lung disease due to *M. kansasii* and *M. szulgai* exhibits similar clinical symptoms and imaging findings as pulmonary TB (e.g., cavities and nodules in apex of the lung).

11.3.2.3 Microbiologic Evaluation

Microbiological confirmation is essential for the diagnosis of NTM infection. Since NTM are ubiquitous organisms in environment, positive sputum culture may be due to environmental contamination or to noninvasive colonization in patients with chronic lung disease, especially in RA patients. Therefore, positive culture results from at least two separate expectorated sputum samples are required for diagnosis [25]. Good-quality sputum is essential for not only diagnosis but also monitoring treatment efficacy. Sputum induction with hypertonic saline is helpful for obtaining good-quality sputum in patients who were unable to expectorate sputum. Bronchial lavage obtained by bronchoscopy is less affected by contamination from the environment; thus, diagnosis can be confirmed with one or more positive culture results. For the prompt diagnosis, smear and cultivation with these samples should be performed at the same time, and if the smear is positive and TB cannot be ruled out, the additional nucleic acid amplification method should be considered.

11.3.2.4 Serodiagnosis

Research on the usefulness of serological diagnostic technology to diagnose MAC disease has been conducted. A serologic diagnostic tool that can detect immunoglobulin A (IgA) antibodies against MAC-specific glycopeptidyl lipid core antigen using an enzyme immunoassay has been available in Japan since 2011. In one study, this assay shows favorable results in terms of sensitivity and specificity and appears to be promising [32]. Further research is needed to verify this technology.

11.3.2.5 Susceptibility Testing

As a drug susceptibility test method of NTM, M24-A2 has been established by the US Clinical and Laboratory Standards Institute (CLSI) [33], and it has been adopted in the guidelines of the United States and Japan. However, in the case of pulmonary MAC disease, the result of the drug susceptibility test is not always along with clinical effect, and its usefulness

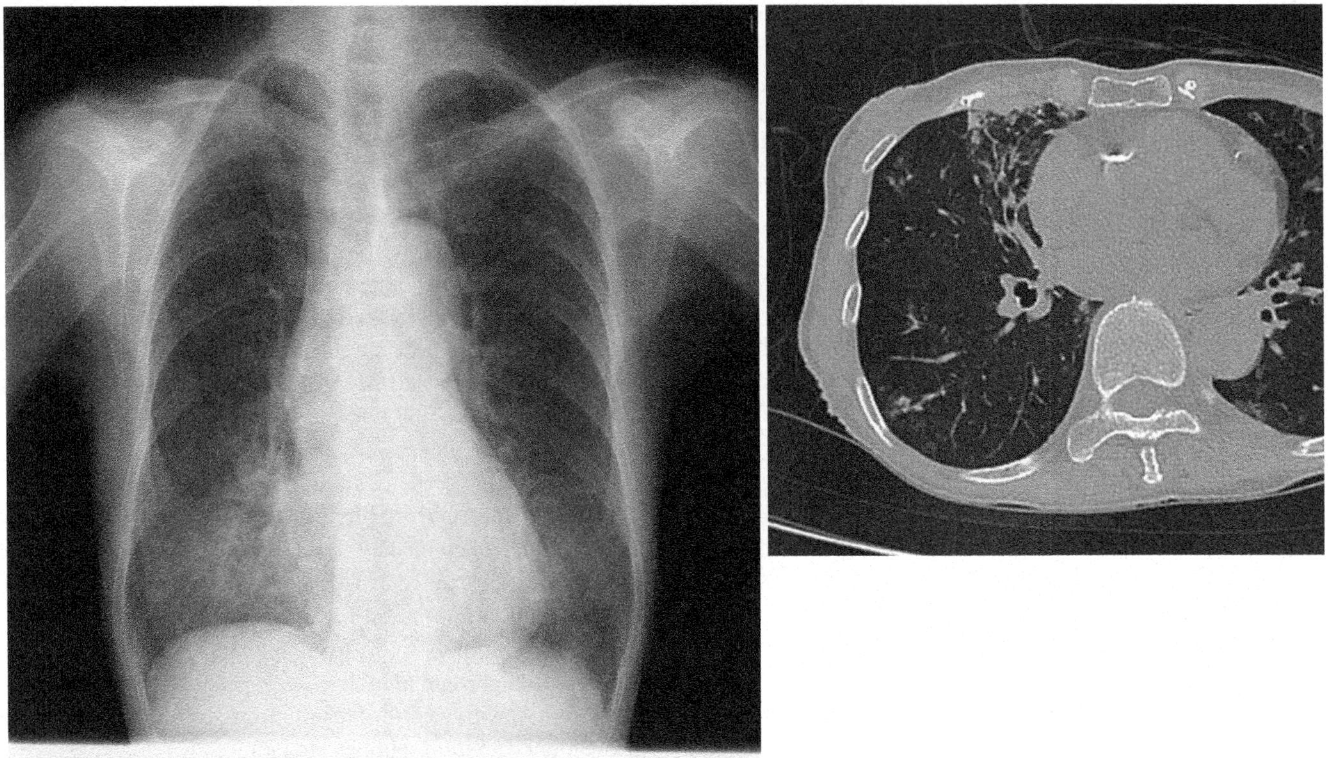

Fig. 11.2 Nodular bronchiectatic form. Case: 77-year-old female with RA

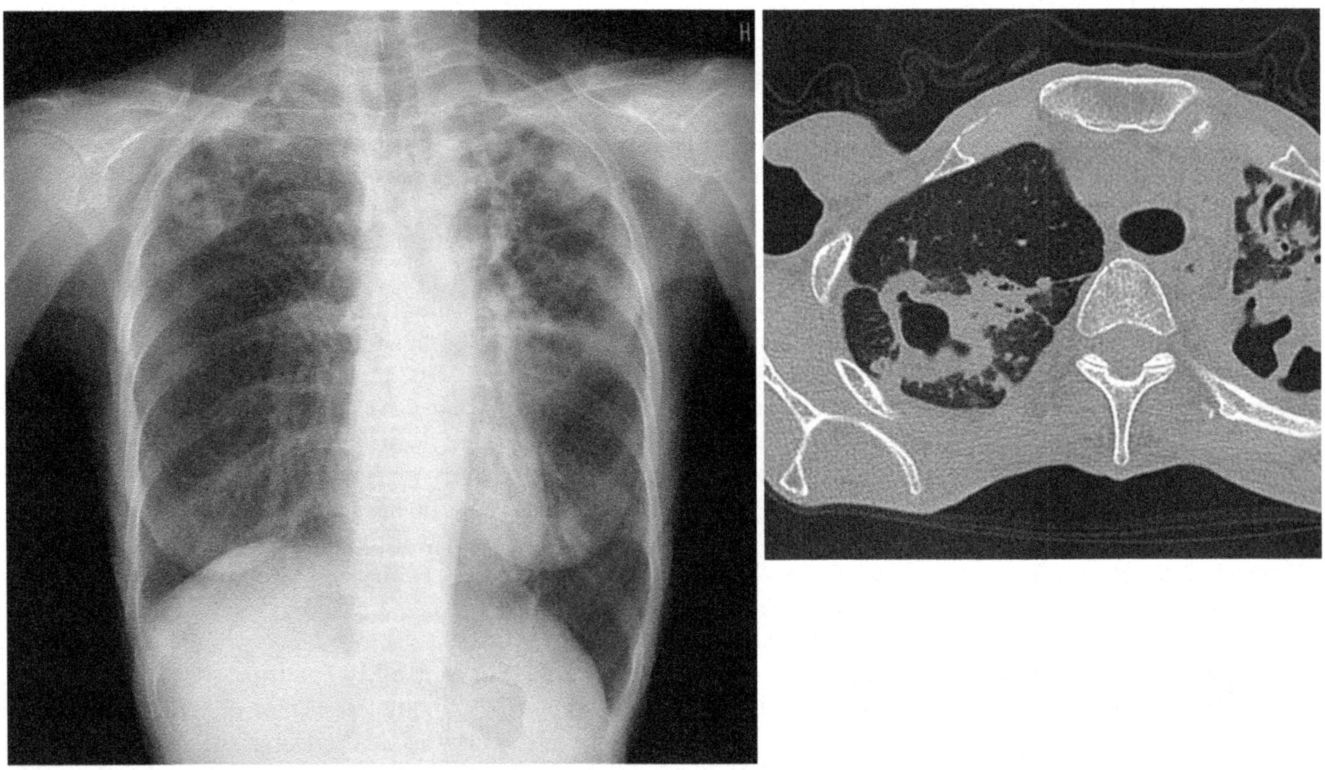

Fig. 11.3 Fibrocavitary form. Case: 73-year-old female

is not established, except for clarithromycin. Clarithromycin is effective to some extent, even for single medication for pulmonary MAC disease [34], and therapeutic effects are obtained in a dose-dependent manner; thus, it is meaningful to perform quantitative susceptibility testing exceptionally. For *M. kansasii*, susceptibility testing for rifampin is considered useful. Since the involvement of resistant strains is extremely rare in untreated cases, it is considered unnecessary to conduct a drug susceptibility test on all cases before the initial treatment.

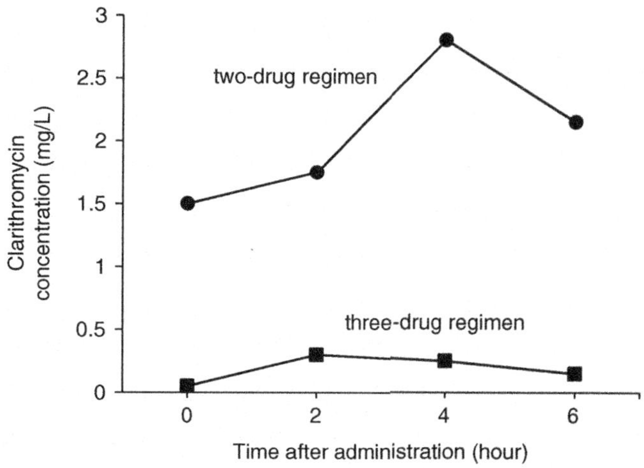

Fig. 11.4 Mean concentration of clarithromycin. Mean serum concentration of clarithromycin after oral administration of the three-drug regimen (clarithromycin, ethambutol, and rifampicin; circles) and the two-drug regimen (clarithromycin and ethambutol; squares) [38]

11.3.3 Treatment

Treatment decisions are made by evaluating the expected risks and benefits of treatment. In immunocompromised hosts, their immune status must also be considered, and close observation is desired. Treatment of pulmonary NTM infection depends on the species of organism. In general, the repertoire of effective drugs is limited, and long-term management with multiple drugs is required.

11.3.3.1 Pulmonary MAC Disease

Timing of treatment is at the discretion of each physician, and key components in the evaluation of patients are the clinical course, manifestation, imaging findings, immune status, and so on. Newer macrolide, clarithromycin, plays a crucial role on the treatment of this disease. Although clarithromycin is effective as a monotherapy, this drug should not be administered alone, because of the concern of selection for drug-resistant strains [34].

The 2007 ATS/IDSA guideline [25] recommends a combination of multiple drugs for nodular bronchiectatic disease, including clarithromycin (1000 mg), ethambutol (25 mg/kg), and rifampin (600 mg) three times per week (Table 11.2). Treatment regimen with clarithromycin (500–1000 mg), ethambutol (15 mg/kg), and rifampin (600 mg) daily is recommended for Cav disease and severe nodular bronchiectatic disease. Additionally, streptomycin or amikacin (10–15 mg/kg, three times per week) for the first 8 weeks should be considered in patients with Cav disease, because streptomycin is especially effective for extracellular bacillus. In these regimens, clarithromycin and rifampin may be replaced by azithromycin and rifabutin, respectively. Dose modification is required for elderly, renal dysfunction, and low body weight to avoid adverse effects [25, 35]. The Japanese guideline recommends a similar treatment regimen, but using a lower dose for clarithromycin (600–800 mg daily), with consideration of a smaller body size [36].

There is no consensus on the best duration of therapy, since there is limited evidence, and biomarker, which can monitor therapeutic effectiveness except for sputum culture, is lacking. The ATS/IDSA guideline recommends the duration of therapy as at least 1 year after sputum culture has consecutively negative. On the other hand, the British Thoracic Society recommends 2 years of therapeutic duration with other regimen (rifampin, ethambutol, with or without isoniazid) [37], and the Japanese guideline described both recommended durations [36]. Further studies are desired to determine the optimum therapeutic duration.

Randomized controlled trials of pulmonary MAC disease treatments have not been conducted in HIV-negative patients, and these treatment recommendations are based upon trials performed in HIV-positive patients [38–40]. Development of new effective antibacterial drugs and better treatment regimens using existing antibacterial drugs are being sought. For example, rifampin reduces the blood concentration levels of clarithromycin (Fig. 11.4) [41, 42], and the decline of therapeutic efficacy is of concern. Additionally, rifampin also modifies the levels of corticosteroids used for some reason, including in RA patients. Because of these points, therapeutic regimens with rifampin are under examination. It was suggested that a two-drug regimen of clarithromycin and ethambutol can achieve clinical effects equivalent to or higher than a three-drug regimen with rifampin [42]. At present, the standard regimen should be maintained; however, such an alternative regimen that is less burdensome for patients should be adopted in the future.

11.3.3.2 *M. kansasii* Disease

In the US treatment guideline, the standard regimen for treating *M. kansasii* disease includes rifampin (600 mg/day), isoniazid (300 mg/day), and ethambutol (600 mg/day) for a duration that includes 12 months of negative sputum culture for *M. kansasii* disease [25]. Generally, better therapeutic effects are expected for this infection, compared with pulmo-

Table 11.2 Chemotherapy for *Mycobacterium avium* complex lung disease (The 2007 ATS/IDSA guideline)

	Nodular bronchiectatic disease	Fibrocavitary disease	Advanced or previously treated disease
Clarithromycin	1000 mg TIW	500–1000 mg/day	500–1000 mg/day
Ethambutol	25 mg/kg TIW	15 mg/kg/day	15 mg/kg/day
Rifampicin	600 mg TIW	450–600 mg/day	450–600 mg/day
Aminoglycoside	None	SM or AM or none	SM or AM

TIW three times weekly

nary MAC disease. Pulmonary *M. kansasii* disease may deteriorate without treatment, and all patients with this disease should receive antimicrobial chemotherapy. As for the treatment period, similar to pulmonary MAC disease, 1 year after negative sputum culture is recommended. Recurrent cases raise concerns about the involvement of rifampin-resistant strains, but since they are very rare at the time of initial treatment, drug susceptibility testing need not be routinely performed.

11.3.3.3 Surgical Management

As described above, conservative treatment with clarithromycin-containing regimen is the mainstay of treatment, but if drug therapy alone does not successfully eradicate the infection, lung resection is still an option for treatment. Retrospective studies in several single institutions, including in a few patients, suggest that surgery may be associated with a good treatment outcome [43, 44]. The ATS/IDSA guideline recommends the surgical resection of limited (focal) disease in a patient with adequate cardiopulmonary reserve to withstand partial or total lung resection, which can be a successful treatment in combination with multidrug treatment regimens [25]. Although there are no established criteria for patient selection, if the patient is refractory to drug therapy, has macrolide-resistant infection, or presents with serious complications including hemoptysis, surgery may be indicated. There are potentially severe perioperative complications, and surgery should be performed in centers with expertise in both medical and surgical management of mycobacterial diseases.

11.3.3.4 Prognosis

A meta-analysis of HIV-negative patients with pulmonary MAC disease reported a treatment success rate of 38% in total [45]. Furthermore, patients with pulmonary MAC disease who have achieved consecutively negative sputum culture with standard regimen are estimated to be about 60% [46]. Taken together, the definitive treatment for pulmonary MAC disease has not been established. Factors predicting a poor prognosis include Cav or Cav+NB disease, low BMI, and anemia [27]. Additionally, associations between the variable number of tandem repeats (VNTR) profiling data and a therapeutic response in patients with pulmonary MAC disease were reported [47]. Thus, it is expected to establish the usefulness of this method in predicting the therapeutic reactivity of pulmonary MAC disease.

11.3.3.5 Special Consideration for RA Patients

As a rule, standard treatments should be conducted as described above, even in RA cases with the use of biological agents. The prognosis of RA-NTM infection was somewhat poorer than NTM infection alone; Yamakawa et al. reported that the 5-year survival rate was 66.1% [48]. In another research conducted in the United States, the mortality rate was 37% in RA-NTM patients who were administered anti-TNF-alpha agents [24]. In general, concomitant use of biological agents is considered a contraindication in cases of RA with confirmed NTM infection. Meanwhile, in a multicenter study conducted in Japan, no death was reported [49]. Also, no deceased case is notified in PMS of biologic agents in Japan. Although the reasons for such differences are unknown, differences in the medical systems of both countries may be an explanation, and frequent chest x-ray imaging and careful monitoring during clinical course are crucial. In this context, the consensus statement of Japan, published in 2014 [50], declared that if the disease activity of RA is severe and requires the use of biological agents, it may be administered in the following situations: (a) MAC disease, (b) nodular bronchiectatic type, (c) mild preexisting lung disease, (d) good general health, (e) antibiotic therapy which can be administered over a long period, and (f) good response to antibiotic treatment. The use of any biological agent for RA patients with NTM infection should be based on whether or not the benefits outweigh the risk, which requires further clinical study.

References

1. Tanoue LT. Pulmonary manifestations of rheumatoid arthritis. Clin Chest Med. 1998;19(4):667–85, viii.
2. Amital A, Shitrit D, Adir Y. The lung in rheumatoid arthritis. Presse Med. 2011;40(1 Pt 2):e31–48.
3. Massey H, Darby M, Edey A. Thoracic complications of rheumatoid disease. Clin Radiol. 2013;68(3):293–301.
4. Pai M, Behr MA, Dowdy D, et al. Tuberculosis. Nat Rev Dis Primers. 2016;2:16076.
5. Gideon HP, Flynn JL. Latent tuberculosis: what the host "sees"? Immunol Res. 2011;50(2–3):202–12.

6. Getahun H, Matteelli A, Abubakar I, et al. Management of latent Mycobacterium tuberculosis infection: WHO guidelines for low tuberculosis burden countries. Eur Respir J. 2015;46(6):1563–76.
7. Carmona L, Hernandez-Garcia C, Vadillo C, et al. Increased risk of tuberculosis in patients with rheumatoid arthritis. J Rheumatol. 2003;30(7):1436–9.
8. Askling J, Fored CM, Brandt L, et al. Risk and case characteristics of tuberculosis in rheumatoid arthritis associated with tumor necrosis factor antagonists in Sweden. Arthritis Rheum. 2005;52(7):1986–92.
9. Arkema EV, Jonsson J, Baecklund E, et al. Are patients with rheumatoid arthritis still at an increased risk of tuberculosis and what is the role of biological treatments? Ann Rheum Dis. 2015;74(6):1212–7.
10. Gardam MA, Keystone EC, Menzies R, et al. Anti-tumour necrosis factor agents and tuberculosis risk: mechanisms of action and clinical management. Lancet Infect Dis. 2003;3(3):148–55.
11. Ehlers S. Role of tumour necrosis factor (TNF) in host defence against tuberculosis: implications for immunotherapies targeting TNF. Ann Rheum Dis. 2003;62(Suppl 2):ii37–42.
12. Lewinsohn DM, Leonard MK, LoBue PA, et al. Official American Thoracic Society/Infectious Diseases Society of America/Centers for Disease Control and Prevention Clinical Practice guidelines: diagnosis of tuberculosis in adults and children. Clin Infect Dis. 2017;64(2):111–5.
13. Geng E, Kreiswirth B, Burzynski J, et al. Clinical and radiographic correlates of primary and reactivation tuberculosis: a molecular epidemiology study. JAMA. 2005;293(22):2740–5.
14. Restrepo CS, Katre R, Mumbower A. Imaging manifestations of thoracic tuberculosis. Radiol Clin N Am. 2016;54(3):453–73.
15. Maartens G, Willcox PA, Benatar SR. Miliary tuberculosis: rapid diagnosis, hematologic abnormalities, and outcome in 109 treated adults. Am J Med. 1990;89(3):291–6.
16. Optican RJ, Ost A, Ravin CE. High-resolution computed tomography in the diagnosis of miliary tuberculosis. Chest. 1992;102(3):941–3.
17. Boehme CC, Nicol MP, Nabeta P, et al. Feasibility, diagnostic accuracy, and effectiveness of decentralised use of the Xpert MTB/RIF test for diagnosis of tuberculosis and multidrug resistance: a multicentre implementation study. Lancet. 2011;377(9776):1495–505.
18. Lein AD, Von Reyn CF. In vitro cellular and cytokine responses to mycobacterial antigens: application to diagnosis of tuberculosis infection and assessment of response to mycobacterial vaccines. Am J Med Sci. 1997;313(6):364–71.
19. Nahid P, Dorman SE, Alipanah N, et al. Official American Thoracic Society/Centers for Disease Control and Prevention/Infectious Diseases Society of America Clinical Practice guidelines: treatment of drug-susceptible tuberculosis. Clin Infect Dis. 2016;63(7):e147–95.
20. Horsburgh CR Jr, Rubin EJ. Clinical practice. Latent tuberculosis infection in the United States. N Engl J Med. 2011;364(15):1441–8.
21. Sterling TR, Villarino ME, Borisov AS, et al. Three months of rifapentine and isoniazid for latent tuberculosis infection. N Engl J Med. 2011;365(23):2155–66.
22. Yeh JJ, Wang YC, Sung FC, et al. Rheumatoid arthritis increases the risk of nontuberculosis mycobacterial disease and active pulmonary tuberculosis. PLoS One. 2014;9(10):e110922.
23. Brode SK, Jamieson FB, Ng R, et al. Risk of mycobacterial infections associated with rheumatoid arthritis in Ontario, Canada. Chest. 2014;146(3):563–72.
24. Winthrop KL, Baxter R, Liu L, et al. Mycobacterial diseases and antitumour necrosis factor therapy in USA. Ann Rheum Dis. 2013;72(1):37–42.
25. Griffith DE, Aksamit T, Brown-Elliott BA, et al. An official ATS/IDSA statement: diagnosis, treatment, and prevention of nontuberculous mycobacterial diseases. Am J Respir Crit Care Med. 2007;175(4):367–416.
26. Moore EH. Atypical mycobacterial infection in the lung: CT appearance. Radiology. 1993;187(3):777–82.
27. Hayashi M, Takayanagi N, Kanauchi T, et al. Prognostic factors of 634 HIV-negative patients with Mycobacterium Avium Complex lung disease. Am J Respir Crit Care Med. 2012;185(5):575–83.
28. Levin DL. Radiology of pulmonary Mycobacterium Avium-Intracellulare Complex. Clin Chest Med. 2002;23(3):603–12.
29. Koh WJ, Lee KS, Kwon OJ, et al. Bilateral bronchiectasis and bronchiolitis at thin-section CT: diagnostic implications in nontuberculous mycobacterial pulmonary infection. Radiology. 2005;235(1):282–8.
30. Christensen EE, Dietz GW, Ahn CH, et al. Initial roentgenographic manifestations of pulmonary Mycobacterium tuberculosis, M kansasii, and M intracellularis infections. Chest. 1981;80(2):132–6.
31. Woodring JH, Vandiviere HM. Pulmonary disease caused by nontuberculous mycobacteria. J Thorac Imaging. 1990;5(2):64–76.
32. Kitada S, Kobayashi K, Ichiyama S, et al. Serodiagnosis of Mycobacterium Avium-Complex pulmonary disease using an enzyme immunoassay kit. Am J Respir Crit Care Med. 2008;177(7):793–7.
33. Institute CaLS. Susceptibility testing of Mycobacteria, Nocardiae and other aerobic Actinomycetes: Clinical and Laboratory Standards Institute; 2011.
34. Wallace RJ Jr, Brown BA, Griffith DE, et al. Initial clarithromycin monotherapy for Mycobacterium Avium-Intracellulare Complex lung disease. Am J Respir Crit Care Med. 1994;149(5):1335–41.
35. Wallace RJ Jr, Brown BA, Griffith DE. Drug intolerance to high-dose clarithromycin among elderly patients. Diagn Microbiol Infect Dis. 1993;16(3):215–21.
36. Guidelines for chemotherapy of pulmonary nontuberculous mycobacterial disease—2012 revised version. Kekkaku. 2013;88(1):29–32.
37. Management of opportunist mycobacterial infections: Joint Tuberculosis Committee Guidelines 1999. Subcommittee of the Joint Tuberculosis Committee of the British Thoracic Society. Thorax. 2000;55(3):210–8.
38. Wallace RJ Jr, Brown BA, Griffith DE, et al. Clarithromycin regimens for pulmonary Mycobacterium Avium Complex. The first 50 patients. Am J Respir Crit Care Med. 1996;153(6 Pt 1):1766–72.
39. Dautzenberg B, Piperno D, Diot P, et al. Clarithromycin in the treatment of Mycobacterium Avium lung infections in patients without AIDS. Clarithromycin Study Group of France. Chest. 1995;107(4):1035–40.
40. Griffith DE, Brown BA, Cegielski P, et al. Early results (at 6 months) with intermittent clarithromycin-including regimens for lung disease due to Mycobacterium Avium Complex. Clin Infect Dis. 2000;30(2):288–92.
41. van Ingen J, Egelund EF, Levin A, et al. The pharmacokinetics and pharmacodynamics of pulmonary Mycobacterium Avium Complex disease treatment. Am J Respir Crit Care Med. 2012;186(6):559–65.
42. Miwa S, Shirai M, Toyoshima M, et al. Efficacy of clarithromycin and ethambutol for Mycobacterium Avium Complex pulmonary disease. A preliminary study. Ann Am Thorac Soc. 2014;11(1):23–9.
43. Nelson KG, Griffith DE, Brown BA, et al. Results of operation in Mycobacterium Avium-intracellulare lung disease. Ann Thorac Surg. 1998;66(2):325–30.
44. Shiraishi Y, Nakajima Y, Takasuna K, et al. Surgery for Mycobacterium Avium Complex lung disease in the clarithromycin era. Eur J Cardiothorac Surg. 2002;21(2):314–8.
45. HB X, Jiang RH, Li L. Treatment outcomes for Mycobacterium Avium Complex: a systematic review and meta-analysis. Eur J Clin Microbiol Infect Dis. 2014;33(3):347–58.
46. van Ingen J, Ferro BE, Hoefsloot W, et al. Drug treatment of pulmonary nontuberculous mycobacterial disease in HIV-negative patients: the evidence. Expert Rev Anti-Infect Ther. 2013;11(10):1065–77.

47. Kikuchi T, Kobashi Y, Hirano T, et al. Mycobacterium Avium genotype is associated with the therapeutic response to lung infection. Clin Microbiol Infect. 2014;20(3):256–62.
48. Yamakawa H, Takayanagi N, Miyahara Y, et al. Prognostic factors and radiographic outcomes of nontuberculous mycobacterial lung disease in rheumatoid arthritis. J Rheumatol. 2013;40(8):1307–15.
49. Mori S, Tokuda H, Sakai F, et al. Radiological features and therapeutic responses of pulmonary nontuberculous mycobacterial disease in rheumatoid arthritis patients receiving biological agents: a retrospective multicenter study in Japan. Mod Rheumatol. 2012;22(5):727–37.
50. Tokuda H, Harigai M, Kameda H, et al. Consensus statements for medical practice: biological agents and lung disease [Abridged English translation by the Japanese Respiratory Society]. Respir Investig. 2017;55(3):229–51.

12 Organizing Pneumonia in Rheumatoid Arthritis

Takahisa Gono

Abstract

Organizing pneumonia (OP) is one of the extra-articular manifestations in rheumatoid arthritis (RA). OP is noninfectious pneumonia with less responsiveness to antibiotics, occasionally mimicking bacterial pneumonia. RA patients with OP typically experience flu-like symptoms and respiratory symptoms such as nonproductive cough and dyspnea at the onset of OP. However, some RA patients do not reveal any respiratory symptoms. The characteristics of chest imaging include bilateral/multiple consolidations or ground-glass opacities with normal lung volumes. The lung lesions are occasionally unilateral/solitary and are frequently observed in the lower zone of the lungs. In the pathophysiology of OP with RA, Th1-dominant response and pro-inflammatory cytokines are associated with the development of OP with RA.

In general, intermediate–high dose of prednisolone ameliorates OP with RA. The prognosis is good for OP with RA, although OP relapse is noted in 10–20% of RA-OP cases. OP is not a direct cause of death in RA.

Keywords

Rheumatoid arthritis • Organizing pneumonia • Fibroblast • Cytokine

12.1 Introduction

Rheumatoid arthritis (RA) is a joint disease that is caused by autoimmune processes. The most common extra-articular manifestation is lung disease, such as usual interstitial pneumonia (UIP), nonspecific IP (NSIP), organizing pneumonia (OP), and airway disease in RA [1]. OP is complicated in several diseases such as infection, connective tissue disease, drug, and radiation therapy, as shown in Table 12.1 [2]. OP associated with these underlying diseases is called secondary OP. By contrast, OP without an underlying disease is called cryptogenic OP (COP). OP is classified as a type of interstitial lung disease (ILD).

The primary affected area is within the alveolar wall in OP. At first, alveolar epithelial cells are injured by some type of factor. Then, the necrosis and sloughing of pneumocytes result in the denudation of the epithelial basal laminae [3]. Interestingly, OP is relatively responsive to treatment with intermediate doses of corticosteroids and can display

Table 12.1 Causes of OP

Infection: Bacteria, virus, fungus, parasite
Connective tissue disease: RA, polymyositis/dermatomyositis
Drug: Amiodarone, carbamazepine, DMARDs, interferon, nitrofurantoin, etc.
Radiation therapy
Organ transplant: Bone marrow transplantation
Aspiration of gastric contents: Gastroesophageal reflux, repeated micro-aspirations

OP organizing pneumonia, *RA* rheumatoid arthritis, *DMARDs* disease-modifying antirheumatic drugs

T. Gono, M.D., Ph.D.
Department of Allergy and Rheumatology, Nippon Medical School, Graduate School of Medicine, Tokyo, Japan
e-mail: t-gono@nms.ac.jp

T. Gono et al. (eds.), *Lung Disease Associated with Rheumatoid Arthritis*, https://doi.org/10.1007/978-981-10-6750-1_12

dramatic reversibility of the lung lesions, despite the fact that the inflammatory exudates are composed of collagen, fibroblasts, and myofibroblasts. By contrast, UIP responds poorly to treatment by corticosteroids and results in progressive irreversible fibrosis. Thus, the prognosis is better in OP than in UIP. However, OP occasionally recurs in RA patients and in COP patients. The detailed pathophysiology of RA-associated OP (RA-OP) remains unknown. The clinical characteristics, diagnosis, treatment, and pathophysiology of RA-OP, including recent findings, are described below.

12.2 Prevalence and Incidence of RA-OP

The accurate prevalence and incidence of RA-OP remain unknown. OP is one type of ILD. ILD is clinically complicated in ~10% of RA patients [4–6]. UIP and nonspecific IP (NSIP) are common in RA-ILD. In a multicenter UK study, OP was revealed in 7 (5%) of 159 RA patients with ILD [7]. In addition, a Japanese study found OP in 19 (4%) of 499 RA patients [8]. Therefore, the complication of OP is not frequently revealed in RA.

12.3 Relationship Between OP Onset and Arthritis Onset in RA

According to the combined results from the two previous reports, OP preceded the onset of arthritis in 12% of the 40 enrolled RA patients, as shown in Fig. 12.1 [8, 9]. The duration between the development of OP and onset of arthritis is 2 weeks to 2 years [9]. In almost all of these cases, rheumatoid factor (RF) and/or anti-citrullinated protein antibody (ACPA) were positive. On the other hand, OP is typically complicated after diagnosis of RA (70%) and occasionally simultaneous development of OP (18%) (Fig. 12.1) [8–10]. When clinicians experience a case with OP in which RF/ACPA is positive in sera and no arthritis is noted, clinicians should be mindful of the development of arthritis in subsequent follow-up appointments.

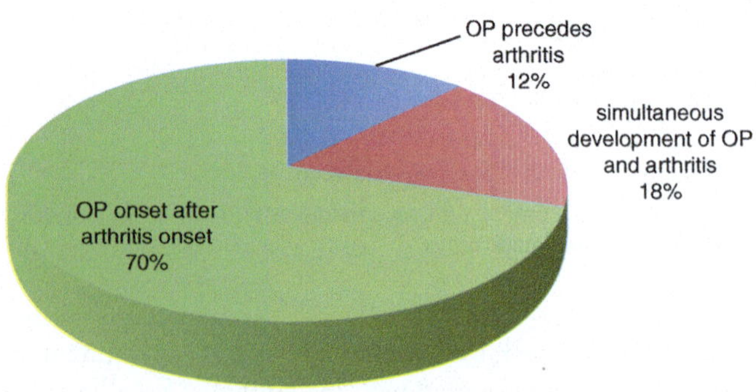

Fig. 12.1 Relationship between OP onset and arthritis onset in RA. *OP* organizing pneumonia. The whole number of enrolled patients is 40

12.4 Clinical Characteristics of OP in RA

The mean age of the development of OP is approximately 60 years. The incidence is twofold greater in females than in males. The disease duration at OP onset is approximately 4–7 years after the onset of RA. There was no significant difference in clinical characteristics, including age, gender, presence of RF/ACPA, smoking history, disease activity, and treatment with DMARDs, between RA-OP patients and RA patients without OP [8, 10]. In some cases with RA-OP, arthritis disease activity is closely associated with the development of OP. However, OP is also complicated in some cases with RA in which disease activity is low or in remission [9, 10]. The difference might depend on the cause of OP in RA. We hypothesized the causes of RA-OP, as shown in Table 12.2. In RA, the causes of OP include RA disease, infections such as from bacteria or viruses, and the use of drugs that include conventional synthetic DMARDs and bDMARDs [3, 9–14].

12.4.1 Clinical Characteristics of OP in RA Patients Treated with bDMARDs

According to a previous report, OP onset was found in 12 RA patients treated with bDMARDs [10]. As shown in Table 12.3, MTX was administered to 9 of these 12 patients. Infliximab, etanercept, and tocilizumab were administered to six, five, and one of the patients, respectively. The selection of which bDMARD was administered could reflect a pharmaceutical market trend at the time of the study. Four patients developed OP within 2 months of initiating their bDMARD treatment. The other eight patients developed OP more than 1 year after commencement of bDMARD treatment. RA disease activity at the onset of OP was low or in remission (DAS28-ESR <3.2) for five patients.

Table 12.2 Presumptive causes of OP associated with RA

RA-itself disease activity
Infection: Bacteria, fungus, virus
Drugs: csDMARDs, bDMARDs, others
Unknown origin

OP organizing pneumonia, *RA* rheumatoid arthritis, *csDMARDs* conventional synthetic disease-modifying antirheumatic drugs, *bDMARDs* biological DMARDs

Table 12.3 Clinical characteristics of OP with RA patients treated with bDMARDs

No.	Age/sex	RA disease duration, month	csDMARD	PSL	bDMARD	Period of bDMARD, month	RF at OP development, IU/mL	DAS28-ESR at OP development
1	53/F	27	MTX	+	IFX	2	6	3.3
2	56/F	35	MTX	–	IFX	12	45	4.3
3	60/F	36	MTX	–	ETN	14	195	4.4
4	31/F	28	MTX	–	ETN	1	45	2.1
5	66/F	102	MTX, TAC	+	TCZ	15	112	2.1
6	66/M	84	MTX	–	IFX	18	122	3.8
7	79/F	144	–	–	ETN	1	<5	2.8
8	78/F	8	SASP	+	ETN	0	307	5.1
9	42/F	106	MTX	+	IFX	62	<5	3.4
10	41/F	258	LEF	+	ETN	60	29	1.4
11	63/M	84	MTX, SASP	–	IFX	26	86	3.0
12	56/M	86	MTX	–	IFX	27	403	4.8

OP organizing pneumonia, *RA* rheumatoid arthritis, *bDMARDs* biological disease-modifying antirheumatic drugs, *csDMARD* conventional synthetic DMARD, *PSL* prednisolone, *RF* rheumatoid factor, *DAS28* disease activity score at joints, *ESR* erythrocyte sedimentation rate, *MTX* methotrexate, *TAC* tacrolimus, *SASP* salazosulfapyridine, *LEF* leflunomide, *IFX* infliximab, *ETN* etanercept, *TCZ* tocilizumab

These results indicate that the initiation of bDMARD treatment might be associated with the onset of OP in some cases and that RA disease activity is not always correlated with the frequency of OP onset. In two cases, OP developed within 1 month of initiating bDMRAD treatment. These two patients were almost 80 years old and had preexisting ILD. Infection or treatment with bDMARDs might induce the onset of OP. Clinicians should be aware of the potential onset of OP in elderly RA patients with preexisting pulmonary disease.

Compared with patients treated with csDMARDs alone, RA disease duration tended to be reduced, and RA disease activity tended to be increased in patients treated with bDMARDs. There was no significant difference in age, gender, prednisolone (PLS) dose, RF titers, and the rate of preexisting pulmonary disease between the two subsets [10].

12.5 Symptoms and Physical Examination

In COP, the following symptoms occur (Table 12.4): persistent nonproductive cough (72%), dyspnea (66%), fever (51%), malaise (48%), and body weight loss [15]. In RA-OP, patients typically feel flu-like symptoms such as fever, malaise, shivering, chills, and body aches [9]. These symptoms in RA-OP are basically the same as those in COP and develop acutely or subacutely across days to weeks. By contrast, some patients with RA-OP occasionally have no respiratory symptoms. According to a previous report, 40% of the RA-OP patients studied had no respiratory symptoms [8], which may be because the disability of physical function caused by RA masks their respiratory symptoms. In these cases, the levels of C-reactive protein (CRP) are higher than usual, although arthritis disease activity is stable compared with previous visits. When the origin of the high levels of CRP is unknown and the arthritis disease activity is the same as previously noted, chest radiography should be assessed to consider any complications of OP. In addition, when treatment with antibiotics is unresponsive or insufficiently responsive to pneumonia in RA patients, clinicians should be mindful in case OP is developing.

Table 12.4 Symptoms of OP

Persistent nonproductive cough
Dyspnea
Fever
Malaise
Weight loss

OP organizing pneumonia

On physical examination, inspiratory crackles are often (74%) revealed in COP patients [15]. There are no respiratory findings on physical examination in one-fourth of patients. Specific findings are also frequently absent in RA-OP. Breath sounds are frequently normal or slightly abnormal in RA-OP patients.

12.6 Evaluation

The main measures to diagnose RA-OP and conduct differential diagnosis are laboratory tests, imaging studies, microorganism tests, and histopathological evaluations, as shown in Table 12.5. Each evaluation is described below.

Table 12.5 Evaluation for diagnosis of RA-OP and differential diagnosis

Laboratory tests: RF, ACPA, CRP, ESR
Imaging studies: Chest radiograph, HRCT
Pulmonary function test: %VC, DL_{CO}
Microorganism test: Gram's stain and culture (blood, sputum, BALF) including mycobacterium and fungus
Cytology/histopathology: BALF (distribution of leukocytes, confirmation of alveolar hemorrhage, cytology), lung biopsy (transbronchial, CT-guided, surgical)

RA rheumatoid arthritis, *OP* organizing pneumonia, *RF* rheumatoid factor, *ACPA* anti-citrullinated protein antibody, *CRP* C-reactive protein, *ESR* erythrocyte sedimentation rate, *HRCT* high-resolution computed tomography, *%VC* vital capacity as percent of predicted, *DLco* diffuse capacity for carbon monoxide, *BALF* bronchoalveolar lavage fluid

12.6.1 Laboratory Tests

No specific laboratory markers are available for the diagnosis of RA-OP. In cases with OP preceding arthritis in RA, RF/ACPA is useful for the consideration of later RA onset. Inflammatory markers such as CRP and erythrocyte sedimentation rate (ESR) increase during the onset of OP. CRP and ESR levels are higher at the OP onset than at the latest visits before the OP onset.

12.6.2 Imaging Studies

12.6.2.1 Chest Radiography

Chest radiography is conventional and appropriate as a screening test for the evaluation of pulmonary disease. As shown in Table 12.6, the characteristics of chest radiography/high-resolution computed tomography (HRCT) are bilateral/multiple consolidations or ground-glass opacities with normal lung volumes. The lung lesions are occasionally unilateral or solitary. In addition, the lung lesions occasionally disappear spontaneously and migrate to another zone. Pleural effusion and shrinking lung are typically not observed in OP.

As shown in Fig. 12.2a, multiple consolidations and ground-glass opacities are observed in the right lobe of the lung. After treatment with prednisolone (PSL), these lesions disappeared. Then, a new ground-glass lesion appeared in the left lower lobe immediately after tapering the PSL dose to 5 mg/day (Fig. 12.2b).

As shown in Figs. 12.3a and 12.4a, a unilateral and solitary lesion is occasionally observed in RA-OP. These lesions are frequently revealed in the lower zone of the lung.

Table 12.6 Characteristics of chest radiography/HRCT in OP

Consolidation/ground-glass opacities
Normal lung volume
Bilateral, occasionally unilateral
Patchy, multiple lesions, occasionally solitary

HRCT high-resolution computed tomography, *OP* organizing pneumonia

12.6.2.2 HRCT

HRCT evaluates pulmonary lesions in greater detail than chest radiography. In general but not especially in RA-OP, the most common radiologic pattern is multifocal peripheral consolidations (Fig. 12.3b). This form is identified in three-quarters of COP patients [16]. The lower zone is preferentially affected. Other zones are also affected in OP. Furthermore, a bronchocentric pattern is also revealed in up to one-third of COP (Fig. 12.5b) [16]. This pattern demonstrates multiple nodules and consolidations in the periphery of the lung and subpleural space. The density of the opacities reflects consolidation with air bronchogram or ground glass (Fig. 12.4b, c). Bronchial wall thickening with dilation is also revealed (Fig. 12.5b).

According to a previous report on RA-OP and as shown in Table 12.7, consolidation/alveolar opacities were observed in all of the 19 RA-OP patients [8]. Multiple consolidation and bilateral lung lesions were noted in 14 (74%) and 8 (42%) patients, respectively. These lesions were frequently revealed in the lower/middle lung zones. The lung lesions disappeared spontaneously in 8 (42%) patients. A reticular shadow was observed in only one patient. This shadow is generally not found in RA-OP.

12.6.3 Pulmonary Function Test

Vital capacity is decreased in OP. Restrictive ventilatory impairment is noted. The severity of the impairment is typically mild to moderate [15, 17]. The diffusing capacity of the lung for carbon monoxide is also reduced in the majority of OP patients [15, 18]. These impairments of pulmonary function usually improve after administration of corticosteroid.

12.6.4 Microorganism Test

To exclude infection in pneumonia, Gram's stain and culture including mycobacterium and fungus in blood, sputum, and bronchoalveolar lavage fluid (BALF) and urinary tests for *pneumococcal* and *Legionella* antigen should be performed. In addition, measurements of β-D-glucan and cytomegalovirus antigenemia also should be considered in RA patients treated with immunosuppressive csDMARDs, bDMRADs, or corticosteroids.

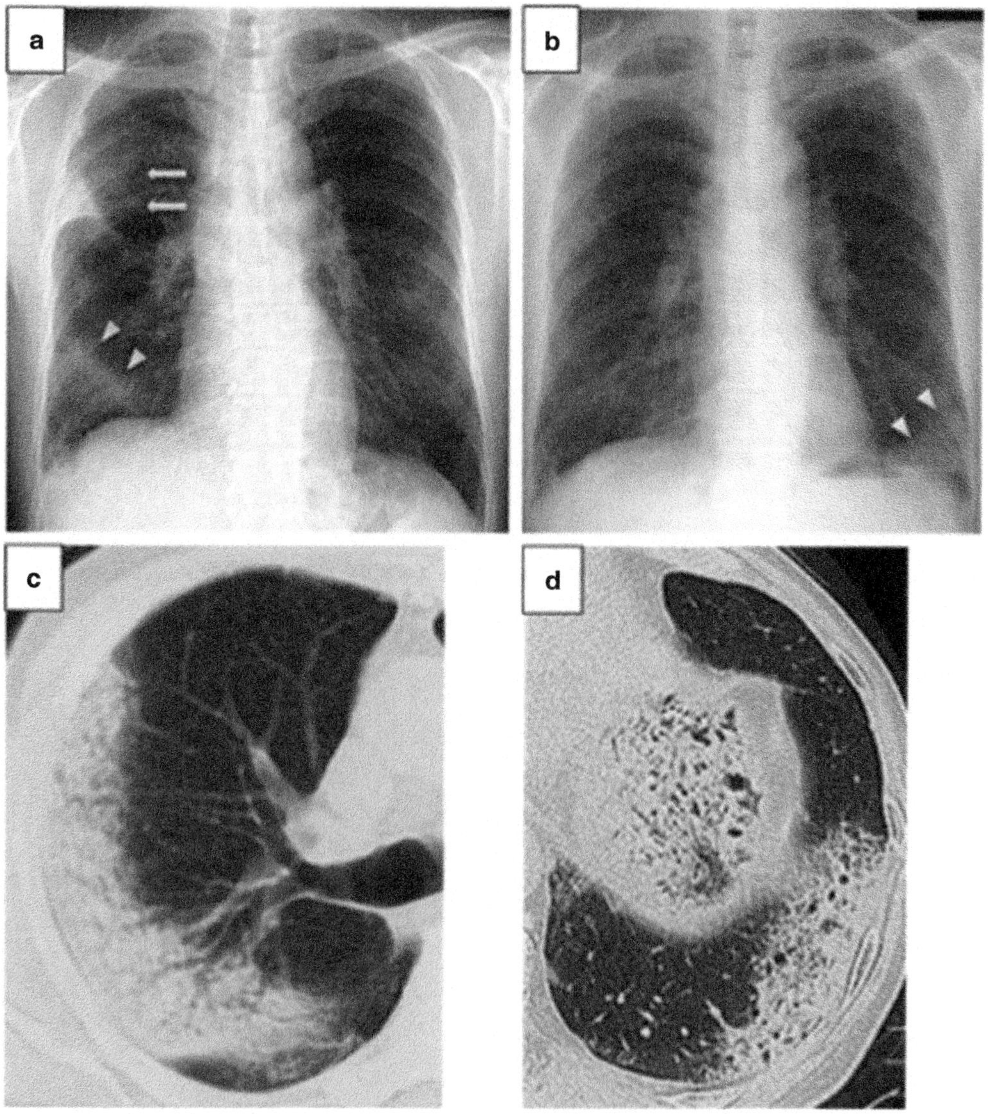

Fig. 12.2 A 67-year-old male with RA developed OP during treatment with bucilamine. (**a**, **c**) Multiple consolidations and ground-glass opacities are found in the right lobe of the lung. (**b**, **d**) A new ground-glass lesion appeared in the left lower lobe just after tapering of PSL dose to 5 mg/day. These images are provided through the courtesy of M. Hanaoka

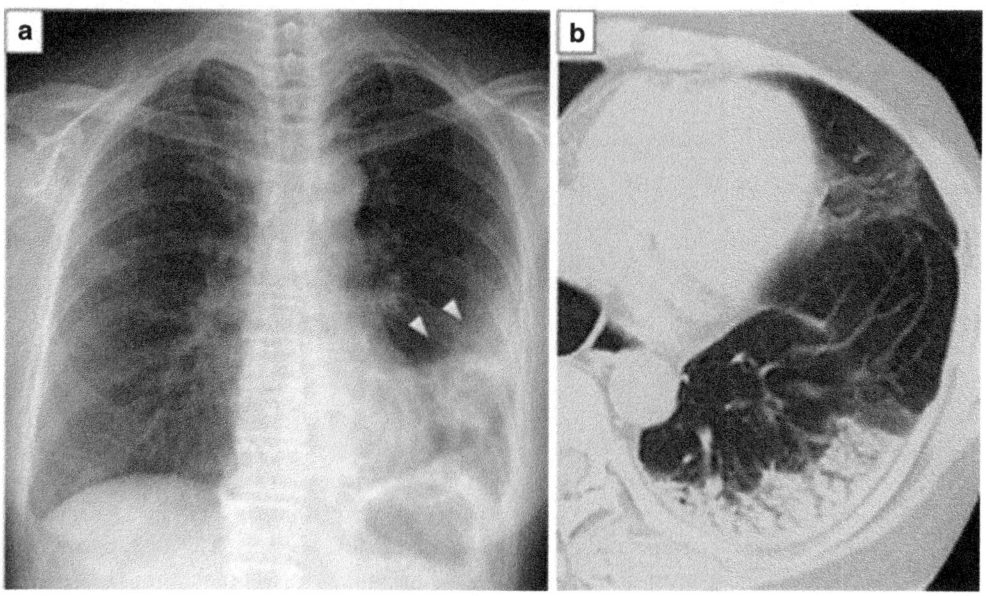

Fig. 12.3 A 55-year-old female developed OP during treatment with infliximab. (**a**) Consolidation is revealed in the middle/lower zone of the lung. (**b**) Air bronchogram is demonstrated in HRCT. These images are provided through the courtesy of M. Hanaoka

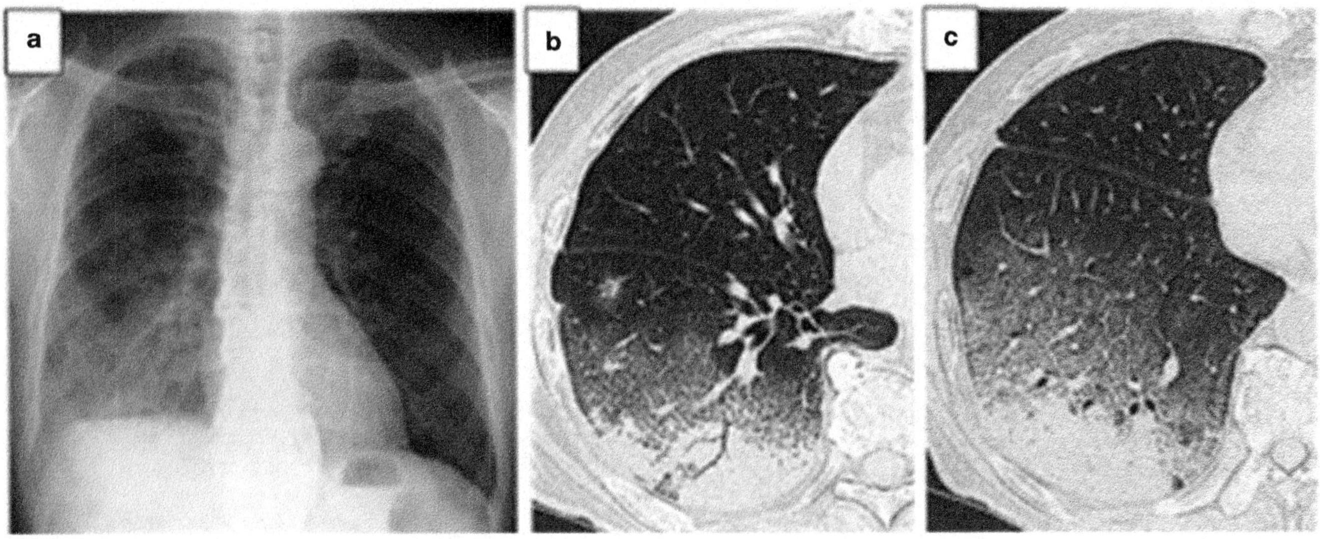

Fig. 12.4 A 70-year-old male developed OP during treatment with methotrexate. (**a**) Consolidation is revealed in the lower zone of the right lung. (**b**, **c**) Air bronchogram and ground-glass opacities are demonstrated in HRCT. These images are provided through the courtesy of M. Hanaoka

Fig. 12.5 A 68-year-old female developed OP during treatment with methotrexate. (**a**, **b**) Multiple nodules and consolidations are found in the periphery lung and subpleural. (**b**) Bronchial wall thickening with dilation is also revealed

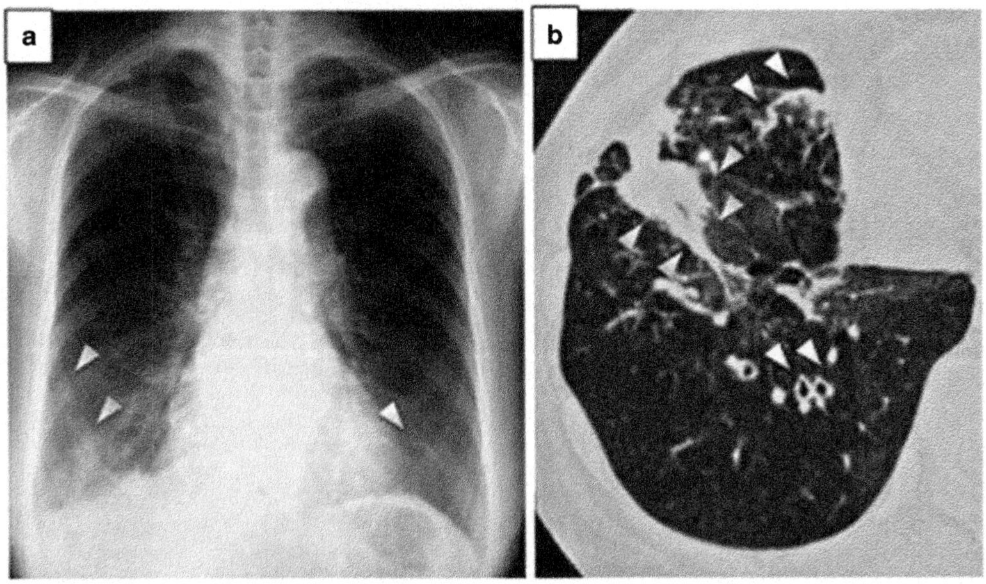

Table 12.7 HRCT findings and frequency in RA-OP (n = 19)

Consolidation/alveolar opacities, 100%
Multiple consolidation, 74%
Ground-glass opacities, 47%
Bilateral lung lesions, 42%
Reticular shadow, 5%

HRCT high-resolution computed tomography, *RA* rheumatoid arthritis, *OP* organizing pneumonia

12.6.5 Cytology/Histopathology

12.6.5.1 BALF

BALF is obtained using bronchoscopy. The evaluation of BALF reveals the distribution of cells such as neutrophils, eosinophils, lymphocytes, and macrophages and detects microorganisms, alveolar hemorrhage, and malignant cells. This investigation is critical for differential diagnosis in lung disease. In OP, increases in lymphocytes are noted; however, this finding is not specific for OP [3, 15, 19]. A decreased ratio of CD4/CD8 and Th1-dominant activation are revealed in BALF with OP [15, 19, 20].

12.6.5.2 Lung Biopsy

To confirm a diagnosis of OP, it could be considered to obtain lung tissues. The measures include transbronchial lung biopsy (TBLB), CT-guided lung biopsy, and surgical lung biopsy. TBLB using bronchoscopy is relatively less invasive as a procedure. However, it is difficult to obtain sufficient tissue for accurate evaluation. By contrast, surgical lung biopsy using video-assisted thoracoscopy makes it possible to obtain sufficient tissue and evaluate it accurately. However, the procedure is invasive and risky for patients with poor general or respiratory health. In a typical case with RA-OP, CT-guided/surgical lung biopsy might not be needed. In these cases, TBLB could be considered. However, CT-guided or surgical lung biopsy should be considered in cases in which the clinical characteristics are inconsistent with those of OP and a more certain differential diagnosis is needed.

12.7 Characteristics of Histopathology

The characteristics of the histopathological findings in OP are shown in Table 12.8. One characteristic is an intraluminal plug of inflammation that consists of buds of granulated tissue (Figs. 12.6 and 12.7). The buds of granulated tissue within the alveolar space are revealed in the area indicated by circles (Fig. 12.6). The granulations are composed of fibroblasts,

Table 12.8 Characteristics of histopathology in OP

Buds of granulated tissue within the alveolar space
Granulated tissue consist of fibroblasts/myofibroblasts embedded in connective tissue
Buds extend into the bronchioles and occasionally obstruct the lumen
Mild interstitial inflammation with lymphocytes/plasma cells, foamy macrophages in alveoli
A uniform appearance within involved area
Patchy distribution without severe disruption of the lung architecture

OP organizing pneumonia

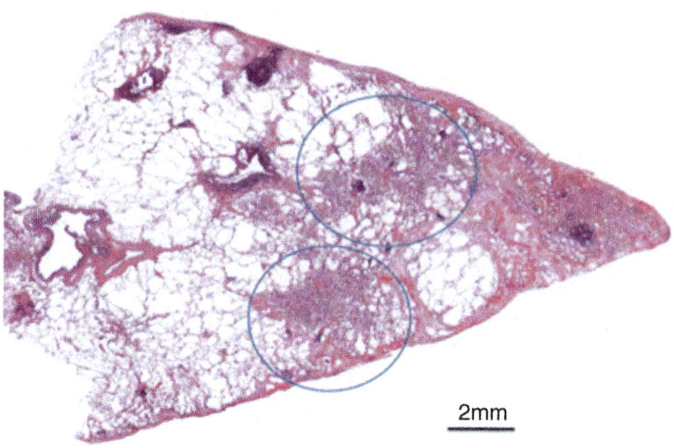

Fig. 12.6 Histopathology of RA-OP in hematoxylin-eosin staining. Buds of granulation tissue within the alveolar space are revealed in the area indicated by circles. A uniform appearance within involved area and a patchy distribution without the disruption of the lung architecture are revealed in this histopathology. This image is provided through the courtesy of T. Takemura

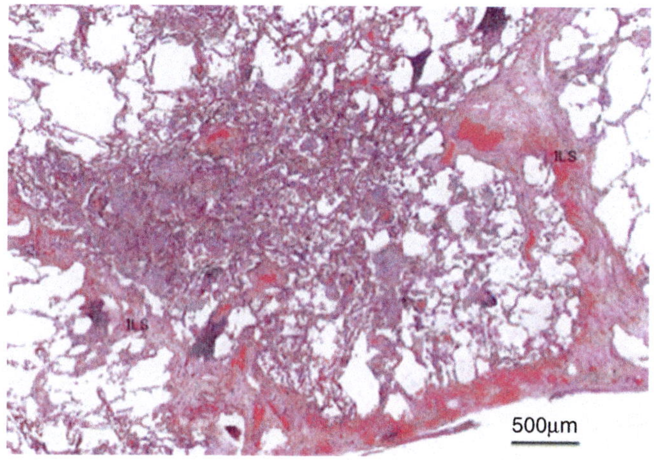

Fig. 12.7 Histopathology of high-power field in the Fig. 12.6 in hematoxylin-eosin staining. Alveolar spaces are filled with granulation tissue. *ILS* interlobular septa. This image is provided through the courtesy of T. Takemura

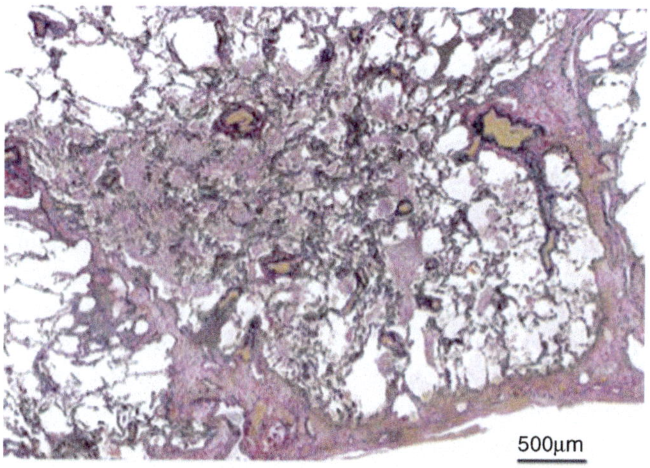

Fig. 12.8 Histopathology in Elastica van Gieson staining. Intra-alveolar buds of granulations and fibrosis were revealed with preserved alveolar structures. This image is provided through the courtesy of T. Takemura

myofibroblasts, and connective tissue matrix within the alveolar ducts and surrounding alveoli (Fig. 12.8) [16]. These buds may extend to adjacent buds through the pore of Kohn [3, 16]. Mild interstitial inflammation is found surrounding the lung (Fig. 12.9). Mononuclear cells are mildly infiltrating into the alveolar walls (indicated by black arrows in Fig. 12.9). Lymphocytes and macrophages are present in the alveolar lumina (indicated by black arrow heads in Fig. 12.9). Foamy macrophages are present in alveoli [16]. A uniform appearance within the involved area and a patchy distribution without severe disruption of the lung architecture are characteristic features in OP (Fig. 12.6). In a typical form of OP, hyaline membranes are absent, as found in diffuse alveolar damage.

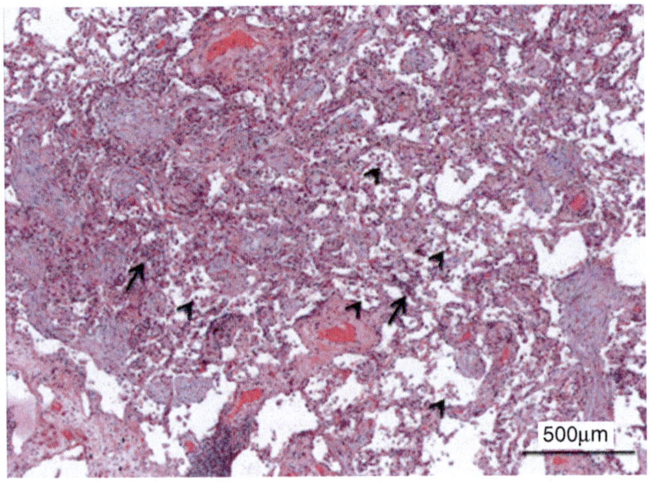

Fig. 12.9 Histopathology of high-power field in the Fig. 12.6 in hematoxylin-eosin staining. Mononuclear cells were mildly infiltrating in the alveolar walls (indicated by black arrows). Lymphocyte and macrophages are present in the alveolar lumina (indicated by black arrow heads). This image is provided through the courtesy of T. Takemura

12.8 Histopathogenesis of OP

In the histopathogenesis of OP, four processes are organized as follows: (1) leakage, (2) coagulation, (3) organization, and (4) resorption [3, 17]. First, alveolar epithelial injury leads to pneumocyte cell death, thus forming gaps in the basal lamina. Plasma proteins containing clotting factors and inflammatory cells such as neutrophils, eosinophils, and lymphocytes leak into the airspace. Then, the activated coagulation cascade causes fibrin deposition. Thereafter, fibroblasts migrate through the gap in the basal lamina. Mature fibrotic buds are formed with concentric rings of myofibroblasts and connective tissue matrix, such as type III collagen, fibronectin, and proteoglycans, into the alveolar space. Finally, inflammation subsides and fibrotic lesions are resorbed.

12.9 Diagnosis

When a typical clinical course, symptoms, imaging findings, and histopathology are observed, it is easy to diagnose RA-OP. In daily practice, histopathology evaluation of the lung is sometimes not conducted because clinicians tend to avoid invasive evaluations such as surgical lung biopsy or because they do not consider any disease other than OP. Otherwise, CT-guided or surgical lung biopsy should be considered in cases in which the clinical characteristics are inconsistent with those of OP in order to more definitively perform a differential diagnosis as described below. In cases that are unresponsive or insufficiently responsive to treatment with corticosteroids for lung lesions mimicking OP, a lung biopsy should be conducted.

Table 12.9 Differential diagnosis for OP

Infection: Coexisting of infection
Malignancy: Invasive mucinous adenocarcinoma, lymphoma
Other forms of ILD: NSIP, DAD
Chronic eosinophilic pneumonia
Hypersensitivity pneumonitis

OP organizing pneumonia, *ILD* interstitial lung disease, *NSIP* nonspecific interstitial pneumonia, *DAD* diffuse alveolar damage

12.10 Differential Diagnosis

For differential diagnosis, several diseases are listed as below and presented in Table 12.9.

12.10.1 Infection

The most important consideration during diagnosis is to exclude the possibility of infection because corticosteroid treatment will be initiated for OP. In some cases, infections can induce OP. When an antibiotic is sufficiently received and a poor response is noted for the lung lesions, the addition of corticosteroid can be considered on conditon that infection is excluded.

12.10.2 Malignancy

In addition, malignancy such as adenocarcinoma(invasive mucinous adenocarcinoma) and lymphoma should be considered when the response to corticosteroid therapy is poor or not sufficient or clinical features and radiological findings are inconsistent with those of typical OP. In these cases, CT-guided or surgical lung biopsy should be conducted.

12.10.3 Other Forms of ILD

In NSIP, OP-like imaging is partly revealed in the peripheral distribution of the lung. In these cases, a reticular shadow is usually found in the lower zone of the bilateral lung. This finding is typically not observed in OP. By contrast, some cases with OP have a fulminant onset, progress rapidly to respiratory failure, and are refractory despite corticosteroid treatment. In those cases, diffuse alveolar damage (DAD) should be considered. Clinicians should pay attention to the development of DAD when OP-like imaging is found, the response to corticosteroids is poor, and the pulmonary function is progressively impaired.

12.10.4 Chronic Eosinophilic Pneumonia

Clinical features of chronic eosinophilic pneumonia (CEP) mimic those of OP. In contrast to OP, the clinical course is more chronic, and eosinophils are more prevalent in peripheral blood, BALF, or lung tissue in CEP.

12.10.5 Hypersensitivity Pneumonia

The clinical manifestation of OP is similar to that of subacute hypersensitivity pneumonia (HP). HP is primarily caused by inhalation of dust. When a known exposure to an etiological agent occurs, a higher percentage of lymphocytes is observed, and the presence of poorly formed granulomas on the lung tissue is found, HP must be diagnosed.

12.11 Treatment

No randomized controlled trial for the treatment of COP or RA-OP has been performed. Corticosteroids have been used traditionally for the treatment of COP or RA-OP. In general, 0.5–1.0 mg/kg of prednisolone (PSL) ameliorates OP in RA [8, 9]. The dose of PSL might depend on the general condition, intensity of inflammation, extent of OP, severity of pulmonary function, and a patient's comorbidity. In some cases, a relatively lower dose of PSL, 15–20 mg/day, would suffice for RA-OP. When an intermediate to high dose of PSL, 30–60 mg/day, is administered as the treatment of OP, most clinicians discontinue csDMARDs or bDMARDs. This might be because they are seeking to avoid excessive immunosuppression or are considering DMARD-induced OP. Whether csDMARDS or bDMARDs should be withdrawn or should be continued at the initiation of PSL treatment remains controversial.

Based on previous clinical experiences, PSL therapy alone is sufficiently responsive to RA-OP. The regimen of PSL therapy has not been determined. The initial dose of PSL is continued for 2–4 weeks until the improvement of OP is obviously confirmed. Then, the dose of PSL should be carefully tapered by 10–20% every 1–2 weeks. If PSL is reduced to less than 10 mg/day, RA patients who are kept in the cessation of DMARDs could begin to suffer from arthralgia again. Therefore, treatment with DMARDs should be reinitiated when the dose of PSL reaches 15–20 mg/day. In relapsing cases with COP or secondly OP, immunosuppressive agents such as tacrolimus, cyclosporine, cyclophosphamide, and azathioprine could be administered, even though RA disease activity primarily needs to be under control upon treatment with DMARDs [21–23]. No reliable evidence supports the usage of these immunosuppressive agents for RA-OP. In addition, upon recommencement of the same DMARDs as previously used, the recurrence of OP should be carefully monitored in cases in which OP developed less than 3 months after the DMARDs were administered.

12.12 Prognosis

The prognosis is good. In typical cases, OP is not a direct cause of death. In 10–20% of cases, OP relapses [8, 9]. In some cases with DAD mimicking the imaging of OP as an initial feature, pulmonary function rapidly and progressively deteriorates regardless of the initiation of PSL. DAD in RA is frequently complicated with preexisting UIP and results in a fatal outcome due to respiratory failure.

12.13 Pathophysiology

12.13.1 Th1-Dominant Response

The pathophysiology of RA-OP remains unclear, as does that of COP. A previous report indicated that a Th1-dominant response was activated [20]. Lymphocytes were increased in BALF with COP. Interleukin (IL)-12, IL-18, and monocyte chemoattractant protein-1 levels were significantly increased in BALF from patients with COP compared with those with UIP or controls [20]. This result is consistent with a study regarding RA-OP. According to the research with serum cytokine profiles in RA-OP, the levels of interferon (IFN)-γ, IL-2, IL-12, and IFN-γ-inducible protein 10 (IP-10) were significantly higher in RA-OP than in RA without OP [10]. Dendritic cells, macrophages, and monocytes synthesize IL-12 [24]. IL-12 differentiates naïve T cells to Th1 cells that produce IL-2 and IFN-γ. IFN-γ activates macrophages and induces leukocytes to produce IP-10 [25]. IP-10 chemoattracts CXCR-3-positive cells including macrophages, dendritic cells, natural killer cells, and activated T lymphocytes toward the inflamed area [10]. These findings indicate that activated innate immune cells such as macrophages and acquired immune cells such as Th1 cells are associated with the development of RA-OP and COP.

12.13.2 High Levels of IFN-α and Pro-inflammatory Cytokines

Serum levels of IFN-α, IL-1β, IL-6, IL-8, and TNF-α were significantly higher than in RA-OP patients than in RA patients without OP [10]. According to a previous report, porcine circovirus type 2 (PCV2) infection caused the development of OP in swine [26]. IFN-α, IL-1β, and IL-6 serum levels were increased in swine infected with PCV2. This

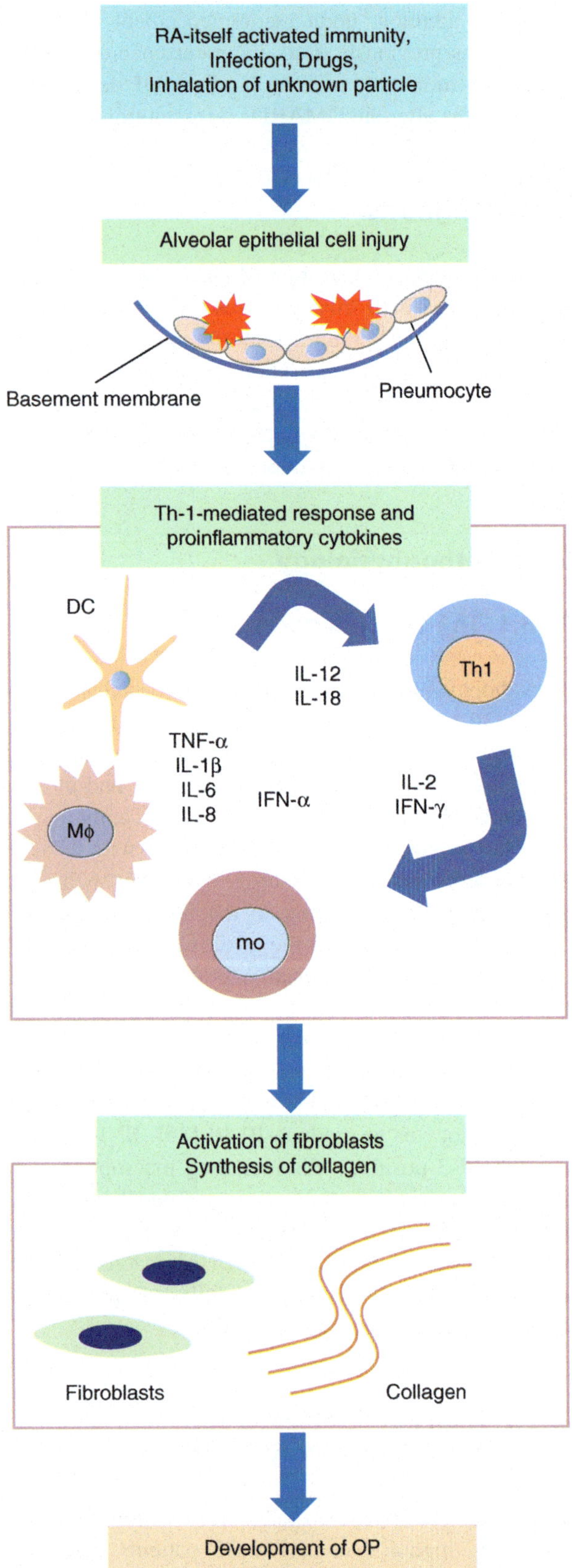

Fig. 12.10 Hypothesis of development of OP in RA

finding is similar to one revealed in RA-OP. It could be hypothesized that viral infection could cause OP in some patients with RA. We present a schema regarding a hypothesis of the development of RA-OP in Fig. 12.10.

Conclusion

OP is occasionally encountered in RA. The important strategies for preventing OP onset are to keep the disease activity of arthritis under control with DMARD treatment and to take precautions against infection as much as possible. If OP develops within 3 months of the initiation of DMARD treatment, it should be considered that the DMARD treatment could be associated with the OP onset. Differential diagnosis should be performed, especially in cases exhibiting a poor response to corticosteroids or progressive impairment of pulmonary function.

Acknowledgments I would like to thank Masanori Hanaoka and Tamiko Takemura for providing the chest imaging and the pulmonary pathology, respectively.

References

1. Kelmenson LB, Demoruelle MK, Deane KD. The complex role of the lung in the pathogenesis and clinical outcomes of rheumatoid arthritis. Curr Rheumatol Rep. 2016;18:69.
2. Baque-Juston M, Pellegrin A, Leroy S, Marquette CH, Padovani B. Organizing pneumonia: what is it? A conceptual approach and pictorial review. Diagn Interv Imaging. 2014;95:771–7.
3. Cordier JF. Cryptogenic organising pneumonia. Eur Respir J. 2006;28:422–46.
4. Doyle TJ, Lee JS, Dellaripa PF, Lederer JA, Matteson EL, Fischer A, Ascherman DP, Glassberg MK, Ryu JH, Danoff SK, Brown KK, Collard HR, Rosas IO. A roadmap to promote clinical and translational research in rheumatoid arthritis-associated interstitial lung disease. Chest. 2014;145:454–63.
5. Gabbay E, Tarala R, Will R, Carroll G, Adler B, Cameron D, Lake FR. Interstitial lung disease in recent onset rheumatoid arthritis. Am J Respir Crit Care Med. 1997;156:528–35.
6. Demoruelle MK, Mittoo S, Solomon JJ. Connective tissue disease-related interstitial lung disease. Best Pract Res Clin Rheumatol. 2016;30:39–52.
7. Kelly CA, Saravanan V, Nisar M, Arthanari S, Woodhead FA, Price-Forbes AN, Dawson J, Sathi N, Ahmad Y, Koduri G, Young A, Network BRILB. Rheumatoid arthritis-related interstitial lung disease: associations, prognostic factors and physiological and radiological characteristics—a large multicentre UK study. Rheumatology (Oxford). 2014;53:1676–82.
8. Okada H, Kurasawa K, Yamazaki R, Tanaka A, Arai S, Owada T, Maezawa R, Ishii Y. Clinical features of organizing pneumonia associated with rheumatoid arthritis. Mod Rheumatol. 2016;1–6.
9. Mori S, Koga Y, Sugimoto M. Organizing pneumonia in rheumatoid arthritis patients: a case-based review. Clin Med Insights Circ Respir Pulm Med. 2015;9:69–80.
10. Kawasumi H, Gono T, Tanaka E, Kaneko H, Kawaguchi Y, Yamanaka H. Clinical characteristics and cytokine profiles of organizing pneumonia in patients with rheumatoid arthritis treated with or without biologics. J Rheumatol. 2016;43:738–44.

11. Ulubaş B, Sahin G, Ozer C, Aydin O, Ozgür E, Apaydin D. Bronchiolitis obliterans organizing pneumonia associated with sulfasalazine in a patient with rheumatoid arthritis. Clin Rheumatol. 2004;23:249–51.
12. Kajiya T, Kuroda A, Hokonohara D, Tei C. Radiographic appearance of bronchiolitis obliterans organizing pneumonia (BOOP) developing during Bucillamine treatment for rheumatoid arthritis. Am J Med Sci. 2006;332:39–42.
13. Cho SK, IH O, Park CK, Bae SC, Sung YK. Etanercept induced organizing pneumonia in a patient with rheumatoid arthritis. Rheumatol Int. 2012;32:1055–7.
14. Ikegawa K, Hanaoka M, Ushiki A, Yamamoto H, Kubo K. A case of organizing pneumonia induced by tocilizumab. Intern Med. 2011;50:2191–3.
15. https://www.uptodate.com/contents/cryptogenic-organizing-pneumonia.
16. Roberton BJ, Hansell DM. Organizing pneumonia: a kaleidoscope of concepts and morphologies. Eur Radiol. 2011;21:2244–54.
17. Cordier JF. Organising pneumonia. Thorax. 2000;55:318–28.
18. King TE, Mortenson RL. Cryptogenic organizing pneumonitis. The North American experience. Chest. 1992;102:8S–13S.
19. Cazzato S, Zompatori M, Baruzzi G, Schiattone ML, Burzi M, Rossi A, Ratta L, Terzuolo G, Falcone F, Poletti V. Bronchiolitis obliterans-organizing pneumonia: an Italian experience. Respir Med. 2000;94:702–8.
20. Forlani S, Ratta L, Bulgheroni A, Cascina A, Paschetto E, Cervio G, Luinetti O, Fietta AM, Meloni F. Cytokine profile of broncho-alveolar lavage in BOOP and UIP. Sarcoidosis Vasc Diffuse Lung Dis. 2002;19:47–53.
21. Aguiar M, Felizardo M, Mendes AC, Moniz D, Sotto-Mayor R, Bugalho de Almeida A. Organising pneumonia—the experience of an outpatient clinic of a central hospital. Rev Port Pneumol. 2010;16:369–89.
22. Katayama H, Yokoyama A, Hamada H, Irita J, Kadowaki T, Ito R, Onishi H, Watanabe A, Mutsukado Y, Kukita H, Hiwada K, Higaki J. [Successful treatment of bronchiolitis obliterans organizing pneumonia with cyclosporin and steroids]. Nihon Kokyuki Gakkai Zasshi. 2003;41: 551–5.
23. Schlesinger C, Koss MN. The organizing pneumonias: a critical review of current concepts and treatment. Treat Respir Med. 2006;5:193–206.
24. Vignali DA, Kuchroo VK. IL-12 family cytokines: immunological playmakers. Nat Immunol. 2012;13:722–8.
25. Romagnani S. The Th1/Th2 paradigm. Immunol Today. 1997;18: 263–6.
26. Cheng CC, Lee YF, Lin NN, CL W, Tung KC, Chiu YT. Bronchiolitis obliterans organizing pneumonia in Swine associated with porcine circovirus type 2 infection. J Biomed Biotechnol. 2011;2011: 245728.

13 Acute Pulmonary Infiltrates in Patients with Rheumatoid Arthritis: Differential Diagnosis and Management

Sadatomo Tasaka

Abstract

Patients with rheumatoid arthritis (RA) sometimes experience acute onset of respiratory symptoms with pulmonary infiltrates on chest roentgenogram, potentially leading to respiratory failure. Because many of RA patients have pre-existing lung complications, such as interstitial lung disease (ILD) and airway disease, and receive various immune-modulating drugs, it is often difficult to make a correct diagnosis. The differential diagnosis includes acute exacerbation of RA-associated ILD, drug-induced occurrence or exacerbation of ILD, and respiratory infection. There are many diagnostic tools, such as radiological examination, laboratory tests, bronchoalveolar lavage, and lung biopsy, but, in most cases, none of these tools has enough power to make a diagnosis by itself, requiring a combined diagnostic approach. Once an RA patient is diagnosed with acute exacerbation of ILD or rapidly progressive ILD, ventilatory management and drug treatment should be initiated immediately in accordance with those of acute exacerbation of idiopathic interstitial pneumonias. In case of bacterial pneumonia in RA patients receiving immune-modulating agents, it should be treated as healthcare-associated pneumonia, considering risk factor for *Pseudomonas aeruginosa* infection. *Pneumocystis jirovecii* pneumonia in RA patients is characterized by an abrupt onset of respiratory insufficiency, requiring a speedy diagnosis using PCR and serum β-D-glucan measurement.

Keywords

Acute exacerbation • Acute pulmonary infiltrates • Drug-induced lung disease • Healthcare-associated pneumonia • *Pneumocystis jirovecii* pneumonia

13.1 Introduction

Most of lung complications in patients with rheumatoid arthritis (RA), such as interstitial lung disease (ILD) and airway disease, develop gradually, but RA patients sometimes experience acute onset of respiratory symptoms with pulmonary infiltrates on chest roentgenogram, potentially leading to respiratory failure [1, 2]. Lung complications of acute or subacute onset (within 3 months) in patients with RA are divided into two categories: (1) acute exacerbation of pre-existing lung complications of RA and (2) those related to RA treatment, including drug-induced lung disease (DILD) and opportunistic infection [3]. Since clinical and radiological features of these two categories are often similar, it may be difficult to make a correct diagnosis.

The incidence of ILD occurring in RA patients was seven times higher than that for other connective tissue diseases [4]. Using high-resolution computed tomography (HRCT), interstitial abnormalities are frequently observed even in patients with early RA, although most of them have no respiratory symptoms [5]. Unless the respiratory system has been precisely evaluated with imaging and pulmonary function tests, pre-existing lung complications may not be recognized, which makes it difficult to discriminate acute exacer-

S. Tasaka, M.D.
Department of Respiratory Medicine, Hirosaki University Graduate School of Medicine, Aomori, Japan
e-mail: tasaka@hirosaki-u.ac.jp

T. Gono et al. (eds.), *Lung Disease Associated with Rheumatoid Arthritis*, https://doi.org/10.1007/978-981-10-6750-1_13

bation from rapid development of lung complications. Furthermore, two or more disease processes may coexist in an RA patient complaining respiratory symptoms. For example, an RA patient with DILD who receives steroid treatment may develop an opportunistic infection. In this chapter, clinical diagnosis and management of acute pulmonary infiltrates in patients with RA will be illustrated.

13.2 Acute Exacerbation of Interstitial Lung Disease

Acute exacerbation of ILD is generally defined as rapidly deteriorating respiratory symptoms within a 30-day period with evidence of new infiltrates and exclusion of an identifiable cause, such as respiratory infection, heart failure, and pneumothorax [6]. An often, overlooked possibility for clinical worsening is environmental or occupational exposures. There are clinical characteristics that increase the likelihood of each of these possibilities in any given patient, and all of these need to be explored before determining that a clinical worsening is attributable to the underlying RA-ILD. The absolute risk of an acute exacerbation is not well established, but based on the limited data of acute exacerbations in collagen vascular diseases (CVD), possibly as many as 20% of patients with RA-ILD will experience an acute exacerbation with a 1-year incidence as high as 2.58% [7]. By the time patients present to the hospital, there may have developed severe hypoxemia, possibly leading to a fatal outcome [7, 8].

Clinical features of acute exacerbation of CVD-associated ILD are characterized by rapidly deteriorating respiratory symptoms, such as dyspnea and cough [7]. Fine crackles are usually evident and coarse crackles may be present. The most conspicuous finding of HRCT at the onset of acute exacerbation was newly developed bilateral ground-glass opacity (GGO) that is observed in 100% of the patients (Fig. 13.1) [7]. GGO is often patchy and distributed with a panlobular pattern, which is rarely observed in acute exacerbation of idiopathic pulmonary fibrosis (IPF). Consolidation, which is superimposed on the bibasilar reticular abnormalities, is also observed in many of the patients [7]. In addition, honeycombing and traction bronchiectasis, which are associated with the underlying ILD, may exist in some of the patients.

In case of acute exacerbation of RA-ILD, serum levels of lactate dehydrogenase (LDH) and C-reactive protein (CRP) are elevated, which may be associated with the severity of lung inflammation and tissue damage. Krebs von den Lungen-6 (KL-6), a glycoprotein expressed by type II pneumocytes and epithelial cells, is a serum marker that can be related to the disease activity of ILD. Serum concentration of surfactant protein-D (SP-D) is another useful marker to detect active ILD. SP-D is elevated in accordance with proliferation of type II pneumocytes and destruction of the basement membrane of alveolar structures in patients with ILD. Both KL-6 and SP-D have been shown to be elevated in patients with RA-ILD [7]. Although KL-6 has relatively poor sensitivity in RA-ILD, it is correlated with reticular opacities and honeycombing on HRCT images [9, 10]. In case of acute exacerbation, further increases in the levels of these serum markers are usually observed. Hypoxemia is apparent in many of those with acute exacerbation of RA-ILD, but it may not be significant in early stage of the disease.

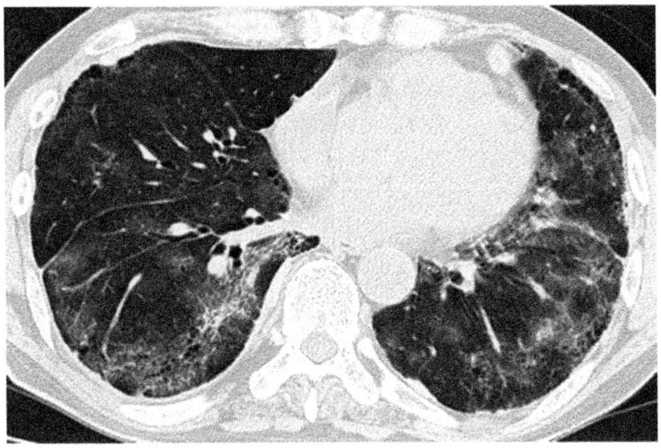

Fig. 13.1 HRCT appearance of acute exacerbation of RA-associated interstitial lung disease. A 61-year-old male patient who is a heavy smoker complained of fever, dry cough, and general fatigue. The findings included ground-glass opacity that was superimposed on preexisting some honeycombing and traction bronchiectasis

Once a patient with RA-ILD develops acute exacerbation, ventilatory management and drug treatment should be initiated immediately in accordance with those of acute exacerbation of idiopathic interstitial pneumonias. Patients with ILD and acute respiratory failure treated by intubation and mechanical ventilation may have an increased risk of ventilator-associated lung injury and pneumonia. Therefore, it is expected that noninvasive ventilation (NIV), which precludes the use of intubation, could lead to decreased rates of complications and mortality among these patients. At present, however, there are no sufficient evidences to support the use of NIV for patients with acute respiratory failure due to RA-ILD. High-flow nasal cannula (HFNC), in which heated and humidified inspired gas with a high flow rate (up to 60 L/min) enables a rise in the fraction of inspired oxygen (FIO_2) to 1.0, has been shown to be useful for the management of acute exacerbation of ILD [11].

In addition to respiratory management, high doses of corticosteroids and immunosuppressant are often administered, although there has been no evidence for the effectiveness of these therapies. In spite of these intensive care and drug treatment, the outcome of acute exacerbation of RA-ILD is usually not favorable [7]. Park and coworkers described three cases of acute exacerbation of biopsy-confirmed RA-ILD, all of whom were deceased [12]. All the three patients had undergone surgical lung biopsy, and pathologic diagnosis was usual interstitial pneumonia (UIP) [12]. Suda and colleagues reported that 6 (7%) of 83 patients with CVD-associated interstitial pneumonia developed acute exacerbation and that 5 (83%) of them expired [7]. In contrast, a recent report by Toyoda and coworkers described better prognosis [13]. They reported a 90-day survival as high as 70% after acute exacerbation of CVD-associated ILD and concluded that immunosuppressant for RA-ILD before onset of acute exacerbation might improve the outcome [13]. Taken together, acute exacerbation of RA-ILD is characterized by poor prognosis, although early introduction of immunosuppressant may exert some beneficial effects. Similar to IPF, RA-ILD with pathological pattern of UIP may be associated with a worse outcome, but it remains to be determined whether the pathological pattern is associated with the frequency of acute exacerbation and its outcome in patients with RA-ILD.

13.3 Drug-Induced Lung Disease

Drug-induced pulmonary disease is an important consideration in the differential diagnosis of RA patients under medical treatment who present with acute respiratory symptoms [14]. For the appropriate diagnosis and management of DILD, we need to understand the characteristics of lung diseases that are associated with the individual agents for RA treatment and the spectrum of potential comorbid disease processes.

Most patients with active RA are on disease-modifying antirheumatic drugs (DMARDs) or immunosuppressant therapy to treat the joint manifestations. Theoretically, these drugs could protect the lungs by reducing production of inflammatory mediators, which are known to be involved in the pathogenesis of various pulmonary complications of RA [14]. In addition, a growing number of RA patients are administered with TNF inhibitors and other biological agents. Although methotrexate (MTX), one of the most frequently prescribed DMARDs, is extensively reported medication associated with pulmonary drug toxicity, almost every medication available for the treatment of RA has been implicated in the development of pneumonitis [14, 15]. It is, however, often difficult to prove causality because patients with RA are prone to lung complications from infection, other medications, and the disease itself. In addition, ILD or airway disease that progresses while on a drug treatment may represent progressive disease rather than an effect of the implicated medication.

The clinical manifestations of DILD are variable, depending upon the type and localization of the pathological changes that can be elucidated by HRCT. DILD with rapidly progressive pulmonary infiltrates is usually characterized by a histopathological pattern of diffuse alveolar damage (DAD) or organizing pneumonia (OP). HRCT in early DAD typically shows heterogeneous foci of consolidation and GGO with a gravitationally dependent gradient (Fig. 13.2). Air bronchograms and small pleural effusions are common. With organization and fibrosis, reticulation and traction bronchiectasis may develop [16]. Typical HRCT findings of OP include airspace consolidation in a subpleural distribution (Fig. 13.3). GGO may also be present, often with a bilateral asymmetric distribution. The reverse halo sign may be present in almost 20% of cases. Centrilobular nodules and GGO suggest pathological changes like hypersensitivity pneumonia.

DILD may be asymptomatic and, when symptomatic, it can develop days to years, possibly leading to respiratory failure. Symptoms include cough, dyspnea, and low-grade fever. Lung auscultation may reveal focal or bibasilar inspiratory crackles but is often normal. Skin eruption may be observed, which is suggestive of drug-induced process.

Due to its diverse clinical presentation, DILD is often a diagnosis of exclusion. The diagnostic approach includes a combination of examinations designed to exclude respiratory infection, RA-ILD, and heart failure. It is also important to elucidate the timing of symptoms relative to drug initiation, eosinophilia in peripheral blood and/or bronchoalveolar lavage (BAL) fluid, and other features suggestive of a drug-induced process. Empiric drug discontinuation is an important diagnostic approach. Pre-existing lung disease, which is not only associated with RA but also independent of RA,

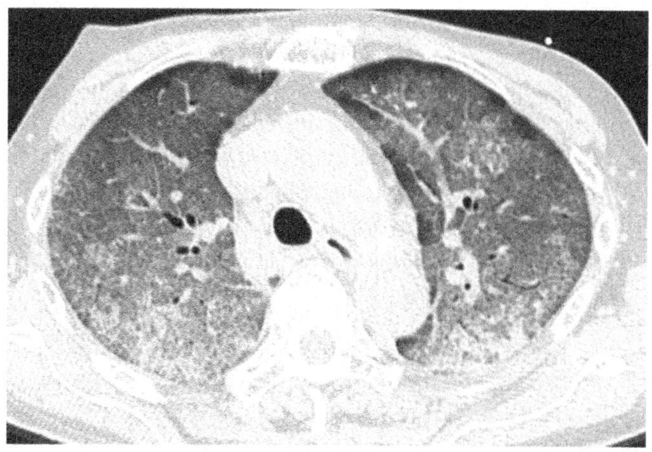

Fig. 13.2 HRCT appearance of drug-induced interstitial lung disease. A 71-year-old female patient who had been receiving methotrexate and etanercept complained of dyspnea. HRCT shows bilateral GGO and consolidation with a gravitationally dependent gradient, suggesting a histopathological pattern of diffuse alveolar damage (DAD). Courtesy of Dr. H. Sakuraba

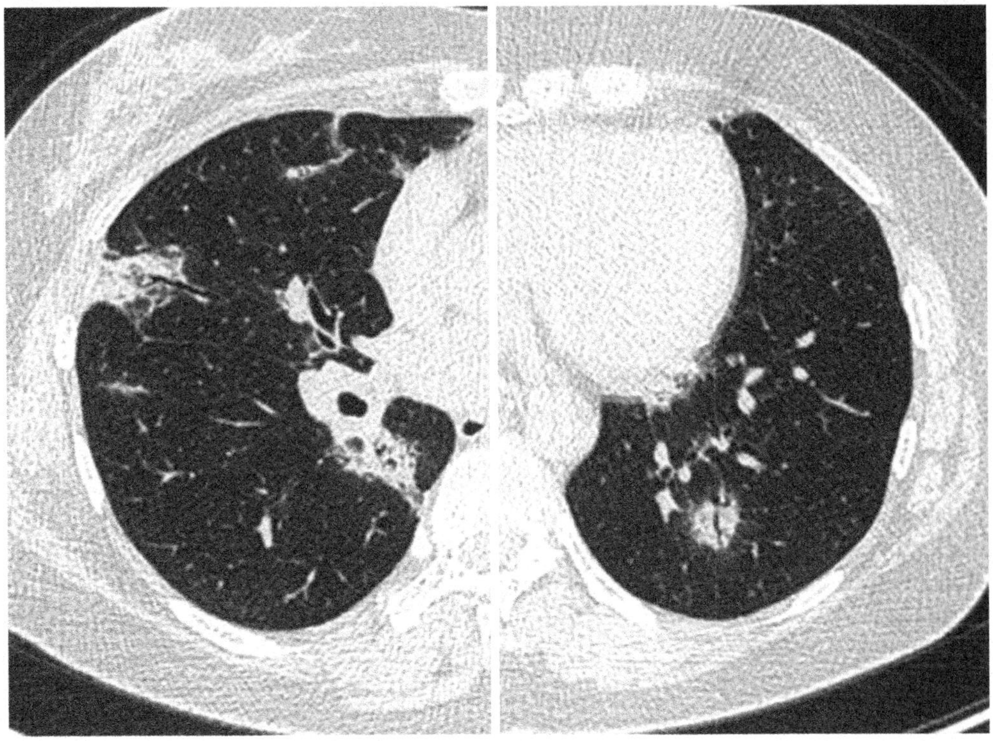

Fig. 13.3 HRCT appearance of drug-induced interstitial lung disease. A 46-year-old female patient who had been receiving etanercept complained of fever. HRCT shows patchy airspace consolidation in a subpleural distribution, suggesting a histopathological pattern of organizing pneumonia (OP). Courtesy of Dr. H. Sakuraba

such as asthma and emphysema, may modify the clinical presentation and results of examination and complicate determination of whether current symptoms are caused by a newly developed process or progression/exacerbation of a pre-existing one.

Laboratory testing is helpful to determine whether other disease processes contribute to the patient's respiratory compromise. Complete blood counts and differentials are informative to identify anemia and neutrophilia, which indicate alveolar hemorrhage and bacterial infection, respectively. Measurement of B-type natriuretic peptide (BNP) can be helpful in exclusion of heart failure as an etiology. Microbiological studies and CRP, procalcitonin, presepsin (soluble CD14 subtype), and other serological markers are also helpful in discriminating infectious causes [17]. Serum β-D-glucan is useful for ruling out *Pneumocystis* pneumonia (PCP) that can occur in RA patients receiving MTX or immunosuppressive agents [18].

Like acute exacerbation of RA-ILD, DILD is often associated with elevated levels of serum LDH, KL-6, and SP-D. Miyata and colleagues reported that monitoring of serum concentrations of KL-6 and SP-D is valuable in detecting the occurrence of MTX-associated ILD, even in RA patients with pre-existing ILD, and in evaluating the response to treatment [19]. Although serial assessment of these markers is informative in evaluating the activity of inflammatory and fibrotic process, it is not useful for discriminating DILD from other disease processes. Drug lymphocyte stimulation test (DLST) is a potentially useful diagnostic test in DILD. DLST verifies the growth of sensitized lymphocytes after a drug is used for antigen stimulation, confirming the presence of drug-sensitized lymphocytes [20]. While DLST has been widely used in the diagnosis of DILD in Japan, this is not the case in other countries. It should be noted that DLST can only detect the presence of sensitization but cannot predict whether the sensitization is associated with the development of DILD [21].

A chest radiograph is obtained to assess the pattern and extent of disease, but HRCT of the chest is much more informative for precise evaluation and differential diagnosis [22, 23]. Various radiological patterns of DILD have been described, including patchy or diffuse, unilateral or bilateral reticular opacities, GGO, consolidation, and pulmonary nodules with or without cavitation [24, 25]. Cleverley and colleagues reported that HRCT interpretation and histological diagnosis were concordant in only 45% of patients with DILD [22]. HRCT may be of limited value in determining the histological pattern and prognosis in many cases of DILD.

After review of clinical findings, laboratory data, and chest imaging, bronchoscopy with BAL may be considered to exclude other processes such as infection, diffuse alveolar hemorrhage, or amyloidosis secondary to RA [26]. In case of opportunistic infection, BAL is also useful in identifying the pathogen, which enables us to initiate optimal antibiotics. Although there are no specific findings of BAL for DILD, cell counts in the lavage fluid are usually increased. The pattern of cellularity is nonspecific. Increased lymphocyte counts in the lavage fluid are common, but eosinophilia or neutrophilia may be observed [26, 27]. Thus, the main role of bronchoscopy is to exclude alternative diagnoses.

Empiric withdrawal of the implicated drug is a key procedure not only for diagnosis but also for treatment. In general, DILD often regresses upon withdrawal of the responsible medication, but lung fibrosis and traction bronchiectasis are usually irreversible. After exclusion of infection, an immediate response to treatment with systemic corticosteroid may be a distinguishing feature of DILD. DILD often responds better to steroid therapy than ILD associated with RA itself.

Lung biopsy is usually not required, and many patients may be too unwell to undergo this invasive procedure. Combination of the clinical picture, radiological appearance, and BAL findings excluding infection are usually robust enough to make a biopsy unnecessary, especially in patients who respond quickly to discontinuation of the suspicious drug. In contrast, a lung biopsy is indicated when the patient has progressive disease and the causes of the pathological changes are uncertain. A lung biopsy is also considered when lymphoproliferative disease, sarcoidosis, or mycobacterial infection remains to be ruled out. Lung biopsy rarely establishes an antirheumatic agent as the definitive cause of the pathological changes of the lungs, because there are no pathognomonic findings for DILD, and histologic criteria for DILD have not been established [28]. However, when available, lung histopathology can characterize the histopathologic pattern, such as lymphocytic, granulomatous, eosinophilic, or organizing pneumonia or DAD, which may help to guide therapy or to predict patient prognosis. For example, lymphocyte-dominant infiltration of the lung suggests better response to steroid treatment.

The differentiation between a drug reaction, underlying RA-ILD, infection, and heart failure may be difficult due to significant overlap in the clinical features. In addition, many of the pulmonary reactions to drugs used for the treatment of RA are rare. An online repository of DILD is available to help identify potential offending medications (Pneumotox.com) [29].

13.3.1 Methotrexate

MTX is the most common first-line agent used to treat RA for prevention of joint destruction. A possible link between this medication and lung disease was first reported in 1983; since then many more cases have been reported [30, 31]. Acute or subacute pneumonitis has been well described in the literature, with a variable incidence ranging from 0.86 to 6.9% in MTX-treated patients, with higher-dose MTX more likely to be associated with pulmonary toxicity [32]. MTX pneumonitis typically occurs within the first year of treatment, suggesting a hypersensitivity reaction as its pathogenesis [33, 34]. Symptoms include dyspnea and nonproductive cough with/without systemic symptoms. Radiological findings are relatively nonspecific, with diffuse pulmonary opacities or patchy consolidation. Typically, HRCT shows bilateral GGO distributed in a panlobular or mosaic pattern (Fig. 13.4) [35]. Chest radiographs may be normal especially in the early stages of disease. New appearance or development of pulmonary nodules has also been shown to be associated with MTX [35]. It was also reported that MTX can be responsible for pleural effusions [30]. It should be noted that these radiological findings can be observed in tuberculosis and other respiratory infections.

BAL and lung biopsy are more helpful in ruling out infection and other alternative causes than in establishing the diagnosis of MTX pneumonitis. In patients with MTX pneumonitis, lung pathology typically reveals poorly formed non-necrotising granulomas and scattered eosinophils, which is rarely observed in RA-ILD [30, 34, 36]. DAD can be observed, which suggests poor prognosis.

Differentiation of MTX pneumonitis from acute respiratory infection is not always easy, even with the widely accepted diagnostic criteria [37]. In case of rapidly progressive disease without eosinophilia, it may be necessary to treat for both conditions, namely, combination of antibiotics and discontinuation of MTX. In patients with unilateral shadows and leukocytosis, infection is more likely, suggesting prompt initiation of antibiotics. In addition, measurement of serum KL-6 and SP-D has been shown to be useful for the detection and monitoring of MTX pneumonitis [19, 38]. Although SP-D levels can be elevated during lung infec-

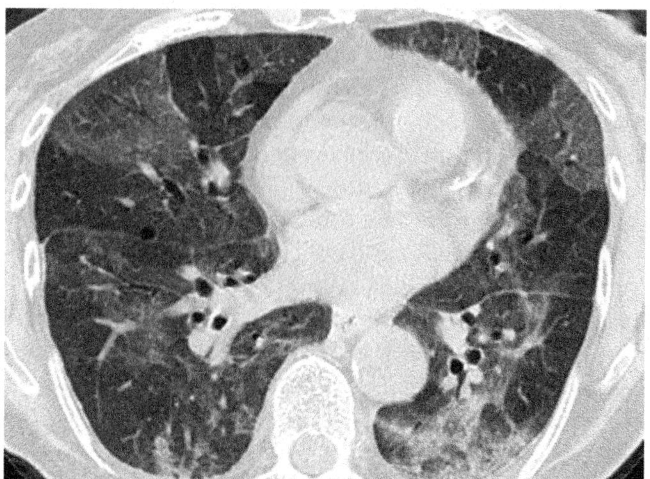

Fig. 13.4 HRCT appearance of methotrexate pneumonitis. A 70-year-old female patient who had been receiving methotrexate and prednisolone complained of fever and dry cough. HRCT shows bilateral GGO distributed in a panlobular manner; that is, GGO was sharply demarcated from the adjacent normal lung by interlobular septa. Courtesy of Dr. H. Tokuda

tion, KL-6 may be useful for discriminating between MTX pneumonitis and respiratory infection [19]. In case radiological findings and elevated KL-6 levels indicate MTX pneumonitis, reversal of the effects of MTX with folinic acid may be useful.

Treatment consists of stopping the medication; most patients will have clinical improvement within days with radiological improvement over the course of several weeks. In case of refractory disease or respiratory insufficiency, corticosteroids may be administered. Unless MTX is necessary for the control of RA, rechallenging with MTX after recovery is generally not recommended. The recurrence rate of MTX pneumonitis has been reported to be around 25% [36]. Mortality estimates from MTX pneumonitis vary but are around 20% [36, 39].

13.3.2 Biological Agents

Biological agents that target and block the actions of cytokines or molecules that play major roles in inflammation have now been widely used in treatment settings of various immune-mediated inflammatory diseases, such as CVD, inflammatory bowel diseases, and autoimmune skin diseases. Although biological agents have remarkable therapeutic effects on joint manifestations of RA, various adverse events have also been documented through a number of clinical studies and the post-marketing surveillances (PMS) [40–46].

Like MTX and other DMARDs, TNF inhibitors and other biological agents have been associated with new onset of ILD or worsening of pre-existing ILD, although clear causality has been difficult to prove. There have been many reports of DILD associated with biologics approved for the treatment of RA [43–52]. Perez-Alvarez and colleagues evaluated 122 cases of new-onset or exacerbated ILD in the setting of TNF inhibitor use, including 108 in those with RA [47]. Of note, 63% of these patients had been treated with MTX, and 38% had pre-existing ILD [47]. Fifteen (29%) patients who died were aged >65 years and had prior ILD, with longer duration of ILD being associated with risk of death [47]. In a recent cohort study, Curtis and colleagues evaluated 11,219 patients with RA who were exposed to biologics and reported the incidence rates of ILD ranging from 4.0 to 12.2 per 1000 person-years [48]. They also revealed that older age, male sex, and another pulmonary condition were associated with increased incidence of ILD [48]. However, it remains controversial whether biological agents are associated with increased risk of new-onset or exacerbated ILD. A large cohort study of 8417 patients with autoimmune disease showed no significant difference in the incidence of ILD between those who were treated with anti-TNF therapy (0.5%) and those who did not (0.3%) [4]. In addition, a systematic literature review revealed that 41.9% of the patients suffered from RA-ILD before experiencing acute worsening of ILD potentially related to TNF inhibitors [30]. These findings may challenge the causal relationship between ILD and the agents.

Nakashita and colleagues evaluated 58 RA patients with pre-existing ILD and revealed that the incidence of exacerbation of RA-ILD was significantly higher with TNF inhibitors (30.4%) compared to tocilizumab and abatacept [53]. In contrast, Curtis and colleagues reported that there were no significant differences in the risk of ILD between TNF inhibitors and other classes of biologics [48]. It remains to be determined whether any specific class of biologics is associated with higher risk of the new occurrence of ILD or worsening of pre-existing ILD in RA patients.

A variety of mechanisms for biologics-induced ILD have been proposed. Theoretically, these agents should even have a therapeutic effect on RA-ILD since TNF and other targeted molecules are known to play an important role in the pathogenesis of ILD [15]. To date, however, no definite etiology has been established.

According to PMS in Japan, the average onset of ILD ranged from 69 to 97 days after initiation of biologics [43–46]. In contrast, a Spanish group reported that ILD appeared a mean of 26 ± 5 weeks after the introduction of TNF inhibitors [47]. Symptoms at presentation of ILD include dyspnea (32–86%), cough (31–38%), and fever (25–44%) [47, 54]. In addition, malaise, pleuritic pain, and hemoptysis may be observed.

In most cases, HRCT shows GGO, but reticular opacity and consolidation can also be seen. Perez-Alvarez and colleagues evaluated HRCT findings in 36 cases of ILD induced or exacerbated by TNF inhibitors and reported that GGO was observed in 31 cases (86%), reticular nodular pattern in 7 (19%), and reticular pattern in 5 (14%) [47]. In case of RA patients with pre-existing ILD, honeycomb changes and reticular opacity can be observed.

Like other types of ILDs, serum levels of KL-6 and SP-D are elevated in most patients with ILD induced or exacerbated by biological agents. However, KL-6 levels were normal in 34% and 31% of RA patients with ILD during treatment with etanercept and adalimumab, respectively [44, 45]. In addition, KL-6 fluctuates in RA patients being treated with TNF inhibitors or MTX, regardless of the emergence or exacerbation of ILD [55]. A diagnosis of active ILD should not be made based solely upon the elevated levels of serum markers. Lung pathology could show a variety of findings, such as UIP, nonspecific interstitial pneumonia (NSIP), OP, DAD, and exacerbation of pre-existing ILD [30, 47, 56, 57].

After the occurrence or exacerbation of ILD, it is important to differentiate between respiratory infection, pulmonary manifestation of RA, and DILD. Particularly, the possibility of PCP should be intensively investigated in

RA patients developing acute-onset diffuse ILD while receiving biologics, partly because HRCT findings are quite similar [58].

When emergence or exacerbation of ILD was considered, the biological agents should be withdrawn immediately. There has been no evidence of treatment effect of corticosteroids on ILD induced or exacerbated by biologics. In case of respiratory insufficiency or poor response to the withdrawal of the biologics, corticosteroids are usually administered [47, 52, 54]. There has been a report of a small number of cases of ILD induced or exacerbated by TNF inhibitors that were treated with adjunctive immunosuppressive agents or intravenous immunoglobulins [47].

According to the British registry, the mortality in patients with RA-ILD is not increased following treatment with anti-TNF therapy compared with traditional DMARDs [59]. Spanish investigators reported a mortality rate ranging from 29 to 32% in patients treated with TNF inhibitors [47]. According to PMS in Japan, the mortality rates range from 7.5 to 20% [43–46]. The reported mortality was higher in patients treated with tocilizumab (20%) compared with those treated with TNF inhibitors. It should be noted that many of the RA patients who receive biologics are already under treatment with MTX and/or corticosteroids, which makes it difficult to estimate the exact impact of biologics-associated ILD on the outcome.

13.4 Infectious Complications

Infection remains the leading cause of death in RA, accounting for 20–30% of the mortality [1, 2]. The respiratory infections in RA patients are now more likely to be acute rather than chronic. Namely, whereas the incidence of bronchiectasis has fallen sharply, up to 2% of the RA population develop an acute respiratory infection requiring hospitalization annually [60]. Bronchiectasis and other comorbidities are found in 92% of RA patients with bacterial pneumonia, indicating that they could contribute to the development of lung infection [61]. In addition to the underlying ILD and airway diseases, the higher incidence of respiratory infection in RA patients could be associated with various therapeutic agents modulating host defense. While patients on MTX or other DMARDs are at no greater risk of developing infection than other RA patients, glucocorticoids have been related to increased risks of lower respiratory tract infections, including influenza [3, 62–64]. Chronic prednisone use increases the risk of hospitalization for pneumonia in a dose-dependent fashion with doses greater than 10 mg/day more than doubling the risk [3]. In addition, an increased incidence of serious infections following the administration of TNF inhibitors and other biologics has been reported [65–68]. The most common sites of infection associated with the administration of biological agents include the respiratory tract (approximately 50%), skin and soft tissue (20–25%), urinary tract, gastrointestinal tract, sepsis, and bone and joints [43–46].

In patients with pneumonia, tachypnea and hypotension are usually markers of severe disease and indicate an increased risk of death [69], often associated with positive blood cultures and raised serum lactate. In case such patients meet criteria of sepsis, they should be promptly referred to an intensive care unit and may need ventilator management. Failure to mount an appropriate leucocytosis is another major risk factor for death [32].

Infectious complications in RA patients treated with immune-modulating agents are not always opportunistic infections. Takayanagi and colleagues evaluated pulmonary infections in 149 RA patients and identified 46 patients with bacterial pneumonia, 5 with PCP, and 9 with lung abscess [70]. In patients under steroid treatment, 65.2% of the pulmonary infections were bacterial pneumonia, including those caused by common pathogens such as *Streptococcus pneumoniae*. In contrast, 80% of the infections were PCP in those receiving MTX [70]. The mechanism of the difference remains unclear.

13.4.1 Bacterial Pneumonia

A higher incidence of pneumonia has been demonstrated in RA patients compared with the general population, although it is difficult to understand the exact prevalence of lung infections related to RA medications as the disease itself is known to be a predisposing risk factor for infection [71]. Pneumonia is the leading cause of death in subjects receiving biological agents, accounting for 21.1% of deaths, while it accounted for 12.1% of deaths in RA patients who were not receiving biological agents in Japan [72]. The standardized mortality rate of pneumonia compared with the general population was 4.19 [72].

In RA patients with pneumonia, *Pseudomonas aeruginosa* was frequently identified, especially in those with pre-existing bronchiectasis. In addition, there have been some reports describing *Legionella pneumophila* as an important causative organism in patients treated with TNF inhibitors [73, 74]. Other pathogens that should be anticipated in RA patients administered biologics include *S. pneumoniae*, *Haemophilus influenzae*, *Staphylococcus aureus*, *Moraxella* spp., *Klebsiella pneumoniae*, and atypical pathogens, such as *Mycoplasma pneumoniae* and *Chlamydophila pneumoniae*. It remains to be determined whether causative bacteria of pneumonia differ between RA patients and population without RA. Risk factors of pneumonia in RA patients receiving biologics include male sex, older age, Steinbrocker stage III or advanced, 10 years or longer of disease duration, comorbid respiratory disease, and concomitant use of corticosteroid [43–46].

Symptoms at presentation of pneumonia include fever, dyspnea, and cough. It should be noted that these symptoms can be masked or mitigated by biologics. For example, patients receiving tocilizumab, humanized antibody against IL-6 receptor, present with only minimal symptoms even when they developed severe pneumonia [75]. It is important to consider that, even if the initial symptoms are negligible or nonspecific, symptoms may rapidly exacerbate following the administration of biologic. In addition, it should be carefully evaluated whether the patient has dehydration, hypotension, or impairment of oxygenation or consciousness especially in the elderly with pneumonia.

The usual radiographic pattern of bacterial pneumonia is an airspace consolidation limited to one lobe or segment. Nevertheless, the pattern may be variable, which may be associated with the causative agent, timing of the examination, and underlying lung disease. If diffuse GGO is observed on chest radiograph or HRCT, PCP should be considered.

Laboratory tests may show leukocytosis and elevated CRP levels in serum. Again, it should be noted that CRP levels are hardly elevated in those receiving tocilizumab, an IL-6 receptor blocker. In such patients, procalcitonin may be preferred as a surrogate marker of bacterial infection [76].

In case of pneumonia in RA patients receiving biologics and other immunosuppressive agents, it should be treated as healthcare-associated pneumonia rather than community-acquired pneumonia. Cases should be classified into four groups (A–D) depending on the preferred setting of management and presence or absence of *P. aeruginosa* risk factors (Fig. 13.5) [77]. Risk factors for *P. aeruginosa* infection include antibiotic therapy within the past 90 days and underlying respiratory diseases. To prevent in-hospital transmis-

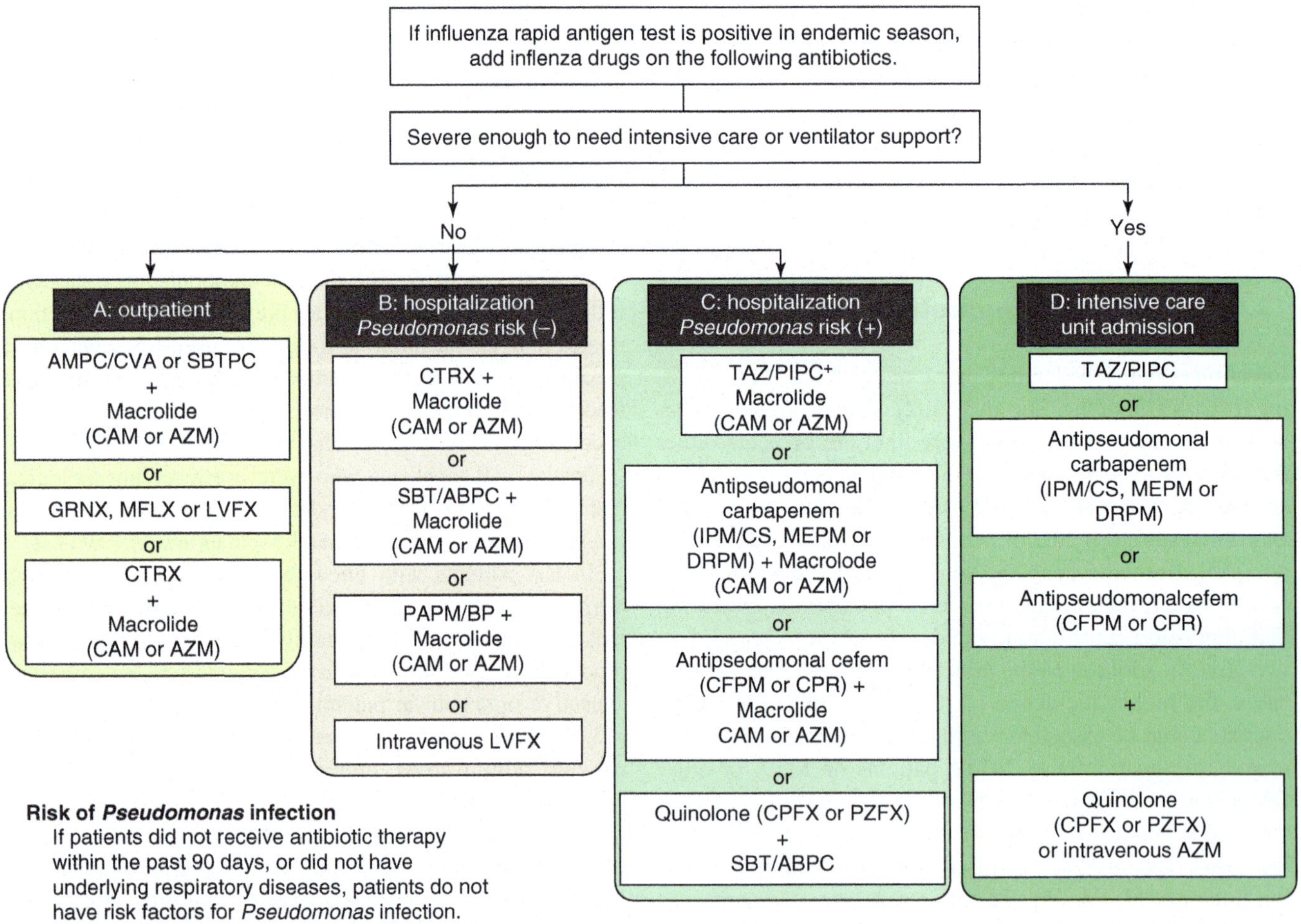

Fig. 13.5 Recommendations of antibiotic therapy against pneumonia under treatment with biological agents. Abbreviations: *AMPC/CVA* amoxicillin clavulanate, *SBTPC* sultamicillin, *CAM* clarithromycin, *AZM* azithromycin, *GRNX* garenoxacin, *MFLX* moxifloxacin, *LVFX* levofloxacin, *CTRX* ceftriaxone, *SBT/ABPC* sulbactam/ampicillin, *PAPM/BP* panipenem/betamipron, *TAZ/PIPC* tazobactam/piperacillin, *IPM/CS* imipenem/cilastatin, *MEPM* meropenem, *DRPM* doripenem, *CFPM* cefepime, *CPR* cefpirome, *CPFX* ciprofloxacin, *PZFX* pazufloxacin; (−), negative; (+), positive; +, add to. Adapted from Consensus statements for medical practice: Biological agents and lung disease by the Japanese Respiratory Society [77]

sion, a rapid test of influenza antigen should be considered in all pneumonia patients, especially when prevalent.

13.4.1.1 Group A: Outpatient Cases

This group consists of mild cases of pneumonia with no preexisting lung disease. Oral quinolones or other drugs against common bacteria, such as *S. pneumoniae*, as well as atypical pathogens, particularly *M. pneumoniae*, should be administered.

13.4.1.2 Group B: Hospitalization Cases without a Risk of *P. aeruginosa* Infection

This group consists of moderate-to-severe cases with no risk factors for *P. aeruginosa* infection. Intravenous levofloxacin or a combination of a macrolide and a broad-spectrum β-lactam antibiotic should be considered.

13.4.1.3 Group C: Hospitalization Cases with a Risk of *P. aeruginosa* Infection

This group consists of moderate-to-severe cases with risk factors for *P. aeruginosa* infection. A combination of an antipseudomonal β-lactam and a macrolide antibiotic or an injectable new quinolone antibiotic and sulbactam/ampicillin should be administered.

13.4.1.4 Group D: Severe and Very Severe Cases That Require Intensive Care Unit Management

Influenza virus was reported as the leading causative agent of very severe pneumonia in Japan, followed by *S. pneumoniae*, *L. pneumophila*, and *P. aeruginosa* [78]. Injectable antibiotics against these three bacterial strains should be chosen. For patients that test positive for influenza using a rapid diagnostic kit, injectable anti-influenza agent should also be administered.

13.4.2 Pneumocystis Pneumonia

PCP is a potentially life-threatening fungal infection that is seen in immunocompromised individuals. PCP used to be uncommon in patients with RA, with reported frequencies of 0.02% in RA patients, until the introduction of low-dose MTX in the 1980s [79]. As novel immune-modulating agents, such as MTX, tacrolimus, and biologics, were introduced for treatment of RA, a rising incidence of PCP has been noticed [80, 81]. In patients with systemic autoimmune diseases and those undergoing immunosuppressive therapy, *P. jirovecii* colonization has been reported [82, 83]. *Pneumocystis*-colonized individuals may not only serve as a reservoir for disease transmission but also pose a risk for developing PCP [84]. Mori and colleagues performed PCR for *P. jirovecii* DNA on respiratory specimens from 82 patients with RA and identified 9 (11%) as asymptomatic carriers [85]. Three among the nine carriers developed PCP within 1 month after the PCR testing, suggesting that a colonized individual can be at risk for rapid development of PCP.

Clinical features of PCP are quite different between HIV-infected patients and those without HIV infection. PCP in non-HIV patients is characterized by an abrupt onset of respiratory insufficiency [81]. In non-HIV patients, it takes about a week from the onset of fever and dry cough until the development of respiratory failure, whereas PCP in HIV-infected patients has a more gradual disease course that lasts for 2 weeks to 2 months. Respiratory insufficiency is usually more severe in non-HIV patients than in HIV-infected population. In non-HIV patients with PCP, the IL-8 levels in BAL fluid were higher than in HIV-infected patients and correlated with the oxygenation index [86]. The mortality rates of PCP range from 30 to 60% among non-HIV patients, whereas the rates are 10–20% among the HIV-infected population [87]. Compared to HIV-infected patients, non-HIV patients including those with RA are characterized by severe lung inflammation, which may be associated with excessive production of inflammatory mediators in the alveolar space, possibly leading to acute respiratory failure and poor prognosis.

Chest radiograph typically reveals bilateral or diffuse GGO, but it can be normal in those with mild disease. HRCT usually shows diffuse GGO with patchy distribution. In some patients with PCP, GGO is distributed in the subpleural lung parenchyma, whereas peripheral sparing of GGO occurs in others [88, 89]. Tokuda and colleagues compared the imaging features of PCP between AIDS patients and RA patients who are not receiving biologics [35]. In half the RA patients with PCP, HRCT revealed diffuse GGO distributed in a panlobular manner; that is, GGO was sharply demarcated from the adjacent normal lung by interlobular septa (Fig. 13.6a). The other half of the RA patients with PCP presented diffuse GGO without sharp demarcation, which is commonly observed in HIV-infected patients with PCP (Fig. 13.6b) [35]. In contrast, diffuse GGO distributed in a panlobular manner was rarely observed in PCP patients who received a biological agent for RA [58]. This difference in the HRCT patterns may result from difference in the host immune response. It should be noted that PCP can have a radiologic appearance that mimics RA-ILD with increased GGO superimposed on interstitial infiltrates, which may make the differential diagnosis difficult.

As *Pneumocystis* cannot readily be cultured in the laboratory, the microscopic demonstration of the organisms in respiratory specimens is required for the diagnosis of PCP. However, PCP patients without HIV infection are char-

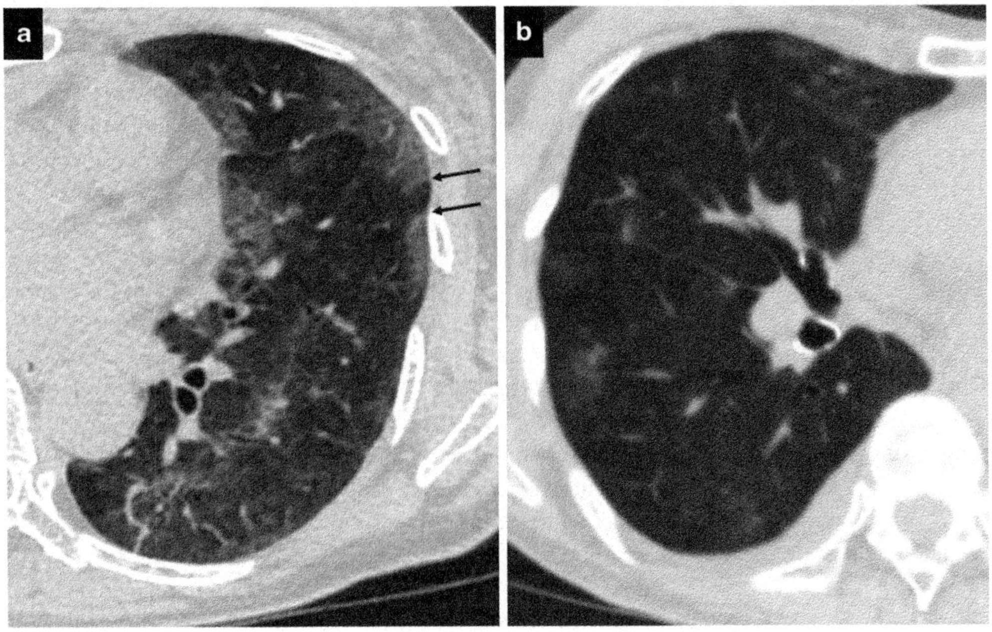

Fig. 13.6 HRCT appearance of *Pneumocystis jirovecii* pneumonia. (**a**) A 70-year-old female patient who had been receiving methotrexate and etanercept complained of fever and dry cough. HRCT shows diffuse GGO distributed in a panlobular manner; that is, GGO was sharply demarcated from the adjacent normal lung by interlobular septa (arrows). (**b**) A 76-year-old female who had been receiving methotrexate and prednisolone complained of fever and dyspnea. HRCT shows diffuse GGO without sharp demarcation

acterized by a lower burden of *Pneumocystis* in the lungs than those with AIDS [90]. In most cases of PCP in RA patients, *Pneumocystis* could not be identified microscopically, requiring PCR for the microbiological diagnosis [35].

Laboratory tests show elevated serum levels of CRP and LDH, as well as β-D-glucan that is derived from the cell wall of several fungi including *Pneumocystis*. Although it is not specific for *Pneumocystis*, measurement of serum β-D-glucan is of great diagnostic value with a sensitivity of 92% and a specificity of 86% [18].

Because of the high efficacy and the availability of oral and parenteral forms, trimethoprim-sulfamethoxazole (TMP-SMX) is the first-line agent for the treatment of mild to severe PCP. The recommended daily dose is TMP 15–20 mg/kg plus SMX 75–100 mg/kg [91]. This therapy is often complicated with adverse events, which include hepatotoxicity, nephrotoxicity, bone marrow depression, and skin rash, that sometimes become an obstacle to the completion of the treatment. Kameda and coworkers reported that 67% of the rheumatic patients treated with TMP-SMX experienced adverse events and 38% could not complete the treatment [58]. Intravenous pentamidine and oral atovaquone are the most studied drugs as alternatives to TMP-SMX.

PCP prophylaxis is often considered in patients taking immune-modulating medications. Harigai and colleagues evaluated 123 RA patients receiving infliximab and identified risk factors for PCP, including an age of at least 65 years, a daily dose of prednisolone of at least 6 mg, and the presence of coexisting pulmonary disease [92]. Patients with two or three risk factors had a significantly higher cumulative probability of PCP than did patients with no risk factors. Although there are no published guidelines, PCP prophylaxis should be considered in RA patients with such risk factors.

Conclusion

In RA patients presenting respiratory symptoms with acute pulmonary infiltrates on the chest images, acute exacerbation of RA-ILD, drug-induced occurrence or exacerbation of ILD, and respiratory infection should be considered. Since many of RA patients have underlying airway diseases or ILD, it could be difficult to make a correct diagnosis without precise evaluation of the respiratory system in advance. There are many diagnostic tools, such as radiological examination, laboratory tests, BAL, and lung biopsy, but, in most cases, none of these tools has enough power to make a diagnosis by itself, requiring a combined diagnostic approach. Also, precise evaluation of the respiratory system with HRCT and pulmonary function test is highly recommended prior to the introduction of DMARDs and biologics and other immunosuppressive agents.

Once an RA patient is diagnosed with acute exacerbation of ILD or rapidly progressive DILD, ventilatory management and drug treatment should be initiated immediately in accordance with those of acute exacerbation of idiopathic interstitial pneumonias. In case of bacterial pneumonia in RA patients receiving immune-modulating agents, it should be treated as health-care-associated pneumonia, considering risk factor for *P. aeruginosa* infection. PCP in non-HIV patients is characterized by an abrupt onset of respiratory insufficiency, requiring a speedy diagnosis using PCR and serum β-D-glucan measurement.

References

1. Turesson C, Jacobsson L, Bergström U. Extra-articular rheumatoid arthritis: prevalence and mortality. Rheumatology. 1999;38(7):668–74.
2. Suzuki A, Ohosone Y, Obana M, Mita S, Matsuoka Y, Irimajiri S, et al. Cause of death in 81 autopsied patients with rheumatoid arthritis. J Rheumatol. 1994;21(1):33–6.
3. Wolfe F, Caplan L, Michaud K. Treatment for rheumatoid arthritis and the risk of hospitalization for pneumonia: associations with prednisone, disease-modifying antirheumatic drugs, and anti-tumor necrosis factor therapy. Arthritis Rheum. 2006;54(2):628–34.
4. Herrinton LJ, Harrold LR, Liu L, Raebel MA, Taharka A, Winthrop KL, et al. Association between anti-TNF-α therapy and interstitial lung disease. Pharmacoepidemiol Drug Saf. 2013;22(4):394–402.
5. Mori S, Cho I, Koga Y, Sugimoto M. Comparison of pulmonary abnormalities on high-resolution computed tomography in patients with early versus longstanding rheumatoid arthritis. J Rheumatol. 2008;35(8):1513–21.
6. Collard HR, Moore BB, Flaherty KR, Brown KK, Kaner RJ, King TE Jr, et al. Acute exacerbations of idiopathic pulmonary fibrosis. Am J Respir Crit Care Med. 2007;176(7):636–43.
7. Suda T, Kaida Y, Nakamura Y, Enomoto N, Fujisawa T, Imokawa S, et al. Acute exacerbation of interstitial pneumonia associated with collagen vascular diseases. Respir Med. 2009;103(6):846–53.
8. Papiris SA, Manali ED, Kolilekas L, Kagouridis K, Triantafillidou C, Tsangaris I, et al. Clinical review: idiopathic pulmonary fibrosis acute exacerbations—unravelling Ariadne's thread. Crit Care. 2010;14(6):246.
9. Kinoshita F, Hamano H, Harada H, Kinoshita T, Igishi T, Hagino H, et al. Role of KL-6 in evaluating the disease severity of rheumatoid lung disease: comparison with HRCT. Respir Med. 2004;98(11):1131–7.
10. Nakajima H, Harigai M, Hara M, Hakoda M, Tokuda H, Sakai F, et al. KL-6 as a novel serum marker for interstitial pneumonia associated with collagen diseases. J Rheumatol. 2000;27(5):1164–70.
11. Horio Y, Takihara T, Niimi K, Komatsu M, Sato M, Tanaka J, et al. High-flow nasal cannula oxygen therapy for acute exacerbation of interstitial pneumonia: a case series. Respir Investig. 2016;54(2):125–9.
12. Park IN, Kim DS, Shim TS, Lim CM, Lee SD, Koh Y, et al. Acute exacerbation of interstitial pneumonia other than idiopathic pulmonary fibrosis. Chest. 2007;132(1):214–20.
13. Toyoda Y, Hanibuchi M, Kishi J, Kawano H, Morizumi S, Sato S, et al. Clinical features and outcome of acute exacerbation of interstitial pneumonia associated with connective tissue disease. J Med Investig. 2016;63(3–4):294–9.
14. Libby D, White DA. Pulmonary toxicity of drugs used to treat systemic autoimmune diseases. Clin Chest Med. 1998;19(4):809–21.
15. Jani M, Hirani N, Matteson EL, Dixon WG. The safety of biologic therapies in RA-associated interstitial lung disease. Nat Rev Rheumatol. 2014;10(5):284–94.
16. Obadina ET, Torrealba JM, Kanne JP. Acute pulmonary injury: high-resolution CT and histopathological spectrum. Br J Radiol. 2013;86(1027):20120614.
17. Tsujimoto K, Hata A, Fujita M, Hatachi S, Yagita M. Presepsin and procalcitonin as biomarkers of systemic bacterial infection in patients with rheumatoid arthritis. Int J Rheum Dis. 2016. https://doi.org/10.1111/1756-185X.12899.
18. Tasaka S, Hasegawa N, Kobayashi S, Yamada W, Nishimura T, Takeuchi T, et al. Serum indicators for the diagnosis of pneumocystis pneumonia. Chest. 2007;131(4):1173–80.
19. Miyata M, Sakuma F, Fukaya E, Kobayashi H, Rai T, Saito H, et al. Detection and monitoring of methotrexate-associated lung injury using serum markers KL-6 and SP-D in rheumatoid arthritis. Intern Med. 2002;41(6):467–73.
20. Pichler WJ, Tilch J. The lymphocyte transformation test in the diagnosis of drug hypersensitivity. Allergy. 2004;59(8):809–20.
21. Matsuno O, Okubo T, Hiroshige S, Takenaka R, Ono E, Ueno T, et al. Drug-induced lymphocyte stimulation test is not useful for the diagnosis of drug-induced pneumonia. Tohoku J Exp Med. 2007;212(1):49–53.
22. Cleverley JR, Screaton NJ, Hiorns MP, Flint JD, Müller NL. Drug-induced lung disease: high-resolution CT and histological findings. Clin Radiol. 2002;57(4):292–9.
23. Padley SP, Adler B, Hansell DM, Müller NL. High-resolution computed tomography of drug-induced lung disease. Clin Radiol. 1992;46(4):232–6.
24. Akira M, Ishikawa H, Yamamoto S. Drug-induced pneumonitis: thin-section CT findings in 60 patients. Radiology. 2002;224(3):852–60.
25. Ellis SJ, Cleverley JR, Müller NL. Drug-induced lung disease: high-resolution CT findings. AJR Am J Roentgenol. 2000;175(4):1019–24.
26. Costabel U, Uzaslan E, Guzman J. Bronchoalveolar lavage in drug-induced lung disease. Clin Chest Med. 2004;25(1):25–35.
27. Akoun GM, Cadranel JL, Milleron BJ, D'Ortho MP, Mayaud CM. Bronchoalveolar lavage cell data in 19 patients with drug-associated pneumonitis (except amiodarone). Chest. 1991;99(1):98–104.
28. Flieder DB, Travis WD. Pathologic characteristics of drug-induced lung disease. Clin Chest Med. 2004;25(1):37–45.
29. Camus P. The Drug-Induced Respiratory Disease Website. www.pneumotox.com. Accessed 7 Jan 2017.
30. Roubille C, Haraoui B. Interstitial lung diseases induced or exacerbated by DMARDS and biologic agents in rheumatoid arthritis: a systematic literature review. Semin Arthritis Rheum. 2014;43(5):613–26.
31. Lateef O, Shakoor N, Balk RA. Methotrexate pulmonary toxicity. Expert Opin Drug Saf. 2005;4(4):723–30.
32. Saravanan V, Kelly C. Drug-related pulmonary problems in patients with rheumatoid arthritis. Rheumatology (Oxford). 2006;45(7):787–9.
33. Cavagna L, Monti S, Grosso V, Boffini N, Scorletti E, Crepaldi G, et al. The multifaceted aspects of interstitial lung disease in rheumatoid arthritis. Biomed Res Int. 2013;2013:759760.
34. Barrera P, Laan RF, van Riel PL, Dekhuijzen PN, Boerbooms AM, van de Putte LB. Methotrexate-related pulmonary complications in rheumatoid arthritis. Ann Rheum Dis. 1994;53(7):434–9.
35. Tokuda H, Sakai F, Yamada H, Johkoh T, Imamura A, Dohi M, et al. Clinical and radiological features of *Pneumocystis* pneumonia in patients with rheumatoid arthritis, in comparison with methotrexate pneumonitis and *Pneumocystis* pneumonia in acquired immunodeficiency syndrome: a multicenter study. Intern Med. 2008;47(10):915–23.
36. Imokawa S, Colby TV, Leslie KO, Helmers RA. Methotrexate pneumonitis: review of the literature and histopathological findings in nine patients. Eur Respir J. 2000;15(2):373–81.
37. Searles G, McKendry RJ. Methotrexate pneumonitis in rheumatoid arthritis: potential risk factors. Four case reports and a review of the literature. J Rheumatol. 1987;14(6):1164–71.
38. Leth-Larsen R, Nordenbaek C, Tornoe I, Moeller V, Schlosser A, Koch C, et al. Surfactant protein D (SP-D) serum levels in patients with community-acquired pneumonia. Clin Immunol. 2003;108(1):29–37.
39. Kinder AJ, Hassell AB, Brand J, Brownfield A, Grove M, Shadforth MF. The treatment of inflammatory arthritis with methotrexate in clinical practice: treatment duration and incidence of adverse drug reactions. Rheumatology. 2005;44(1):61–6.
40. Picchianti Diamanti A, Germano V, Bizzi E, Laganà B, Migliore A. Interstitial lung disease in rheumatoid arthritis in the era of biologics. Pulm Med. 2011;2011:931342.

41. Roubille C, Martel-Pelletier J, Haraoui B, Tardif JC, Pelletier JP. Biologics and the cardiovascular system: a double-edged sword. Antiinflamm Antiallergy Agents Med Chem. 2013;12(1):68–82.
42. Hadjinicolaou AV, Nisar MK, Bhagat S, Parfrey H, Chilvers ER, Ostör AJ. Non-infectious pulmonary complications of newer biological agents for rheumatic diseases—a systematic literature review. Rheumatology (Oxford). 2011;50(12):2297–305.
43. Takeuchi T, Tatsuki Y, Nogami Y, Ishiguro N, Tanaka Y, Yamanaka H, et al. Postmarketing surveillance of the safety profile of infliximab in 5000 Japanese patients with rheumatoid arthritis. Ann Rheum Dis. 2008;67(2):189–94.
44. Koike T, Harigai M, Inokuma S, Inoue K, Ishiguro N, Ryu J, et al. Postmarketing surveillance of the safety and efectiveness of etanercept in Japan. J Rheumatol. 2009;36(5):898–906.
45. Koike T, Harigai M, Ishiguro N, Inokuma S, Takei S, Takeuchi T, et al. Safety and effectiveness of adalimumab in Japanese rheumatoid arthritis patients: postmarketing surveillance report of the first 3,000 patients. Mod Rheumatol. 2012;22(4):498–508.
46. Koike T, Harigai M, Inokuma S, Ishiguro N, Ryu J, Takeuchi T, et al. Postmarketing surveillance of tocilizumab for rheumatoid arthritis in Japan: interim analysis of 3881 patients. Ann Rheum Dis. 2011;70(12):2148–51.
47. Perez-Alvarez R, Perez-de-Lis M, Diaz-Lagares C, Pego-Reigosa JM, Retamozo S, Bove A, et al. Interstitial lung disease induced or exacerbated by TNF-targeted therapies: analysis of 122 cases. Semin Arthritis Rheum. 2011;41(2):256–64.
48. Curtis JR, Sarsour K, Napalkov P, Costa LA, Schulman KL. Incidence and complications of interstitial lung disease in users of tocilizumab, rituximab, abatacept and anti-tumor necrosis factor α agents, a retrospective cohort study. Arthritis Res Ther. 2015;17:319.
49. Kawashiri SY, Kawakami A, Sakamoto N, Ishimatsu Y, Eguchi K. A fatal case of acute exacerbation of interstitial lung disease in a patient with rheumatoid arthritis during treatment with tocilizumab. Rheumatol Int. 2012;32(12):4023–6.
50. Lager J, Hilberg O, Løkke A, Bendstrup E. Severe interstitial lung disease following treatment with certolizumab pegol: a case report. Eur Respir Rev. 2013;22(129):414–6.
51. Hagiwara K, Sato T, Takagi-Kobayashi S, Hasegawa S, Shigihara N, Akiyama O. Acute exacerbation of preexisting interstitial lung disease after administration of etanercept for rheumatoid arthritis. J Rheumatol. 2007;34(5):1151–4.
52. Sen S, Peltz C, Jordan K, Boes TJ. Infliximab-induced nonspecific interstitial pneumonia. Am J Med Sci. 2012;344(1):75–8.
53. Nakashita T, Motojima S, Fujio N, Jibatake A. The incidence of exacerbation of pre-existing interstitial lung disease (ILD) is higher in TNF blockers than in non-TNF blockers in RA. Arthritis Rheum. 2012;64(Suppl 10):1332. https://doi.org/10.1002/art.39064.
54. Ramos-Casals M, Perez-Alvarez R, Perez-de-Lis M, Xaubet A, Bosch X, BIOGEAS Study Group. Pulmonary disorders induced by monoclonal antibodies in patients with rheumatologic autoimmune diseases. Am J Med. 2011;124(5):386–94.
55. Harigai M, Takamura A, Atsumi T, Dohi M, Hirata S, Kameda H, et al. Elevation of KL-6 serum levels in clinical trials of tumor necrosis factor inhibitors in patients with rheumatoid arthritis: a report from the Japan College of Rheumatology Ad Hoc Committee for Safety of Biological DMARDs. Mod Rheumatol. 2013;23(2):284–96.
56. de Lauretis A, Veeraraghavan S, Renzoni E. Review series: aspects of interstitial lung disease: connective tissue disease-associated interstitial lung disease: how does it differ from IPF? How should the clinical approach differ? Chron Respir Dis. 2011;8(1):53–82.
57. Hallowell RW, Horton MR. Interstitial lung disease in patients with rheumatoid arthritis: spontaneous and drug induced. Drugs. 2014;74(4):443–50.
58. Kameda H, Tokuda H, Sakai F, Johkoh T, Mori S, Yoshida Y, et al. Clinical and radiological features of acute-onset diffuse interstitial lung diseases in patients with rheumatoid arthritis receiving treatment with biological agents: importance of *Pneumocystis* pneumonia in Japan revealed by a multicenter study. Intern Med. 2011;50(4):305–13.
59. Dixon WG, Hyrich KL, Watson KD, Lunt M, Symmons DP. Influence of anti-TNF therapy on mortality in patients with rheumatoid arthritis-associated interstitial lung disease: results from the British Society for Rheumatology Biologics Register. Ann Rheum Dis. 2010;69(6):1086–91.
60. Coyne P, Doe S, Saravanan V, Heycock C, Hamilton J, Kelly CA. Is respiratory infection in patients with rheumatoid arthritis caused by disease modifying drugs? Rheumatology. 2005;i74(A42):44.
61. Takayanagi N. Biological agents and respiratory infections: causative mechanisms and practice management. Respir Investig. 2015;53(5):185–200.
62. Coyne P, Hamilton J, Heycock C, Saravanan V, Coulson E, Kelly CA. Acute lower respiratory tract infection in patients with rheumatoid arthritis. J Rheumatol. 2007;34(9):1832–6.
63. Blumentals WA, Arreglado A, Napalkov P, Toovey S. Rheumatoid arthritis and the incidence of influenza and influenza related complications: a retrospective cohort study. BMC Musculoskelet Disord. 2012;13:158.
64. Dixon WG, Suissa S, Hudson M. The association between systemic glucocorticoid therapy and the risk of infection inpatients with rheumatoid arthritis: systematic review and meta-analyses. Arthritis Res Ther. 2011;13(4):R139.
65. Gardam MA, Keystone EC, Menzies R, Manners S, Skamene E, Long R, et al. Anti-tumour necrosis factor agents and tuberculosis risk: mechanisms of action and clinical management. Lancet Infect Dis. 2003;3(3):148–55.
66. Keane J, Gershon S, Wise RP, Mirabile-Levens E, Kasznica J, Schwieterman WD, et al. Tuberculosis associated with infliximab, a tumor necrosis factor alpha-neutralizing agent. N Engl J Med. 2001;345(15):1098–104.
67. Komano Y, Tanaka M, Nanki T, Koike R, Sakai R, Kameda H, et al. Incidence and risk factors for serious infection in patients with rheumatoid arthritis treated with tumor necrosis factor inhibitors: a report from the Registry of Japanese Rheumatoid Arthritis Patients for Longterm Safety. J Rheumatol. 2011;38(7):1258–64.
68. Winthrop KL, Baxter R, Liu L, Varley CD, Curtis JR, Baddley JW, et al. Mycobacterial diseases and antitumour necrosis factor therapy in the USA. Ann Rheum Dis. 2013;72(1):37–42.
69. Macfarlane JT, Boldy D. 2004 update of BTS pneumonia guidelines: what's new? Thorax. 2004;59(5):364–6.
70. Takayanagi N, Tsuchiya Y, Tokunaga D, Miyahara Y, Yamaguchi S, Saito H, et al. [Pulmonary infections in patients with rheumatoid arthritis]. Nihon Kokyuki Gakkai Zasshi. 2007;45(6):465–73.
71. Doran MF, Crowson CS, Pond GR, O'Fallon WM, Gabriel SE. Frequency of infection in patients with rheumatoid arthritis compared with controls: a population based study. Arthritis Rheum. 2002;46(9):2287–93.
72. Nakajima A, Saito K, Kojima T, Amano K, Yoshio T, Fukuda W, et al. No increased mortality in patients with rheumatoid arthritis treated with biologics: results from the biologics register of six rheumatology institutes in Japan. Mod Rheumatol. 2013;23(5):945–52.
73. Hansen RA, Gartlehner G, Powell GE, Sandler RS. Serious adverse events with infliximab: analysis of spontaneously reported adverse events. Clin Gastroenterol Hepatol. 2007;5(6):729–35.
74. Tubach F, Ravaud P, Salmon-Céron D, Petitpain N, Brocq O, Grados F, et al. Emergence of *Legionella pneumophila* pneumonia in patients receiving tumor necrosis factor–α antagonists. Clin Infect Dis. 2006;43(10):e95–100.
75. Fujiwara H, Nishimoto N, Hamano Y, Asanuma N, Miki S, Kasayama S, et al. Masked early symptoms of pneumonia in

patients with rheumatoid arthritis during tocilizumab treatment: a report of two cases. Mod Rheumatol. 2009;19(1):64–8.
76. Gaensbauer JT, Press CA, Hollister JR, Asturias EJ. Procalcitonin: a marker of infection not subverted by treatment with interleukin-6 receptor inhibition. Pediatr Infect Dis J. 2013;32(9):1040.
77. Tokuda H, Harigai M, Kameda H, Tomono K, Takayanagi N, Watanabe A, et al. Consensus statements for medical practice: biological agents and lung disease. Respir Investig. 2017;55(3):229–51.
78. Takayanagi N, Hara K, Tokunaga D, Takaku Y, Minagawa S, Tsuchiya Y, et al. [Etiology and outcome of community-acquired pneumonia in relation to age and severity in hospitalized adult patients]. Nihon Kokyuki Gakkai Zasshi. 2006;44(12):906–15.
79. Ward MM, Donald F. *Pneumocystis carinii* pneumonia in patients with connective tissue diseases: the role of hospital experience in diagnosis and mortality. Arthritis Rheum. 1999;42(4):780–9.
80. Carmona EM, Limper AH. Update on the diagnosis and treatment of *Pneumocystis* pneumonia. Ther Adv Respir Dis. 2011;5(1):41–59.
81. Tasaka S, Tokuda H. *Pneumocystis jirovecii* pneumonia in non-HIV-infected patients in the era of novel immunosuppressive therapies. J Infect Chemother. 2012;18(6):793–806.
82. Mekinian A, Durand-Joly I, Hatron PY, Moranne O, Denis G, Dei-Cas E, et al. *Pneumocystis jirovecii* colonization in patients with systemic autoimmune diseases: prevalence, risk factors of colonization and outcome. Rheumatology. 2011;50(3):569–77.
83. Wissmann G, Morilla R, Martín-Garrido I, Friaza V, Respaldiza N, Povedano J, et al. *Pneumocystis jirovecii* colonization in patients treated with infliximab. Eur J Clin Investig. 2011;41(3):343–8.
84. Morris A, Wei K, Afshar K, Huang L. Epidemiology and clinical significance of *Pneumocystis* colonization. J Infect Dis. 2008;197(1):10–7.
85. Mori S, Cho I, Sugimoto M. A follow-up study of asymptomatic carriers of *Pneumocystis jiroveci* during immunosuppressive therapy for rheumatoid arthritis. J Rheumatol. 2009;36(8):1600–5.
86. Tasaka S, Kobayashi S, Kamata H, Kimizuka Y, Fujiwara H, Funatsu Y, et al. Cytokine profiles of bronchoalveolar lavage fluid in patients with *Pneumocystis* pneumonia. Microbiol Immunol. 2010;54(7):425–33.
87. Kovacs JA, Hiemenz JW, Macher AM, Stover D, Murray HW, Shelhamer J, et al. *Pneumocystis carinii* pneumonia: a comparison between patients with the acquired immunodeficiency syndrome and patients with other immunodeficiencies. Ann Intern Med. 1984;100(5):663–71.
88. Kuhlman JE, Kavuru M, Fishman EK, Siegelman SS. *Pneumocystis carinii* pneumonia: spectrum of parenchymal CT findings. Radiology. 1990;175(3):711–4.
89. Fujii T, Nakamura T, Iwamoto A. *Pneumocystis* pneumonia in patients with HIV infection: clinical manifestations, laboratory findings, and radiological features. J Infect Chemother. 2007;13(1):1–7.
90. Reid AB, Chen SC, Worth LJ. *Pneumocystis jirovecii* pneumonia in non-HIV-infected patients: new risks and diagnostic tools. Curr Opin Infect Dis. 2011;24(6):534–44.
91. Kaplan JE, Benson C, Holmes KK, Brooks JT, Pau A, Masur H. Guidelines for prevention and treatment of opportunistic infections in HIV-infected adults and adolescents: recommendations from CDC, the National Institutes of Health, and the HIV Medicine Association of the Infectious Diseases Society of America. MMWR Recomm Rep. 2009;58(RR-4):1–207.
92. Harigai M, Koike R, Miyasaka N. *Pneumocystis* pneumonia associated with infliximab in Japan. N Engl J Med. 2007;357(18):1874–6.

The manufacturer's authorised representative in the EU is Springer Nature Customer Service Centre GmbH, Europaplatz 3, 69115 Heidelberg, Germany. If you have any concerns regarding our products, please contact ProductSafety@springernature.com

Printed and bound by CPI Group (UK) Ltd, Croydon, CR0 4YY
26/09/2026
02222871-0007